Bioethics
An Introduction

Providing readers with the confidence needed to debate key issues in bioethics, this introductory text clearly explains bioethical theories and their philosophical foundations.

Over 250 activities introduce topics for personal reflection, and discussion points encourage students to think for themselves and build their own arguments. Highlighting the potential pitfalls for those new to bioethics, each chapter features boxes providing factual information and outlining the philosophical background, along with detailed case studies that offer an insight into real-life examples of bioethical problems. Within-chapter essay questions and quizzes, along with end-of-chapter review questions, allow students to check their understanding and to broaden their thinking about the topics discussed.

The accompanying podcasts by the author (two of whose podcasts on iTunesU^{TM} have attracted over 3 million downloads) explain points that might be difficult for beginners. These, along with a range of extra resources for students and instructors, are available at www.cambridge.org/bioethics.

Marianne Talbot has been Director of Studies in Philosophy at Oxford University's Department For Continuing Education since 2001, where she is responsible for the university's lifelong learning in philosophy. Talbot pioneered Oxford's popular online short courses, and has more recently specialised in teaching ethics to scientists. She teaches ethics for Doctoral Training Centres in Oxford and in London, has trained the EPSRC itself in ethics and has written two online courses in bioethics for Oxford University.

Bioethics

An Introduction

MARIANNE TALBOT

University of Oxford

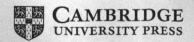

CAMBRIDGE
UNIVERSITY PRESS

University Printing House, Cambridge CB2 8BS, United Kingdom

One Liberty Plaza, 20th Floor, New York, NY 10006, USA

477 Williamstown Road, Port Melbourne, VIC 3207, Australia

314-321, 3rd Floor, Plot 3, Splendor Forum, Jasola District Centre, New Delhi - 110025, India

79 Anson Road, #06-04/06, Singapore 079906

Cambridge University Press is part of the University of Cambridge.

It furthers the University's mission by disseminating knowledge in the pursuit of education, learning and research at the highest international levels of excellence.

www.cambridge.org
Information on this title: www.cambridge.org/9780521714594

First published 2012
8th printing 2018

A catalogue record for this publication is available from the British Library

Library of Congress Cataloging in Publication data
Talbot, Marianne.
Bioethics : an introduction / Marianne Talbot.
     p.   cm.
ISBN 978-0-521-88833-2 (Hardback) – ISBN 978-0-521-71459-4 (Paperback)
1. Medical ethics.   2. Bioethics.   I. Title.
R724.T35 2012
174.2–dc23   2011027886

ISBN 978-0-521-88833-2 Hardback
ISBN 978-0-521-71459-4 Paperback

Additional resources for this publication at www.cambridge.org/bioethics

CONTENTS

PREFACE

If you are reading this you must have at least a passing interest in the ethical and social issues generated by biotechnology. Maybe a newspaper article or television programme has made you worry about cloning, bio-security or human–animal hybrids? Perhaps you have found yourself embroiled in a bioethical problem at work or as the result of needing IVF? Or perhaps you are a student required to do bioethics as part of your course? Or a school teacher, or college or university lecturer charged with teaching bioethics? If you are an instructor there are special notes for you at the end of this section.

I have written this book to help anyone with an interest in the ethical and social problems thrown up by our fastest moving areas of science and technology. The book will help its readers:

- understand the key issues in bioethics and the different positions people take on them;
- appreciate the arguments for and against the differing positions;
- discuss the issues with confidence;
- think productively about the issues that might arise in the future;
- come to their own considered positions on various issues, understanding the arguments for and against those positions.

I am a philosopher not a scientist.[1] This is an advantage because ethics is a philosophical discipline, not a scientific one. Both philosophers and scientists aim to discern truth, but the truths they aim to discern are different, as are the methods they use to discern them.

Philosophical background: science and philosophy

Scientists rely on observation, reason and empirical experiment to acquire an understanding of how the world is governed by the laws of nature.

Philosophers rely on reason, argument and thought experiment[2] to acquire an understanding of how the world is governed by the laws of logic.

The remit of a philosopher is wider than the remit of the scientist. The scientist is concerned only with:

- empirical possibilities (events consistent with the laws of nature),
- what *is* the case.

Philosophers are also concerned with:

- logical possibilities (events consistent with the laws of logic),
- what *ought* to be the case.

No amount of experimentation in the laboratory, or even in the field, will generate an adequate account of right and wrong. Observation and experiment will only tell us how things *are*, not how things *ought to be*. To determine right and wrong it is necessary to invoke the methodology of the philosopher.

I have been teaching bioethics for many years. I started by writing activities for the Labnotes' series for the Wellcome Trust. I regularly teach bioethics to students of the doctoral training centres funded by the Engineering and Physical Sciences Research Council (EPSRC[3]) at Oxford, Imperial College, London, Sheffield and Manchester Universities. I wrote two of Oxford University's popular online courses on bioethics, one for students of the MSc in bioinformatics and one for the public. I like to think I know the pitfalls that intelligent people can fall into in thinking about ethics, and that reading this book will help you to avoid them.

I have started from the assumption that readers will not have a philosophical background. For this reason I have included a chapter on how to construct, analyse and evaluate arguments. Readers will practise these reasoning skills as they work through the activities in this book. A lot of these activities are discussions. This is because argument – the life-blood of the philosophical method – might best be seen as the *collaborative* pursuit of truth. Although we can engage in solitary argument by playing devil's advocate to ourselves, an activity encouraged in this book, there is no substitute for arguing with others.

I have kept philosophical background to a minimum directing readers to additional resources to follow up anything of particular interest.

Factual information: The devil's advocate

When the Roman Catholic Church is considering a candidate for sainthood, his or her case is made by The Promoter of the Cause, otherwise known as God's Advocate (Advocatus Dei). In 1587 Pope Sixtus V appointed a Devil's Advocate (Advocatus Diaboli), whose job it would be to argue against the canonisation.

The title 'devil's advocate' is used in everyday conversation to mean a person who, irrespective of his own position, argues against a position being considered.

If the devil's advocate's arguments succeed, the argument under consideration is not a good one. If his arguments fail, they will strengthen the argument being considered.[4]

This book is about the ethics of biotechnology. This means we shall not be discussing issues such as patient confidentiality or autonomy, nor those involving scientific misconduct or arising from the pressure to publish. These are issues of medical ethics or the ethics of science more generally. We shall discuss issues common to bioethics and these other disciplines – for example euthanasia, animal rights and open source publishing – but always from a biotechnological perspective.

It is always difficult to decide how to structure a book like this. A field as broad as bioethics does not fall neatly into pigeonholes. Here is a description of the way this book is structured:

Part I introduces the reader to biotechnology and bioethics, to ethics in general, ethics in the context of society and the most important ethical theories. It also considers the nature of argument and how to evaluate arguments, and some general arguments that arise with respect to all the issues discussed in the book and that will certainly be familiar to you.

In Part II we will consider the ethical decisions we face, collectively and individually, as (and for) potential parents and their children, and those who are aging and dying. These include human cloning, both therapeutic and reproductive, reproductive freedom, the shortage of reproductive resources and how it might be alleviated, embryo selection and its relation to eugenics, the nature of death, the moral acceptability of 'curing' it, and finally the moral acceptability of assisted suicide and euthanasia.

In Part III we will turn to the issues that, in the midst of life, we have a duty collectively and individually to consider as citizens and subjects with duties to ourselves, each other and to nature. Under *our duties to ourselves* we will consider biological enhancement, bioinformation, 'garage' biology and biological warfare. In *our duties to each other* we will discuss food and energy security, bio-ownership, and justice between the developed and developing worlds. Finally we'll discuss *our duties to nature*, including our duties to non-human animals and the non-living environment.

It might be objected that this structure is anthropomorphic because the focus is on us and the decisions we face. I accept this, but believe it can be justified: it is largely the decisions *we* make that will shape the future, for ourselves and the generations to come, for the environment and for non-human animals. This book aims to make some contribution to ensuring that these decisions are informed by reason and reflection.

That's it with the preliminaries. I hope you enjoy reading this book as much as I have enjoyed writing it.

Notes

1 http://www.philosophy.ox.ac.uk/members/marianne_talbot (the author's website at the Faculty Of Philosophy, University of Oxford); www.mariannetalbot.co.uk (the author's official website).

2 http://www.philosophybites.libsyn.com/category/Julian%20Baggini (Philosopher Julian Baggini on thought experiments for Philosophy Bites). See also: http://www.practicalethics. ox.ac.uk/audio/analysis_280609.mp3. Janet Radcliffe-Richards on the same topic.

3 http://www.epsrc.ac.uk/Pages/default.aspx.

4 http://www.newadvent.org/cathen/01168b.htm (The Catholic Encyclopedia entry on the Devil's Advocate).

USING THIS BOOK

Each chapter of this book:

1. Starts with a list of objectives to be met by reading the chapter;

2. Includes boxes containing:

 Activities to deepen thinking, stimulate discussion, and enhance analytical skills;

 Case studies to illustrate issues under discussion;

 Factual information about the issue being discussed;

 Philosophical background on the issue under discussion;

 Definitions.

To avoid possible misunderstandings the definition boxes should always be read. The other boxes are not usually necessary for the understanding of the text (it will be made clear when it is necessary), but reading them will take readers just that bit further on matters of particular interest.

3. Ends with:
   (a) A **summary** of its content;
   (b) A series of **questions** to stimulate reflection;
   (c) A list of **additional activities** by which to enhance understanding;
   (d) A list of **further reading** and **useful websites**.

Ideally the book should be read in the order in which it is presented. If this is too much philosophy too soon, the book can be read in the order that appeals to the reader who will be directed, when necessary, to other parts of the book to glean the background information needed.

The book is accompanied by a dedicated website (www.cambridge.org/bioethics) on which readers will find:

   (a) Links to all the references in the book that are available on the web;
   (b) Updates on issues in bioethics since the writing of the book;
   (c) Short podcasts by the author explaining concepts, distinctions and issues she knows to be particularly difficult for those new to the area.

Much of the additional reading to which readers will be directed is available online. This makes it easier for references regularly to be updated. Many references will be to newspaper articles or television or radio pieces on the issues under discussion.

Some might think this use of the media discredits bioethics as a discipline. I disagree. Most people reading this book will have no intention of becoming professional bioethicists. They do not need scholarly articles or worthy books, nor do they have time to read them, they just need a grasp of the issues in question. They will usually find it easier, quicker and more enjoyable to acquire such a grasp from the sort of references I have included. At the end of the book, and on the website, I have included a list of places to go and books to read for those who do wish to study further.

NOTE FOR INSTRUCTORS

If you are using this book to teach bioethics to classes at any level you will find the activity boxes, and the boxes of *additional activities* you'll find at the end of every chapter, useful for setting students tasks inside or outside the classroom.

Many of these activities involve discussions for pairs of students, or for groups (small or large). They can be used in different ways, for example:

1. You might allocate students sides in the discussion irrespective of their own views (this is useful to encourage them to consider the side of the argument other than their own);
2. You might use the discussion during class without the students preparing, or ask them to prepare by setting work for them to do outside the classroom;
3. If you have the luxury of time you could ask students to organise a formal debate to which others might be invited.

The 'questions to stimulate reflection', also found at the end of each chapter, will be useful for triggering discussion in class, for setting essays, or just to give students something to think about.

The author's podcasts, available on the website, have been designed to help people acquire difficult and/or unfamiliar concepts, distinctions and ideas. None of them is more than 10 minutes in length, and some instructors may find them useful in the classroom, or for students to watch outside the classroom.

Many of those who teach bioethics are specialists who have been properly trained in bioethics. These people will be able to use this book without any special preparation. I hope they will find the book accessible to their students and enjoyable to use.

Some of those tasked with teaching bioethics, however, are not specialists in this area. Some, indeed, have relatively little experience of the area, but having expressed an interest find themselves teaching it, often without having been given much time to acquire the understanding they need to plan lessons and teach with confidence. There is a special area of the website (www.cambridge.org/bioethics) devoted to those in this position, which is accessible by getting a password from the publisher of this book. In this area of the website you will find:

1. Course and lesson plans for various course lengths and depths;
2. References to help you acquire – as efficiently as possible – a deeper background understanding of the issues discussed in each chapter;
3. Figure files, along with files for the activity and case study boxes and the discussion questions.

Even those most experienced in teaching bioethics, of course, may find themselves short of time for lesson planning and preparation. You might also find this part of the website of interest.

If you have any ideas the implementation of which would make the website more helpful to you as an instructor, I should be grateful if you could let me know by leaving your comments on the website, I appreciate your willingness to help.

ACKNOWLEDGEMENTS

I should like to thank all the directors and administrators at the Life Sciences Interface Doctoral Training Centre at the University of Oxford, and at the Chemical Biology Doctoral Training Centre at Imperial College London. Thank you also to the people at Technology Assisted Lifelong Learning (TALL) and the Department for Continuing Education at the University of Oxford, especially those who were instrumental in putting together the online courses in bioethics for public programmes and the MSc in bioinformatics. Thank you also to the people at the Engineering and Physical Sciences Research Council: I greatly enjoyed the session I held with you. Katie Fletcher and Reuben Thorley, thank you for reading drafts of the books and for your useful corrections.

In particular though I should like to thank all the students to whom I have taught bioethics, both face to face and online: your questions were brilliant and your disagreements instructive. I am privileged to have taught you.

Thank you also to everyone at Cambridge University Press.

Part I Bioethics and Ethics

1 Biotechnology and bioethics: what it's all about

Objectives

In reading this chapter you will:

- reflect on the nature of bioethics;
- familiarise yourself with the definition of biotechnology that we will use in this book;
- reflect on the interdisciplinary and multi-disciplinary nature of biotechnology;
- consider the place of biology in biotechnology;
- consider briefly the history of biotechnology;
- reflect on how bioethics is generated by biotechnology;
- acquire an understanding of the different biotechnologies that generate social and ethical issues.

Bioethics is the study of the ethical and social issues generated by biotechnology.[1] In Box 1.1 you will find the definition of biotechnology that we will use in this book.

Box 1.1 **Definition: Biotechnology**

Biotechnology is the application of science and technology to living organisms and their parts, or to products and models of living organisms, in the hope of producing understanding, goods or services.

Examples of work in biotechnology:

- physicists and engineers working together to produce nano-vehicles, vehicles small enough to enter the bloodstream and deliver drugs to cure various diseases;
- geneticists and information technologists helping to eliminate adverse drug effects and make personalised medicine a reality;
- engineers and biologists working together to engineer organisms that will alert us to, and even remove, pollutants from the environment.[2]

This definition of biotechnology makes it clear that the 'bio' of biotechnology refers to the subject matter of biotechnology, not the disciplines involved. Biotechnology is *multidisciplinary* in that it involves many different disciplines, all the pure and applied sciences in fact, and *interdisciplinary* in that all these sciences and technologies work together to achieve biotechnological ends.

The 'bio' bit is important because in biotechnology, these different sciences and technologies are all applied to biological organisms: to living organisms, their parts and products, and to models of such organisms. Biology is central to the pursuit of biotechnological ends because biotechnology is the application of science and technology to biological organisms.

Box 1.2 **Activity: Conceptual analysis**

Put 'Def: "biotechnology"' into a search engine. Choose two definitions that differ from the one in Box 1.1, and compare and contrast the three definitions.

Can you think of a situation in which the definition of 'biotechnology' would be important?

Biotechnology, arguably, has been practised continuously since the Sumerians discovered how to use yeast to brew beer in 1750 BC. Modern biotechnology emerged in the twentieth century as we acquired the understanding and ability to manipulate organisms at the molecular level, specifically as we acquired the understanding and skills needed to manipulate an organism's genes.[3]

This understanding, and the skills we have developed as a result of it, enables us to do many things our ancestors never dreamed of. Our ability to manipulate the characteristics of plants and animals, for example, no longer depends on the techniques of selective breeding. We can directly engineer the genes of organisms to produce the traits that interest us, clone animals that possess these traits, or even create synthetic organisms capable of performing desired functions.

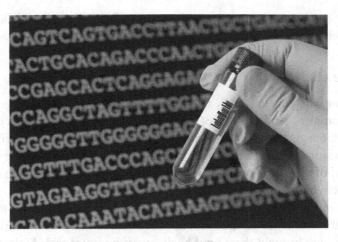

Figure 1.1 Sequencing human DNA. © iStockphoto.com/dra_schwartz.

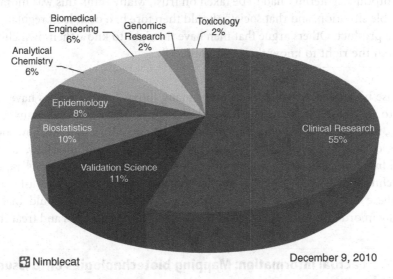

Figure 1.2 The people that biotechnology companies in the USA were hiring in November 2010. Image courtesy of nimblecat.com. (http://nimblecat.typepad.com/thecareerists/2010/12/55-of-new-biotech-jobs-in-clinical-research.html).

Biotechnology in relation to human beings received a huge boost from the completion in 2003 of the Human Genome Project,[4] which sequenced and mapped the 25–26 000 genes in the human genome.

Current projects involve attempts (many already very successful) to:

- discover the function of the various genes;
- map the locations of common variations between individuals;
- correlate these bio-markers with phenotypical traits of interest;
- develop techniques to detect the presence of important bio-markers;
- develop techniques by which to manipulate gene expression.

Biotechnology is advancing at a breathtaking pace, facilitating the development of numerous potentially life-enhancing and life-saving techniques.[5]

Box 1.3 **Case study**

In 2009 a private company in the UK started marketing an 'over-the-counter' paternity testing kit. Customers send samples of their own DNA and that of the child whose paternity is in doubt and, for a fee, get results within 5 days (or 24 hours for a higher fee).

Two adults must consent to the procedure: the putative father and the mother of the child. Proof of identity is required and one adult will be telephoned to check that the consequences of possible test results have been considered.

Many have argued that such kits should be banned on the grounds that the consent requirements are too easy to get around, and that children may be summarily rejected by the man who has brought them up if he discovers he is not their biological father.

Until biotechnology came up with the techniques facilitating the development of such products paternity had to be taken on trust. Many think this was morally a more desirable situation, and that society should therefore ban or at least regulate the use of such a product. Others argue that men have the right to know their own children, and children the right to know their own fathers.[6]

Because biotechnology enables us to do many things human beings have never been able to do before, it has generated and will continue to generate many new ethical issues, issues concerning what we *should* and *shouldn't* do, and many new social issues, issues concerning what we as a society should and shouldn't allow, or should or shouldn't fund. Bioethics is the discipline that studies the actions permitted by biotechnology – actions like cloning or genetic engineering – and asks whether or not these actions are morally acceptable, and if so how we should manage them socially in order to promote citizens' welfare, protect their rights and treat them fairly.

Box 1.4 **Factual information: Mapping biotechnologies onto issues in this book**

The techniques of biotechnology do not map neatly onto the ethical issues that are generated by biotechnology. For example, genetic engineering produces ethical issues in respect of designer babies, GM foods and our use of animals.

If you are interested in a particular biotechnological technique this will help you find the chapter(s) in which you'll find a discussion of the ethical issues generated by it.

The techniques of assisted reproduction[7]
Under this heading fall all the techniques by which individuals and couples having trouble conceiving can be helped to achieve a healthy baby. There are many such techniques of which in vitro fertilisation – the mixing, in a Petri dish, of sperm and egg in such a way as to ensure the fertilisation of the egg – is probably the best known. The social and ethical issues generated by such techniques are discussed in Chapters 9, 10 and 11.

Cloning[8]

Every time a cutting of a plant successfully roots the plant is cloned. We have been cloning plants by such means for centuries. In the late twentieth century, however, a mammal – Dolly the sheep – was cloned for the first time by means of somatic cell nuclear transfer. The social and ethical issues generated by cloning are discussed in Chapters 7 and 8.

Genetic screening/testing[9]

The techniques of genetic screening/testing include any means by which we can identify (some part of) the genetic inheritance of an individual. The most controversial of these techniques is pre-implantation genetic diagnosis. This involves taking an eight cell embryo and removing just one cell for analysis. The social and ethical issues such techniques engender are discussed in Chapter 11.

The technology of life support[10]

These technologies include techniques by which to maintain circulation when the heart no longer beats spontaneously and nutrition and hydration when a patient is unable to eat or drink. The social and ethical issues generated by such technologies are discussed in Chapters 12 and 13.

Genetic engineering[11]

Sometimes called genetic modification, genetic engineering involves the introduction, elimination and modification of genes in such a way as to affect the properties or behaviour of an individual human, plant or non-human animal (and perhaps the properties and behaviours of its progeny). Such techniques and the issues surrounding them are discussed in Chapter 17.

Bioinformatics[12]

Bioinformatics involves the application of information technology to the various fields of molecular biology. Specifically, it involves developing methods for storing, retrieving, comparing and analysing biological data. It generates social and ethical issues that are discussed in Chapter 18.

Pharmacogenetics/pharmacogenomics[13]

The techniques grouped under these names, for all practical purposes interchangeable, comprise the study of the genetic variations that determine an individual's metabolism and response to various drugs. The social and ethical issues that arise from such techniques are discussed in Chapter 19.

Synthetic biology[14]

A relative newcomer to the discipline of biotechnology, synthetic biology involves the re-design and fabrication of existing organisms, and the design and fabrication of organisms that don't exist in nature. Such activities generate social and ethical issues that are discussed in Chapter 18.

Nanotechnology[15]

A 'nanometre' is one billionth of a metre (1×10^{-9}). Nanotechnology exploits the properties and behaviours of the very small.[16] Nanotechnology is sometimes characterised as 'soft' or 'hard' depending on whether it exploits a biological system ('soft') or a mechanical system ('hard'). The social and ethical issues generated by soft nanotechnology will be discussed in Chapter 18.

Before we can consider specific issues in bioethics we need to acquire some understanding of the nature of ethics in general. We will do this in the next chapter.

Summary

In this chapter we have considered:

- the fact that bioethics is the study of the ethical and social issues generated by biotechnology;

- the definition of biotechnology that we will be using in this book;

- a brief account of the history of biotechnology;

- the fact that biotechnology generates ethical and social issues by enabling us to perform actions we have never been able to perform before;

- the fact that biotechnological techniques do not map neatly onto the ethical issues;

- a list of techniques and indications of where in the book discussions of them will be found.

Questions to stimulate reflection

What is the difference between biotechnology's being *interdisciplinary* and *multidisciplinary*?

Can you think of a few of the advantages and disadvantages to be derived from biotechnology's being interdisciplinary?

What do you think might be advantageous and disadvantageous about biotechnology's being multidisciplinary?

How do advances in biotechnology generate ethical problems?

What do you think might be the difference between an *ethical* problem and a *social* problem?

Can you think of two examples each of (1) an ethical problem generated by biotechnology, and (2) a social problem generated by biotechnology?

Additional activities

Make a list of actions that are now possible thanks to biotechnology but which weren't possible 100 years ago.

Using your list identify at least one ethical or social problem that is generated by this action.

Put 'bioethics' into a search engine and follow up anything that interests you.

Conduct an informal opinion poll amongst your friends, family and fellow students on what they understand by 'bioethics' (you might find yourself having to explain it quite often: be prepared!).

Buy yourself an exercise book in which to write your thoughts as you work through this book. Start by writing down your own understanding of the nature of bioethics.

Identify from the list in Box 1.4 a biotechnology that particularly interests you. In your diary jot down the ethical and social issues you think might be generated by it.

Put 'ethics' into the search facility of the website of the agency that funds biotechnological research in your country, and see if you can find anything interesting.

Notes

1 'Bioethics' can also be used more widely to cover the biomedical sciences, but we are concentrating on this aspect of bioethics (see Preface, p. viii).

2 http://www.biotechinstitute.org/careers/career_profiles.html. Biotechnologists talk about their careers on the website of the Biotechnology Institute.

3 http://www.biotechinstitute.org/what_is/timeline.html. A timeline of biotechnology from the Institute of Biotechnology in the United States.

4 http://www.ornl.gov/sci/techresources/Human_Genome/home.shtml. Information pages from the Human Genome Project.

5 http://www.wellcome.ac.uk/Funding/Biomedical-science/Funded-projects/Major-initiatives/WTDV029748.htm. Information about the 1000 Genomes Project from the Wellcome Trust.

6 http://www.dailymail.co.uk/health/article-1200420/Fathers-30-DNA-paternity-test-counter-cost-119-results-back.html. An article from the UK's *Daily Mail* on the introduction of paternity testing kits.

7 http://www.fertilityexpert.co.uk/chapter-three-assisted-reproduction-techniques.html. An article on the techniques of assisted reproduction from the website of Fertility Expert in the UK.

8 http://www.reuters.com/article/idUSN1551320720080115. Facts and a timeline on cloning from the Reuters website.

9 http://www.ukgtn.nhs.uk/gtn/Home. Information about genetic testing in the UK from the UK Genetic Testing Network.

10 http://www.deathreference.com/Ke-Ma/Life-Support-System.html. Definition of 'Life Support' from the Encyclopedia of Death and Dying.
11 http://www.eurekascience.com/ICanDoThat/gen_eng.htm. A simple explanation of genetic engineering from Eureka Science.
12 http://www.bioinformatics.org/wiki/Bioinformatics_FAQ. Information about bioinformatics from the Bioinformatics Organization in the United States.
13 http://ghr.nlm.nih.gov/handbook/genomicresearch/pharmacogenomics. An account of pharmacogenomics from the US National Library of Medical Information.
14 http://www.youtube.com/watch?v=XIuh7KDRzLk&feature=related. YouTube video of Drew Endy (an assistant professor at Palo Alto) explaining synthetic biology.
15 http://www.nano.gov/nanotech-101/nanotechnology-facts. FAQ from the national Nanotechnology Initiative in the United States.
16 http://cpd.conted.ox.ac.uk/nanotechnology/nanobasics/nano/accessweb/history.html. The basics of nanotechnology from the University of Oxford.

Further reading and useful websites

Okasha, S. (2002) *A Very Short Introduction to Philosophy of Science*. Oxford: Oxford University Press.
Smith, J. E. (2009) *Biotechnology*. Cambridge: Cambridge University Press.
Stephansson, H. (ed.) (2002) *Life Sciences in Transition: A Special Edition of the JMB*. London: Academic Press.
Walker, S. (2006) *Biotechnology Demystified*. New York: McGraw-Hill Professional.

http://wings.buffalo.edu/faculty/research/bioethics/osce.html. Standardised Patient Scenarios for teaching bioethics from the University of Toronto.
http://www.bbsrc.ac.uk/. The website of the UK's Biotechnology and Biological Sciences Research Council.
http://www.beep.ac.uk/content/46.0.html. The website of the Bioethics Education Project funded by the Wellcome Trust and based at the Graduate School of Education, University of Bristol.
http://www.bioethics.ac.uk/index.php. The Biocentre, a site which examines new biotechniques from a social and ethical perspective.
http://www.nsf.gov/about/. The website of the National Science Foundation, who fund research in the United States.

2   Ethics in general: ethics, action and freedom

Objectives

In reading this chapter you will:

- reflect on the practical nature of ethics;
- consider the place of rules in ethical decision-making;
- acquire an understanding of why ethical dilemmas arise;
- learn how to distinguish *first order* ethics and *second order* ethics;
- consider the relation between ethics and truth;
- learn how to distinguish epistemology from metaphysics;
- reflect on the importance of free will to ethics and on the possibility we do not have free will;
- think about how religion is related to ethics.

People can be surprised to discover that ethics is primarily a practical discipline. But if ethics didn't link with action it would be useless. Ethics, after all, is concerned with what we should and shouldn't *do*. Should we clone human beings (Chapters 7 and 8)? Should we pursue immortality (Chapter 12)? Should we produce genetically modified crops (Chapter 17) or 'engineer' our genes (Chapter 14) or those of animals (Chapters 17 and 20)? All these decisions are ethical decisions.

Ethics and rules

Ethical decision-making would be easy if all we had to do was follow the small set of rules – 'do not lie', 'keep promises' and so on – we were given as we grew up. But there is more to moral decision-making than this. Consider the following situation:

Your friend comes home from the hairdresser's, strikes a pose and says: 'what do you think?' You think: 'yuk!'

You have a problem. It is not a problem you can solve by invoking the rules you were given as a child. Those would certainly have included both 'be honest' and 'be kind' and your problem is that in this situation it seems impossible to be both honest *and* kind.

You might respond by being honest (and taking the risk of hurting your friend) or by being kind (risking your friend later discovering you weren't honest). Either response is justifiable. But both seem to involve breaking one of the rules with which you were brought up.

You might find yourself arguing that sometimes it is necessary to be cruel to be kind. Telling your friend you like her hair might lead to her going around looking awful. If you are right then being honest does not necessarily involve being unkind, and your problem dissolves.

Or you might argue that telling your friend she looks fine would only be a *white* lie. Telling a white lie, you might claim, doesn't really involve being dishonest. If you are right then again your problem dissolves: being kind doesn't involve being dishonest.

Box 2.1 **Activity: Paired discussion**

What would you do in the situation described? How would you justify your action?

Do you think the fact that there are different actions that could be counted as *right* in this situation means that nothing could count as wrong in this situation? Describe two actions that you think might be wrong in this situation.

Participants should have 10 minutes for discussion before being asked for feedback.

Hint: a person could act wrongly

- by doing *what* they do (if you told your friend she was stupid for asking you, many would think this was rude),
- by *the way in which they do it* (if you told your friend she looked fine, but in a sarcastic manner many would deem this wrong),
- in *the reason* for doing what they do (if you told your friend the truth, but only out of spite, your action would arguably be wrong).

But notice how moral decision-making forces us to reflect on our values, on what exactly we believe to be right and wrong. Kindness might involve hurting people. Honesty might not always mean telling the truth.

But there must be limits. At some point we have to ask ourselves what those limits are. At this point our dilemma will arise again.

Some people try to escape such dilemmas by giving themselves additional rules. They might decide that when honesty and kindness conflict they will always tell the truth (do you know anyone like this?) or that they will always be kind (do you know anyone like this?). By ordering their values, they hope to avoid moral dilemmas.

But is this wise? Imagine that when your friend comes home from the hairdressers it is the first time you have seen her smile for 6 months. Should honesty trump kindness here? Or imagine your friend's hair is so bad it will make her a laughing stock. Should you still put kindness before honesty? Devising a strict ordering of values may often lead to the wrong action.

Box 2.2 Activity: Playing devil's advocate

Imagine an ordering of values that *always* puts kindness before honesty. Can you come up with examples of situations in which this would produce the wrong action?

Variations might include orderings that always put:

- honesty before kindness;
- loyalty before honesty;
- honesty before loyalty.[1]

Ethics and truth

It seems that there is more to moral decision-making than following the rules you were given as a child, even supplemented by an ordering of these rules. But what is this 'more'? If there are no rules to guide our moral reasoning how can we be sure our moral reasoning is correct?

Some people believe that moral reasoning is not the sort of reasoning that *can* be correct, that moral judgements are not the sort of judgements that can be true (or false). We shall consider why some people think this when, in Chapter 6, we consider the argument entitled 'it's a matter of opinion'.

Other people – and this includes most philosophers – believe that moral judgements can be both correct and incorrect, and that it is possible to say something about what makes our moral reasoning correct or incorrect, our moral judgements true or false.

Theorising about ethics

To think about such issues, however, is to start *theorising* about morality, it is to start thinking not about whether a given type of action is right or wrong ('first order' moral issues), but about whether moral judgements can be true or false at all, and if they are, about what *makes* them true or false ('second order' moral issues).

Box 2.3 Activity: Personal reflection

Lying is wrong.

Do you think this statement is always true, sometimes true or never true?

If you think it is sometimes or always true, what do you think *makes* it true (when it is true)? If some sort of fact, *what* sort of fact?

If you think it is never true how would you explain why most people generally think of this statement as true (at least sometimes).

Once participants have had time to reflect on these questions, they could be used to stimulate group discussion.

Just as there are disagreements between scientists about almost any scientific theory, so there are disagreements between philosophers about the correct theory of morality. In Chapter 4 we shall be introduced to some of these theories.

As we work through the ethical and social issues generated by biotechnology we shall see these theories being applied in our attempts to deal with different dilemmas. We will also see why none of these theories can currently be considered to be the final word on ethics.

Box 2.4 Activity: Conceptual analysis

Can you sort the following questions into 'first order' (practical) questions, and 'second order' (theoretical) questions:

(i)   Is reproductive cloning morally acceptable?
(ii)   Should drug addicts be allowed to use IVF?
(iii)   How can we know that a given moral judgement is true?
(iv)   Should clinical trials be run according to different rules in developed and undeveloped countries?
(v)   Could it ever be right to kill an innocent human being?
(vi)   What makes a moral judgement true or false?
(vii)   Is it morally permissible to discard embryos with the gene for Huntington's disease?
(viii) What sort of evidence can we cite for the claim that something is right or wrong?

Answers:
First order: (i), (ii), (iv), (v), (vii)
Second order: (iii), (vi), (viii).

Knowledge of right and wrong

One of the first things every student of philosophy has to learn is the difference between *metaphysics* and *epistemology*. In a nutshell metaphysics has to do what *is* the case. Epistemology has to do with how we *know* what is the case. To see the difference between these two consider the difference between the following two questions:

(i)   Is it morally wrong to rob elderly ladies?

(ii)   How do we know it is morally wrong to rob elderly ladies?

The first question is a 'yes or no' question about the ethics of a particular type of action: robbing elderly ladies. The second question demands our justification for the answer we give to the first question.

It might be thought that metaphysical questions are first order questions, and epistemological questions second order questions. But this is not the case. Consider the following questions:

(i)   Is utilitarianism the correct account of morality?

(ii)   How do we know that utilitarianism is the correct account of morality?

(Utilitarianism is one of the moral theories we shall be learning about in Chapter 4.) Here the metaphysical question is itself a second order question. The metaphysical/ epistemological distinction appears in relation to this second order question in exactly the way it did in relation to the first order question. The fact is that we can always ask a question (ask what is true), and then ask how we can know we have the right answer to that question (ask how we can justify the claim that it *is* true).

The metaphysical/epistemological distinction doesn't just arise for questions, of course, there are also metaphysical claims such as 'lying is wrong', and epistemological claims such as 'I believe it is wrong to tell lies'. The first claim is a claim about lying, the second a claim about yourself and your beliefs.

If this seems double-dutch don't worry. The best way of acquiring an understanding of the metaphysics/epistemology distinction is to make use of it. You will be doing this throughout this book.

Box 2.5 Definitions: Metaphysics, ontology and epistemology

Metaphysics and ontology: Metaphysics is the study of what exists and what its nature is. Ontology[2] is the branch of metaphysics concerned with what exists.

   For example: a metaphysician will take the belief that there are physical objects (a belief that must be assumed by scientists if they are to get anything done) and subject it to rational scrutiny, asking what we are really saying when we say that physical objects exist. He will ask, for example, whether physical objects have some essential characteristic (four-dimensionality?) and what that characteristic really is.[3]

Epistemology: is the study of knowledge and justification.

   For example: an epistemologist will take any claim to the effect that physical objects exist, and he will ask what our reasons are for believing this, how conclusive those reasons are and whether those reasons could hold true even if physical objects didn't exist.[4]

Ethics, intentional action and free will

Because ethics is a practical subject, in thinking about ethics we are never far from thinking about action. In thinking about action, however, it is important to note that we are not thinking about everything we *do*, we are thinking only of the things we do *intentionally*, those we *choose* to do.

Consider coming into a room and tripping over a mat. Now consider coming into the room and *pretending* to trip over the mat. Although the things you do on each occasion seem identical, only the latter is an action, something you do intentionally, the former is not an action at all, it is something that *happens* to you.

When we talk about actions in talking about ethics, we are talking only of the things we do intentionally. The reason for this is that it is only the things we choose to do that can be counted as right or wrong. You cannot be either praised or blamed for something that happens to you.

The importance of intentional action to ethics is underpinned by the importance, to ethics, of the notion of free will. It is believed that only mature human beings can act morally (and immorally) because only mature human beings are capable of:

(i)   understanding the difference between right and wrong;

and

(ii) freely choosing to perform actions *because* they are right or *despite* their being wrong.

Only human adults, in other words, are deemed capable of choosing freely to act for *moral* reasons.

Very young children are not usually considered to be full moral agents. This is because although they are believed to be capable of acting intentionally, they are not deemed capable of understanding the difference between right and wrong. They can't do something therefore *because* it is right. Nor can they prevent themselves from doing something *because* it is wrong. In many countries the law recognises this by not holding children fully responsible should they break the law.

Non-human animals are not usually accorded the status of moral agents at all.[5] This is partly because they are not believed to be capable of understanding the difference between right and wrong. It is also partly because many think they are incapable of acting intentionally, of freely choosing how to act. Many have believed that all the behaviour of non-human animals is determined by the laws of nature, by the physical state the animal is in and by the environmental conditions in which it finds itself. Behaviour that is determined by such things, not being freely chosen, is not believed to be morally evaluable. How, after all, can an animal (human *or* non-human) be held responsible for a behaviour it could not *but* perform given the laws of nature and the totality of the physical circumstances in which it was in?

Table 2.1 Age of criminal responsibility
Minimum age at which children are subject to penal law in countries with 10 million or more children under 18 years old

Mexico	6–12[a]
Bangladesh	7
India	7
Myanmar	7
Nigeria	7
Pakistan	7
South Africa	7
Sudan	7
Tanzania	7
Thailand	7
United States	7[b]
Indonesia	8
Kenya	8
UK (Scotland)	8
Ethiopia	9
Iran	9[c]
Philippines	9
Nepal	10
UK (England)	10
UK (Wales)	10
Ukraine	10
Turkey	11
Korea, Rep.	12
Morocco	12
Uganda	12
Algeria	13
France	13
Poland	13
Uzbekistan	13
China	14
Germany	14
Italy	14
Japan	14
Russian Federation	14
Viet Nam	14
Egypt	15
Argentina	16
Brazil	18[d]
Colombia	18[d]
Peru	18[d]
Congo, Dem. Rep.	–

[a] Most states 11 or 12 years; age 11 for federal crimes.
[b] Age determined by state, minimum age is 7 in most states under common law.
[c] Age 9 for girls, 15 for boys.
[d] Official age of criminal responsibility, from age 12 children's actions are subject to juvenile legal proceedings.
Sources: CRC Country Reports (1992–1996); Juvenile Justice and Juvenile Delinquency in Central and Eastern Europe, 1995; United Nations, Implementation of UN Mandates on Juvenile Justice in ESCAP, 1994; Geert Cappelaere, Children's Rights Centre, University of Gent, Belgium. http://www.unicef.org/pon97/p56a.htm.

Box 2.6 Philosophical background: Understanding right and wrong

You might object that your dog *does* understand the difference between right and wrong. You know this every time he looks guiltily at you when caught in some heinous act.[6]

Arguably though what your dog understands is the difference between behaviours that attract punishment and those that don't. This is a very different difference.

If you doubt this ask yourself which of these reasons would prevent you from stealing someone's purse:

(i) you might be caught and punished
(ii) it would be wrong.

One who understands the difference between right and wrong is one who wouldn't steal the purse even if there were no chance of being caught or punished.

They don't steal the purse because they recognise that it would be *wrong*. Even if this is some sort of internalisation of the fear of punishment it seems different in kind from anything of which animals are capable.

Free will and determinism

Many people would insist that non-human animals *do* act freely even if they can't understand the difference between right and wrong. But a more interesting claim for our purposes is the claim that human beings *can't* act freely. Hard determinists claim that all human behaviour is determined by the laws of nature, the physical states of the agent and the environmental conditions in which he finds himself.

If determinism is true, but free will is a necessary condition for acting morally, it would seem that no one *ever* acts morally. Just as you cannot reasonably be convicted of a crime if it is discovered you have a condition – kleptomania perhaps – that means you could not help yourself from doing what you did, if it is discovered that *all* our behaviour is determined, we cannot be praised or blamed for anything we do. Morality will have been shown to be an illusion.

Clearly it goes beyond the remit of this book to decide whether or not hard determinism is true. Instead we will simply assume that hard determinism is false, that morality exists and that the concepts of right and wrong have application. The justification for this is that if morality does exist then it is extremely important to think about it. If it doesn't then we may be wasting our time, but as we cannot do anything else nothing is lost.

Box 2.7 Philosophical background: Free will and determinism

There are (at least) three possible positions to adopt on the question of free will and determinism:[7]

Hard determinism: according to which all behaviour is causally determined. None of us actually chooses to do anything.

Soft determinism: according to which behaviours can be both determined *and* free.

Libertarian: according to which *some* behaviours – intentional actions – really are freely chosen and *not* causally determined at all.

Faced with this choice many people would go straight for soft determinism (SD) because it allows us to insist:

(i)   everything is causally determined, which seems to be required by our scientific theories, *and* simultaneously:

(ii) to recognise as accurate the very strong intuition we all have that we are free to act as we choose.

On the other hand it would seem that a soft determinist must believe of a given behaviour – a single action – that it is *both* causally determined (such that the agent could *not* have chosen otherwise) *and* freely chosen (such that the agent *could* have chosen otherwise).

If you think this involves a logical inconsistency (and many have) then you will have to be either a hard determinist or a libertarian or find some other way of answering our question.

Ethics and religion

The very first philosophers – in Greek 'lovers of wisdom' – were distinguished by their refusal to accept supernatural explanations. They didn't believe that the explanation for *everything* would be found in God's will: they always looked first for a logical or natural explanation. This was not because they weren't religious; it seems certain that many of them were. What they didn't believe in was religion as the *only* explanation.

Over the centuries these philosophers have been shown to be right: even if God created the universe, it would seem that He chose various laws and mechanisms to govern events in that universe. It is these laws and mechanisms that are studied by science. The discovery of these laws and mechanisms enables us to predict and explain events and, often, to manipulate them according to our own will.

Many, however, have thought that there is one phenomenon that cannot possibly be explained without appeal to God: morality. Without God to ordain the absolute rules that govern morality, to make Divine judgements, and to punish wrongdoers, many believe there could be no such thing as morality.

Others, especially in recent years, have demurred. It is entirely possible, they argue, to explain morality by appeal to Darwinian evolutionary forces: altruistic behaviour, they argue, has been selected for by nature because it facilitates survival and reproduction, especially amongst social animals like human beings.[8]

Again it is not part of the remit of this book to take a stance on the metaphysical question of whether or not morality could exist without God. It is relevant to the remit of this book, however, to point out that even if God *is* the source of morality, this does not relieve us of our responsibility to engage in moral decision-making. We need to do this for several reasons:

(i)   even if we think we know God's will we need a common ground for discussion;
(ii) many believers disagree about right and wrong;
(iii) we can all be wrong even about things we hold very dear;
(iv) many people will not accept religious justifications for anything;
(v)   religion has been appealed to in justification of deeds many find appalling.

In this book we will not be appealing to God or religion to justify any claim. This is wholly consistent with recognising the possibility that God exists, that He created the universe, that without him morality wouldn't exist, and that many people are motivated in their moral behaviour by belief in Him.[9]

> ### Box 2.8 Activity: Conceptual analysis
>
> 1. If the question: 'could there be morality without God?' is a metaphysical question, which epistemological question would be associated with it?
> 2. If the question: 'How do we justify the claim that lying is wrong?' is an epistemological question, what is the metaphysical question associated with it?
>
> Answers:
> 1. How do we know there is morality without God?
> 2. Is lying wrong?

Ethical and moral

Throughout the book words like 'ethics' and 'ethical, 'moral' and 'morality' appear in various forms. Strictly speaking 'morality' is properly used of first order questions and decisions, and 'ethical' of second order questions and decisions. Ethics is the systematic study of morality, which is itself constituted of the everyday decisions we make about right and wrong. Notwithstanding this, we shall not be making hard and fast distinctions between the two clusters of terms. We shall, for example, speak interchangeably of 'ethical decisions' and 'moral decisions'. This accords with our everyday use of these terms and should not, therefore, cause misunderstanding.

This completes our discussion of how the study of ethics is related to our everyday moral decision-making, and of some of the pre-suppositions and consequences of our ethical thinking.

Summary

In this chapter we have considered:

- the practical nature of ethics;
- that there is more to ethical decision-making than following rules;
- the distinction between first order moral thinking (thinking about which actions are right and wrong) and second order moral thinking (thinking about what makes an action right and wrong);
- the distinction between metaphysics (questions about what is the case) and epistemology (questions about how we can justify our claim to know what is the case);
- the existence of different theories about what makes our actions right and wrong;
- that the only actions that are morally evaluable are intentional ones, and that some people – the hard determinists – deny that there are any such actions;
- that as philosophers we can and should attempt to separate our ethical thinking from our thinking about religion.

Questions to stimulate reflection

What role is played by rules in moral decision-making?

Are moral claims such as 'lying is wrong' true or false? If so are they *always* true or false?

What makes an action morally acceptable or unacceptable?

What is the difference between first order and second order ethics?

How does metaphysics differ from epistemology?

Why is intentional action and free will of such importance to ethics?

If every action is a function of the physical states of the agent and his environment plus the laws of nature, do we really *have* free will?

Can we think about morality without thinking about religion?

Additional activities

Prepare a brief description of the moral dilemma about your friend and her hair. Ask your friends, family or fellow students what they would do and why.

Put 'moral dilemma' into a search engine and see if you can find some more moral dilemmas.

Get from the library an introduction to moral philosophy (you'll find a few suggestions below) and write a review of it.

Listen to the podcast 'An Introduction to Ethics' by the author of this book (reference below).

Listen to this video by philosopher Daniel Dennett on his views on free will: http://www.youtube.com/watch?v=Utai74HjPJE.

Use Dennett's video to stimulate a discussion on free will.

Notes

1 http://news.bbc.co.uk/1/hi/magazine/4954856.stm. A BBC website offering four moral dilemmas with poll results from readers.
2 'Ontology' has been borrowed by the computing world (and by science in general), to mean something more like standardising word usage, as in: 'we need to define ontologies for the physiology' meaning, e.g. 'when we're talking about a "hand" are we including the thumb or not?' Beware of confusing the two meanings.
3 http://plato.stanford.edu/entries/metaphysics/. Information on metaphysics from the *Stanford Encyclopedia of Philosophy*.
4 http://plato.stanford.edu/entries/epistemology/. Information on epistemology from the *Stanford Encyclopedia of Philosophy*.
5 http://ezinearticles.com/?A-Pardons-Process-for-a-Moose:-Animal-Trials&id=5954369. An 'Ezine' article about animals facing trial.
6 http://news.bbc.co.uk/1/hi/education/8096912.stm. A BBC report of research on the 'guilty look' of dogs.
7 http://www.rep.routledge.com/article/V014. The entry on free will from the *Routledge Encyclopedia of Philosophy*.
8 Ridley, M. (1997) *The Origins of Virtue*. London: Penguin Press.
9 This claim can be modified appropriately for pantheists, polytheists, etc.

Further reading and useful websites

Blackburn, S. (2003) *A Very Short Introduction to Ethics*. Oxford: Oxford University Press.
LaFolette, H. (2005) *The Oxford Handbook of Practical Ethics*. Oxford: Oxford University Press.
Pink, T. (2004) *Free Will: A Very Short Introduction*. Oxford: Oxford University Press.

http://plato.stanford.edu/. The *Stanford Encyclopedia of Philosophy* – an invaluable online resource. A bit hard-going for non-philosophers.
http://bioethics.od.nih.gov/casestudies.html. A series of bioethics resources from the US NIH.
http://www.mariannetalbot.co.uk. The author's podcasts on ethics.
http://www.philosophy.ox.ac.uk/podcasts. A series of podcasts on moral philosophy given by the author.
http://www.rep.routledge.com/about. The *Routledge Online Encyclopedia of Philosophy*.
http://www.scu.edu/ethics/practicing/decision/. A series of ethics resources from the Santa Clare University, a Jesuit University in Silicon Valley.

3 Ethics in the context of society: ethics, society and the law

Objectives

In reading this chapter you will:

- learn to distinguish ethical issues from social issues;
- reflect on the requirements for the smooth running of society;
- consider the nature of social decision-making;
- learn to distinguish the moral and the legal;
- consider the principles that govern just societies;
- briefly consider the nature of political authority.

In thinking ethically we are trying to decide which actions are right and wrong, which actions we should or shouldn't perform. But no man is an island, and the decisions we make about how to act must be made in the context of the laws of the land in which we live. Some of the most important ethical decisions, therefore, are not primarily decisions about how individuals should or shouldn't act, but rather decisions about whether a given action:

- **should or shouldn't be illegal**

Nearly every country in the world has made it illegal to clone a human being for reproductive purposes. Even if an individual believes that human cloning is morally acceptable, therefore, he cannot rationally clone a human being without taking into account the fact it is illegal and that the state will punish him if it discovers what he is doing. (We shall be considering reproductive cloning in Chapter 8.)

- **should or shouldn't be regulated by law**

In Britain and in some US states (e.g. Rhode Island, California and New Jersey) it is legal to clone a human being as far as the blastocyst stage of embryo development for the purposes of research (so-called 'therapeutic' cloning). Anyone wanting to clone a human being for such purposes, however, must jump through the myriad hoops by which such activities are regulated by the law. They will, for example, in the UK, need a licence from the Human Fertilisation and Embryology Authority (HFEA),[1] whose job it is to subject requests for licences to close examination, then they will need to obey the various regulations governing the activity itself, then finally they will have to destroy the clone by the 14th day. (We shall be considering therapeutic cloning in Chapter 7.)

- **should or shouldn't be funded by the public purse**

In the United States, under President Bush, therapeutic cloning, though legal, could not be carried out by anybody needing public funding. It was forbidden to use money from the public purse for such activities. Only private organisations able to fund their own research were therefore able to take advantage of the legality of therapeutic cloning in the United States.

Such decisions cannot be made by ordinary individuals, they must be made by the nation-states to which individuals belong as citizens or as subjects, or by the parts of those nation-states to which the nation-state has delegated decision-making power.

Box 3.1 **Philosophical background: The state of nature**

In deciding the principles by which the state should be governed political philosophers talk about the 'state of nature'. This is the condition human beings were in before governments came into existence. The questions asked about the state of nature include: how did humans act? Were there any rules all human beings followed? Why did humans bring states into existence?[2]

There are different views about what life was like in the state of nature. Some, for example British Philosopher **John Locke** (who was instrumental in writing the US constitution), believed that in the state of nature human beings would be naturally sympathetic and co-operative. He also believed there'd be a natural morality which he called the 'law of nature'. This law gave us, in Locke's opinion, the right to self-defence and to own those goods with which we 'mixed our labour' (for example, if we plough some land, we become the owner of that land). Locke believed the state would come into existence because we would soon see that this would be a better way of making sure the law of nature is imposed fairly and in accordance with majority rule.

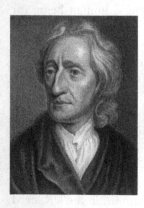

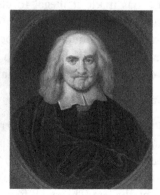

Another British philosopher, **Thomas Hobbes**, rejected Locke's benign view of human nature. He believed that in the state of nature we would be constantly at war with each other and that life would be 'solitary, poore, nasty, brutish and short'. Hobbes believed our motivation for introducing the state would be our need to protect ourselves from each other: we would want a single leader, one strong enough to put down the insurrections, disagreements and infighting that would inevitably arise without the rule of such a leader.

Figure 3.1 John Locke. © Photolibrary.com.

Figure 3.2 Thomas Hobbes. © Photolibrary.com.

In making these decisions the state sometimes has a very difficult task. In every society there are issues, often moral, that cause huge controversy. On such issues most citizens believe themselves to be right, but they disagree with each other on exactly *what* is right. Sometimes these disagreements can become very bitter. Those who believe that experimentation on animals, or abortion, is wrong, for example, have resorted to extreme violence to make their case (as we'll see in Chapter 20).

Most people who believe such things are wrong do not act so unreasonably. But when reasonable people disagree the state cannot adjudicate.[3] All it can do is to take account of that controversy in making its decisions.

The decisions made by the state or its agents all involve the allocation of important social resources such as freedom, power and public money. It is the state that decides what its citizens are free to do and not to do, who should have the authority to act on behalf of the state, and how state-sponsored activities should be funded.

Different nation-states have different decision-making processes. Some states are dictatorships. In Zimbabwe, until recently, decisions have largely been made by one man, Robert Mugabe,[4] and by those he has appointed. The same is true in North Korea.[5] Other states, including most of those in the west, are democracies in which decisions are made by those who have been elected by the people to represent them. Different democracies go about the process of decision-making in different ways. The decisions they make are sometimes very different.

Box 3.2 Activity: Group activity

There are two parts to this activity, one could be carried out as an individual activity (an essay perhaps), the other as a group discussion. Or both could be done as group discussions (perhaps at different times) or as individual activities.

Everyone in the group should imagine that they are in the state of nature (see Box 3.1) and must therefore look out for themselves and their family group. There is no law and therefore no protection from the law for individuals.

1. In small groups participants should:
    (i) try to identify the advantages and disadvantages of their situation;
    (ii) decide whether they would like to continue to live without benefit of the law or whether they'd prefer to agree to live together according to the rule of law.

Each group should appoint a spokesperson to explain the group's view and the reasoning behind it.

2. Participants should discuss the type of government they think would be best. They might choose from (some combination of):
    (i) anointing a hereditary monarchy;
    (ii) electing a representative government;
    (iii) appointing a leader for life;

(iv) appointing a short-term leader;

(v) anything else they can think of.[6]

Again each group should appoint a spokesperson to explain the group's view and the reasoning behind it.

In a democracy individuals are able to participate in the process of deciding what their government should or shouldn't do. Some participate only to the extent of voting for a representative, others don't even do this. Some do far more than this. It is clear that the more concerned one is about the decisions that the state makes (and about the laws that one will therefore have to obey) the more one should engage actively in the process of making these decisions.

In order to participate effectively in such decision-making, individuals must be informed about the decisions to be made, must have reflected on the decisions they think *should* be made and, ideally, will have put their reflections to the test by engaging in debate with those whose views differ. Such debates provide an opportunity for those involved to attempt to achieve a 'reflective equilibrium' between their different beliefs.[7] This can be achieved by listening to others' arguments and taking good arguments into account in their own thinking.

Democracies, ideally, will try to provide forums to help citizens participate in such activities, expect schools to prepare citizens for participation, and perhaps provide incentives for citizens to participate.[8]

As biotechnology advances and makes it possible for us to engage in many activities that have previously been impossible, it is not just individuals who must decide for themselves whether or not the activities made possible are morally permissible, required or forbidden: states must also make such decisions. The decisions made by states will, of course, interact importantly with the decisions of individuals.

Morality and the law of the land

That the law of the land is quite different from what many have called the 'moral law' can be seen in the fact that there are actions that are immoral but not illegal and vice versa.

Lying, for example, is not illegal, though most people would agree that lying is – usually – morally wrong. There are types of lie, of course, that *are* illegal (fraud is usually against the law and fraud is a type of lying), but no state would pass a law forbidding you from falsely telling your friend you think she looks nice.

Box 3.3 Activity: Personal reflection

Why do you think no (sensible) state would pass a law against lying to your friend about her hair?

> Reflect on the different ways we punish those who have broken the law and those who have acted immorally. Why should there be such different sorts of punishment?

There are also actions that are illegal but not obviously immoral. In Britain it is illegal to drive on the right, for example, in the United States it is illegal to drive on the left. Morality, however, says nothing about the side of the road on which one should drive. At least it doesn't until a law is passed, then it might be argued that as morality *would* say 'obey the law', then morality also says 'drive on the left when in Britain and on the right when in the United States'. Nevertheless it is easy to see that here there is an arbitrary element to the law: this law is needed to co-ordinate behaviour not to enforce morality.

Other laws, for example 'do not kill', seem to have a clear moral element. If human beings have the right to life then morality would say 'you must not kill', and the law of the land merely gives state expression to the moral requirement. In doing so the state gives itself (or its agents) the power to punish anyone who kills another human being. In deciding whether or not to kill someone, an individual who is not dissuaded by the immorality of doing so, might be dissuaded by the illegality of it. If not, and he is caught, he will be punished.

Another indication that the law of the land is not the same as the moral law is given in the fact that morality can seem to require the making of, or the abolition of, a law. Many people in the United States, for example, believe that the death penalty is immoral. How could a law be immoral if there was no more to morality than the law of the land? In Britain many people believe that morality demands that a law should be passed permitting assisted dying. How could morality demand a law that doesn't exist if there was no more to morality than the law?

Box 3.4 **Factual information: Civil disobedience**

Civil disobedience involves disobeying the law openly and with every intention of taking due punishment in the hope of changing the law. Mahatma Ghandi famously used civil disobedience in his dealings with the British Empire. He proposed the following rules for those engaged in campaigns of civil disobedience:[9]

1. harbour no anger
2. suffer the anger of the opponent
3. never retaliate to assaults or punishment; but do not submit, out of fear of punishment or assault, to an order given in anger
4. voluntarily submit to arrest or confiscation of your own property
5. if you are a trustee of property, defend that property (non-violently) from confiscation with your life
6. do not curse or swear

7. do not insult the opponent

8. neither salute nor insult the flag of your opponent or your opponent's leaders

9. if anyone attempts to insult or assault your opponent, defend your opponent (non-violently) with your life

10. as a prisoner, behave courteously and obey prison regulations (except any that are contrary to self-respect)

11. as a prisoner, do not ask for special favourable treatment

12. as a prisoner, do not fast in an attempt to gain conveniences whose deprivation does not involve any injury to your self-respect

13. joyfully obey the orders of the leaders of the civil disobedience action

14. do not pick and choose amongst the orders you obey; if you find the action as a whole improper or immoral, sever your connection with the action entirely

15. do not make your participation conditional on your comrades taking care of your dependents while you are engaging in the campaign or are in prison; do not expect them to provide such support

16. do not become a cause of communal quarrels

17. do not take sides in such quarrels, but assist only that party which is demonstrably in the right; in the case of inter-religious conflict, give your life to protect (non-violently) those in danger on either side

18. avoid occasions that may give rise to communal quarrels

19. do not take part in processions that would wound the religious sensibilities of any community.

The making of the law, as an activity, is itself governed by morality. There are three important moral considerations that must be taken into account in every decision the state makes:

- public welfare;
- individual rights;
- justice between individuals.

As we work through this book we will see that it can be hugely difficult to balance these considerations against each other: just as the values that guide the conduct of individuals conflict, so the values that guide the decision-making of states conflict: hard decisions cannot be avoided.

Box 3.5 Activity: Creative writing

It is 2020. Scientists have discovered a procedure that used once will reliably add 10 healthy years to our lives. Used a second time it produces 10 extra years, but not healthy ones. Unfortunately, each use of the procedure is very costly. But the news is out: people everywhere badly want to be able to use the procedure once to gain those extra 10 years.

Write a short piece (about 500 words) describing the thoughts of a person (the President? The Prime Minister?) who will be involved in making the government's final decision.

We will think more about this in Chapter 12.

This completes our discussion of ethics in the context of society, and of the relation between the 'moral law' and the laws of the land.

Summary

In this chapter we have considered:

- that many ethical decisions must be made by governments rather than individuals;
- that individual ethical decision-making always takes place in the context of a society governed by laws that will have to be taken into account;
- that in a democracy individuals are able to contribute to the governmental decision-making process;
- that advances in biotechnology will generate many moral decisions that must be addressed by governments as well as individuals;
- that the laws of the land are distinct from the rules of morality, though ideally they are constrained by these rules;
- that in making moral decisions good governments are constrained by concern for welfare, rights and justice.

Questions to stimulate reflection

What is the difference between an 'ethical issue' and a 'social issue'?

How are the rules that are the laws of the land related to the rules of morality?

What is the 'state of nature' and why is it important to political philosophers? Are we morally obliged to obey the law? Why?

Is rebellion against the law ever justified? If so, when? What form might this rebellion take if it is to be morally acceptable?

What are the principles that guide decision-making in the context of the state?

Should citizens and subjects of a democracy contribute to the decision-making process? Why?

Additional activities

Put 'Hart–Fuller debate' into a search engine, and find out about this famous debate about the extent to which morality and the law go together.

With a partner, role-play a discussion between John Locke and Thomas Hobbes on what life would be like in the state of nature.

Access this website: http://www.wgp.cf.ac.uk/CitizensJury.htm and learn about the Citizens' Jury on Designer Babies conducted by the Wales Gene Park with the University of Glamorgan and Techniquest.

Consider setting up a citizens' jury of your own on a social issue generated by biotechnology.

Access this website: http://webarchive.nationalarchives.gov.uk/20100824180635/ http://yourfreedom.hmg.gov.uk/ and learn about a British government's attempt to discover which laws British citizens believe should be scrapped.

Conduct an opinion poll amongst your family, friends and fellow students on the laws that local people believe should be repealed.

Access this website: http://www.pbs.org/wnet/religionandethics/episodes/march-20–2009/civil-disobedience/2473/ and decide whether or not you think Tim DeChristopher should go to jail.

Can you find any famous cases of civil disobedience in your country?

Notes

1 http://www.hfea.gov.uk. The website of the HFEA.
2 http://www.open2.net/historyandthearts/philosophy_ethics/state_of_nature_p.html. The state of nature from the BBC with the Open University.
3 http://www.procon.org/. A US website offering the pros and cons on many controversial issues. The website: http://www.sac.edu/students/library/nealley/websites/controversial.htm contains many useful resources on controversial issues.
4 http://www.guardian.co.uk/world/robert-mugabe. Articles on Robert Mugabe from the UK's *Guardian* newspaper.
5 http://www.bbc.co.uk/news/world-asia-pacific-15256929. A BBC Country Profile on North Korea.
6 http://news.bbc.co.uk/cbbcnews/hi/find_out/guides/world/united_nations/types_of_government/newsid_2151000/2151570.stm. A BBC website on different types of government.
7 http://philosophy.hku.hk/think/value/reflect.php. An OpenCourseWare website on the type of critical thinking known as striving for 'reflective equilibrium'.
8 http://www.ncl.ac.uk/peals/dialogues/juries.htm. A website from PEALS (Policy, Ethics and the Life Sciences) describing its 'Citizens' Jury' project.
9 Gandhi, M.K. (23 February 1930) 'Some Rules of Satyagraha'. Young India (Navajivan) (*The Collected Works of Mahatma Gandhi*, vol. 48, p. 340).

Further reading and useful websites

Boucher, D. and Kelly, P. (eds.) (2009) *Political Thinkers from Socrates to the Present*. Oxford: Oxford University Press.

Haldane, J. (2009) *Practical Philosophy: Ethics, Society and Culture*. St Andrews: St Andrews Studies in Philosophy and Public Affairs, Imprint Academic.

Miller, D. (2003) *Political Philosophy: A Very Short Introduction*. Oxford: Oxford University Press.

http://www.citizen.org.uk/. The website of the UK's Institute for Citizenship offering plenty of resources and activities to promote citizenship.

http://www.changemakers.org.uk/. A website aimed at encouraging young people to engage in active citizenship.

http://www.youtube.com/watch?v=nmVtdFLzlvI. A lecture on the history of political philosophy by John Rawls, a highly influential contemporary political philosopher.

4 | Ethical theories: virtue, duty and happiness

Objectives

In reading this chapter you will:

- reflect on the metaphysics and epistemology of morality;
- learn about Aristotle and virtue ethics;
- reflect on the advantages and disadvantages of virtue ethics;
- acquire an understanding of Immanuel Kant and deontology;
- reflect on the advantages and disadvantages of deontology;
- reflect on John Stuart Mill and utilitarianism;
- reflect on the advantages and disadvantages of utilitarianism;
- consider how to balance the three theories against each other in approaching moral dilemmas.

If we were to consider every ethical theory, this book would be too long. Instead we shall consider the three theories that command most followers. These are:

Virtue Theory: according to which the right action is the action that would be performed by a virtuous person.

Deontology: according to which the right action is the action that is performed out of duty (or 'reverence for the moral law').

Utilitarianism: according to which the right action is the one that would produce the greatest happiness of the greatest number.

Each of these theories postulates an account of the metaphysics of morality (what makes an action morally right or wrong) and the epistemology of morality (an account of how we know an action is morally right or wrong).

As you read about these theories and as, throughout the book, you apply them to specific problems, you will probably find yourself drawn to first one, then the other. Each theory has strengths and weaknesses which must be balanced against each other as we decide how to act.

We shall start by considering the theory of greatest longevity, the theory with its origins in the writings of Aristotle, one of the greatest philosophers of all time.

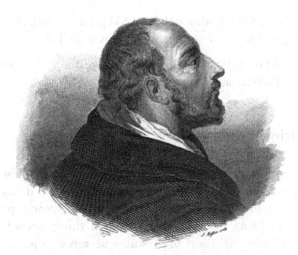

Figure 4.1 St Thomas Aquinas (*c.* 1225–1274), italian philosopher and theologian. © Photolibrary.com.

Amongst the philosophers who have adopted (and adapted) his theory are St Thomas Aquinas, Elizabeth Anscombe and Alisdair Macintyre.

Virtue ethics[1]

The virtue ethicist argues that what matters morally is not what we *do at a time*, but what we *become over time*. We all make mistakes, but so long as we recognise and learn from our mistakes, we will be on the way to acquiring a good character. To the virtue ethicist it is the acquisition of a good character that is – or should be – our moral aim, everything else will flow from this.

Here are some situations that might prompt you to agree with this:

- Despite his fear a fireman judges that running again into the burning house might enable him to save a child without injury to himself. He springs into action. Sadly he fails to save the child and injures himself in the attempt.

Virtue ethicists would argue that the fireman's action expressed the virtue of courage, and was therefore the right action, even if the consequences were other than those for which he acted.

- A poverty-stricken scientist is offered money by a rival company to share details of her work. The scientist knows these details will soon be in the public domain, so no harm would be done by accepting. Nevertheless she rejects the offer, unable to betray her company.

The virtue ethicist would say that the scientist's action expresses the virtue of loyalty and is therefore the right action, even though in performing it she arguably acts against her own interests without obvious benefit to anyone else.

- An unemployed biologist is interviewed for his dream job. The interview goes well until he discovers the company is funded by a Christian organisation that expects employees to be Christian. Although he could get away with claiming to be a Christian, the biologist doesn't want to lie and so loses the job.

The biologist's action might be thought to be self-defeating. But to the virtue ethicist it manifests the virtue of honesty and is the right action.

Virtues as dispositions

The virtue ethicist believes there is no set of rules such that if we follow them we will do the right thing. He also believes that we will not succeed in doing the right thing if we simply try to produce some consequence – happiness perhaps, or equality. The only way of being sure of doing the right thing, according to the virtue ethicist, is to become the right sort of person, a person who possesses all the virtues. Such a person cannot *but* act morally because his actions are the expression of a virtuous character.

Central to this account of morality is the notion of a *virtue*. A virtue is a disposition to act in a certain way, courageously, for example, honestly or benevolently. Acquiring the virtues is not an easy matter. It is a matter of becoming honest, courageous, wise, temperate, kind and loyal. It is a matter of obeying the 'golden mean', so that you do not go to extremes in anything you do. In facing danger, for example, you do not act in either a rash or a cowardly way, but rather courageously, in your interactions with others you avoid being either obsequious or surly and instead act with friendliness.

In order to acquire a virtue it is necessary to reflect on that virtue, to learn its true character and what it requires of one. It is also necessary to act in accordance with that

DEFICIENCY	MEAN VIRTUE	EXCESS
Cowardice	Courage	Rash
Insensible	Temperance	Dissipation
Stinginess	Generosity	Wastefulness
Chintziness	Magnificence	Vulgar
Smallness of Soul	Greatness of Soul	Vanity
Unambitious	(no name)	Ambitious
Spiritlessness	Gentleness	Irascibility, Irritable
Self-deprecation: Pretense as understatement	Truthfulness	Boastfulness: pretense as exaggeration
Boorishness	Wittiness, Charming	Buffoonery
Quarrelsome, Sultry	Friendliness	Obsequious if for no purpose Flatterer if for own advantage

Figure 4.2. Aristotelian Virtues: the mean and the two extremes. From the Moral Premise Blog based on 'The Moral Premise: Harnessing Virtue and Vice for Box Office Success' by Stanley D. Williams, PhD published by Michael Wiese Productions Books, Studio City, 2006 (http://moralpremise.blogspot.com/2010/07/aristotles-nicomachean-ethics-mean.html).

virtue: it is no good knowing what honesty is and what it requires if one doesn't *do* what honesty requires. Finally, it is necessary to do what a virtue requires *because* that virtue requires it. Telling the truth out of momentary spite or because one is unable to think of a convincing lie is not a manifestation of the virtue of honesty.

Box 4.1 Philosophical background: Aristotle (384–322 BC)

For Aristotle[2] a virtuous person is a person who:

- knows what the right action is;
- performs the right action;
- performs the right action because it is the right action.

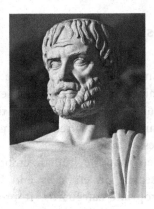

Figure 4.3 Aristotle.
©iStockphoto.com/
Panagiotis Karapanagiotis.

Being virtuous, for Aristotle, is a matter of acquiring the right habits. Just as an athlete must acquire the right habits so his natural strength will flourish, so human beings must habitually act in accordance with virtue to avoid becoming morally flabby.

Aristotle believed that human beings are unique in having a potential they can fulfil by their own efforts. The only way to fulfil this potential, and achieve happiness,[3] he argued, is to acquire the virtues.

Of course no one whose child is killed in an accident will be happy however virtuous he is. Luck and money are also required for happiness. For Aristotle, virtue is *necessary* for happiness, but not sufficient.

Importantly, acquiring the virtues cannot be understood as a *means* to happiness. Anyone who attempts to be virtuous because they want their own happiness has missed the point. Virtue is its own reward.[4]

Virtue ethics and epistemology

It has seemed to some that there is an uncomfortable whiff of circularity about virtue ethics. It claims that a person is virtuous if he performs virtuous acts for virtuous reasons, and then that a virtuous act is one that would be performed by a virtuous person for virtuous reasons. What is the use, it might be asked, of a theory of ethics that gives us no guidance on what to do?

To this charge a virtue theorist would reply that there is no such thing as a manual that will tell us how to act morally. The only way we can learn how to act morally is by emulating those who already act morally. If we do this until we can ourselves see how we should act in order to act morally, and acting morally has become a habit with us, we will ourselves have become virtuous. Even then the knowledge we have acquired will not be the sort of knowledge that could be encapsulated in any manual: there is no set of rules that will help us when it comes to morality. Moral knowledge is practical, not theoretical, knowledge.

The only guidance virtue theory offers us when it comes to our own actions, therefore, is to advise us to seek out virtuous people and emulate them. But such advice is not empty. It is a good description of what we usually do when faced with a moral dilemma: we ask the advice of those we respect.

It is not only individuals that follow this decision-procedure in facing moral dilemmas. Governments do this whenever they put together committees of the 'great and good'. In the field of bioethics such committees are very common.[5] The best of these committees will draw members with proven track-records from a wide range of backgrounds and views, the better to ensure that every perspective is covered, and no position will simply be assumed.

Box 4.2 Factual information: Committees of the great and the good

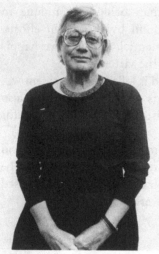

In 1982 the British government formed a committee of enquiry to develop principles by which to regulate IVF and embryology, and in particular to determine the moral status of the embryo (see Chapter 7). The committee was chaired by the philosopher Mary Warnock, later Baroness Warnock.

The committee concluded that the human embryo should be protected, but that research on embryos and IVF would be permissible, given appropriate safeguards. It proposed the establishment of a regulatory authority to license the use in treatment, storage and research of human embryos. This body became the Human Fertilisation and Embryology Authority (HFEA).

The findings of the committee were published in the Warnock Report in 1984 which formed the basis for the Human Fertilisation and Embryology Act.[6]

Figure 4.4 Mary Warnock, 1990. © Steve Pyke/Premium Archive/Getty Images.

Problems for virtue ethics

There are several problems with which the virtue ethicist must grapple:

How do we know who is virtuous?

Isn't it possible for someone to pretend to be virtuous? A dishonest person, for example, will want us to trust him. This gives him reason to tell the truth most of the time. But he will hold himself ready to lie to us when it will benefit him. How can we distinguish such a person from a person who really is honest?

Are there any virtuous people?

Human beings can be ignorant (they often don't know what to do), weak (they often do not do what they should) and dishonest (they sometimes do what they should but for the wrong reasons). If no one is virtuous surely virtue theory is impractical?

Is an act virtuous because a virtuous person performs it, or does the virtuous person perform it because it is a virtuous act?

Which comes first, the virtuous person or the virtuous act? Could there be an act such that it was (i) virtuous and (ii) no virtuous person could perform it?

What are the virtues?

Is Aristotle's list the definitive list? What about that of the Catholic Church?

> **Box 4.3 Activity: Paired discussion**
>
> In pairs imagine two Mother Teresas:
>
> Mother Teresa number one longs to dance in scarlet silk, but believing it is right to help the poor she suppresses her desire.
>
> Mother Teresa number two has never considered any life other than that of helping the poor.
>
> Aristotle would argue that the first Mother Teresa is more virtuous because she does what she does because she believes it is the right thing rather than because she is naturally altruistic. Do you agree?
>
> After 10 minutes of discussion participants should be asked for feedback.

Virtue ethics in this book

You will find virtue ethics discussed in:

Chapter 7 (in connection with the discussion about the moral status of the embryo);
Chapter 4 (in connection with human genetic enhancement).

Deontology

There are strong intuitions to the effect that certain actions are morally required or forbidden.[7] These situations might trigger these intuitions in you:

- A doctor saves the lives of seven of his dying patients by gently killing a healthy tramp and using his organs for the transplants his patients need.

Deontologists (the word stems from the Greek for 'duty') argue that killing the tramp is wrong, however, gently it is done and even if by killing him seven lives could be saved.

- A government official, desperate to avert a food crisis and believing the fear of genetically modified food to be overblown, orders his underlings to remove the labels and distribute GM food as non-GM.

Deontologists argue that lying to get people to do something you want them to do is wrong, even if their own beliefs are false and you might, by lying to them, be saving their lives.

- A father of two daughters, believing the family will starve if they have to pay another dowry, forces his unwilling wife to abort a pregnancy when he discovers it is another daughter.

Deontologists believe that it is wrong to force someone to do something they don't want to do even if it is for their own benefit.

Rules as constraints on our freedom

For the deontologist, the end cannot justify the means: if a given action is intrinsically wrong, then it doesn't matter how good its consequences, the act is forbidden. Similarly if a given action is intrinsically good then it is morally required whatever the consequences.

There are different types of deontologist according to the different types of actions they believe to be intrinsically right and wrong. Those who embrace the 10 commandments are deontologists, for example, as are those who embrace the Kantian 'Categorical Imperative' (see Box 4.4). Central to deontology are rules that forbid or enjoin certain types of action. Unlike the virtue ethicist, the deontologist thinks morality is all about rules, though not all these rules are the simple ones you were taught as a child.

Box 4.4 **Philosophical background: Immanuel Kant (1724–1804)**

To Kant each of us takes ourselves to have a right to decide what to believe and how to live our lives.[8] He argued that in recognising others are like ourselves, we must also recognise others' right to self-determination. From this, according to Kant, follows the whole of the 'moral law'.

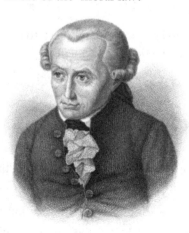

Figure 4.5 Immanuel Kant.
©iStockphoto.com/Steven Wynn.

Kant offered several formulations of the moral law – the 'categorical imperative' – the two most important of which are:

The principle of humanity: always treat humanity whether in yourself or in another, as an end (in itself), never solely as a means.

Kant believed that it is our possession of reason and free will that generates our right to be treated as self-determining, as 'ends in ourselves'. It is always wrong, according to Kant, to use others as nothing more than tools by which to achieve your own ends.

The principle of universalisability: Act only on that maxim you could will to be universal law.[9]

We make choices about our actions on the basis of reasons. Kant calls these 'maxims'. He argues that before we act for a given reason we should always ask ourselves 'what if everyone were to do this?'

Imagine you are about to tell a lie to get someone to do something for you but then ask yourself 'what if everyone were to lie in order to get someone to do something for them?' An honest answer would involve recognising that it would make trust impossible. But without trust no society could survive. Recognition of this, says Kant, gives you reason not to treat yourself as a special case: if you have reason to lie to get someone to do what you want, so has everyone else.

For Kant, the moral law binds us absolutely in virtue of our capacity for reason: to act immorally is to act irrationally.

Deontology and absolutism

Many people are put off deontology because deontologists are absolutists: they believe that there are moral rules that are true everywhere, at every time, for everyone. If you deny this you will reject deontology.

But there are different types of rule. There are rules like 'do not lie' and 'keep promises', and then there are rules like 'do as you would be done by' and 'never treat others solely as means to your own ends'.

Many people dismiss absolutism believing that no rule of the first kind is true absolutely. But this does not show that no rule of the second kind is true absolutely. There are reasons for thinking moral rules of this kind *are* true absolutely. If you want to be treated in the way you like being treated, then it seems reasonable to think that everyone else would want to be treated as *they* want to be treated. They might want to be treated in a way that you wouldn't want to be treated, but they have as much right to being treated as *they* want as you have to being treated as *you* want.

Many people think that because different cultures (or indeed different individuals) have different moral beliefs this means that moral truth must be relative. It is certainly the case that one explanation for differences in belief is that truth in that area of discourse is relative: a Frenchman might believe it is 5 p.m., for example, whilst an American believes it is 11 a.m. Yet both are right because temporal truth is relative to a time zone.

But there are other explanations for differences in belief that do not appeal to relativism. Here are two non-relativistic explanations for differences in moral belief:

(i) there is a 'higher level' belief that generates different 'lower level' beliefs in different circumstances;
(ii) the fact that one belief may be false.

The Inuit used to put their elderly gently to death. We keep ours alive as long as possible. But given the differences between the lives the Inuit used to live, and the lives we live, the shared belief 'we should respect the elderly' might express itself differently for the Inuit and for ourselves. An analogy would be the fact that two genetically identical seeds, raised in different circumstances, may be phenotypically very different.

That a 'lower level' belief like 'the elderly should be put gently to death' should be true only relative to a culture, does not show that absolutism is false because it doesn't show that a higher level belief like 'everyone should be treated as an end in themselves' isn't an absolute truth.

Differences in moral belief might also be the result of error. Could it be that those societies that claim to honour women by circumcising them have simply got it wrong? Could it be that we are wrong not to put the elderly gently to death? When we learn that other people's beliefs are different from our own this might tell us nothing more than that at least one of us is wrong (we will consider this again in Chapter 5, pages 67–69 when we discuss the principle of charity). In particular, it doesn't, in and of itself, tell us that absolutism is false.

Box 4.5 Philosophical background: Vulgar relativism

Some people reject moral absolutism because of a common logical error. They think everyone's moral beliefs should be respected, and this means that moral relativism *must* be true.

This is the argument offered:

Premise one: everyone's moral beliefs should be respected
Conclusion: therefore no moral belief is absolutely true.

The philosopher Bernard Williams calls this 'vulgar relativism' because:

- if the premise is true then the conclusion is false (because the premise is a moral belief that is absolutely true);
- if the conclusion is true then the premise is false (because *no* moral belief can be absolutely true).

Vulgar moral relativism is self-defeating.

Even if we must respect everyone's moral beliefs, this does not mean that we need to insist that they are true. It is entirely possible to respect someone whilst believing that they have a false belief. It is even possible to respect someone whilst *saying* they have a false belief – what matters is *how* you say this.[10]

For further discussion of this see the principle of charity in Chapter 5, and 'It's all a Matter of Opinion' in Chapter 6.

Problems for deontology

There are several problems the deontologist must grapple with:

How do we know which actions are intrinsically right or wrong?

Some deontologists believe that we have a special moral faculty: just as we see a leaf is green, so we *see* an action is wrong. Other deontologists believe God reveals to us which actions are right or wrong. Other deontologists believe that reason tells us which acts are right or wrong (see the Box 4.4).

Are there any actions that are intrinsically right or wrong?

Many people deny the existence of actions that are intrinsically right or wrong. Consequentialists, for example, believe that it is only the consequences of an action that make it right or wrong.

How could blindly following a set of rules make us moral?

What reason is there to think that there is a 'rulebook' for morality, when everyday moral rules conflict so easily?

Do rules like 'do as you would be done by' provide any guidance on action?

If a deontologist insists we should follow rules like this or like 'always treat others as ends in themselves' is he giving us any guidance at all?

Aren't there sometimes moral reasons for breaking moral rules?

If we can by killing one person prevent the killing of several, would the deontologist still insist we shouldn't kill?

> ## Box 4.6 Activity: Small group work
>
> Imagine we could save the life of five people by diverting a train from one track onto another on which one person is working. If we divert the train we kill one person, if we do not five people die.
>
> Some deontologists would argue that we should not divert the train. This may lead to the death of the five, but no *action* of ours led to their death and we are not morally responsible for what we *don't* do. Such a deontologist is relying on the 'act–omission distinction'.[11]
>
> Other deontologists would argue that we should divert the train with the intention of saving the five. This makes the death of the one a foreseen *but unintended* outcome of our action. We are not morally responsible, this deontologist will say, for the unintended consequences of our actions. Such a deontologist is relying on the 'doctrine of double effect'.[12]
>
> In small groups, participants should discuss whether the act–omission distinction and/or the doctrine of double effect can save the deontologist from having to insist that we do things we shouldn't do, or not do things we should do.
>
> A spokesperson from each group should present the group's conclusions to the rest of the class.
>
> The discussion of euthanasia and assisted killing in Chapter 13 applies these two distinctions to a particular problem. Participants might be asked to read that discussion before they do this activity. Alternatively *half* the groups might be asked to read that discussion before they do this activity.

Deontology in this book

You will find deontology discussed in:

  Chapter 5 (where deontological arguments against therapeutic cloning are used as
      examples in our discussion of evaluating arguments);
  Chapter 7 (in connection with the discussion about the moral status of the embryo);
  Chapter 19 (in connection with the requirement of informed consent).

Consequentialism

Many people have strong intuitions to the effect that it is only the consequences of an
action that matter morally.[13] Here are some actions that might trigger these intuitions
in you:

- A patient with a terminal and painful illness desperately wants to die. His family are
  exhausted and beg their doctor to help him. The doctor gives him a dose of
  morphine intending it to kill him.

Consequentialists would argue that in helping the man to die the doctor acts morally
even though generally speaking it is wrong to kill people.

- A high ranking officer, knowing the enemy will attack a particular hotel, tells the
  hotel manager to close the hotel on the grounds of an outbreak of food poisoning.
  The manager does so.

Consequentialists would argue that although it is usually wrong to lie, there are times
when the consequences of not lying would be disastrous and must be avoided.

- A father, knowing his unemployed son is depressed, forces him to work in the
  family business in order to regain his self-esteem.

Consequentialists would not normally force people to do something, but accept that the
consequences of doing so are sometimes better than the consequences of not doing so.

Rules as rules of thumb

Consequentialists do not believe that any actions are good or bad in and of themselves. The only thing that makes an action good or bad, according to a consequentialist, is the consequences of that action.

   If the consequences of a given action are better than those of any other action, then
the action should be performed even if such actions usually shouldn't be performed.
If an action is such that its consequences are worse than those of another action then
it shouldn't be performed, even if it is the sort of action that could usually be expected
to have good consequences.

   For the consequentialist, unlike the deontologist, the end *does* justify the means.
There is no action at all that cannot be performed so long as performing it would have
consequences better than those of any other action available at the time.

There are different types of consequentialist according to the different types of consequences – happiness, liberty, equality, etc. – that are believed to be the proper end of our actions. We will look in Chapter 21, p. 420, at a type of consequentialism that deems *life* to be the only thing of intrinsic value. The best known type of consequentialism is utilitarianism. The utilitarian believes that the right action is the one that produces the greatest happiness of the greatest number (GHGN). It is utilitarianism we shall be discussing in this book.

Box 4.7 Philosophical background: John Stuart Mill (1806–1873)

John Stuart Mill[14] believed that the fact we all desire our own happiness (or 'utility') is sufficient to show that the right action is the one that 'tends to' produce the greatest happiness of the greatest number. He claimed that all the other things we desire – liberty, equality, love – we desire as part of happiness.

For Mill, to be happy is to feel pleasure and not to feel pain. Our moral duty is to act in such a way as to maximise pleasure and to minimise pain.

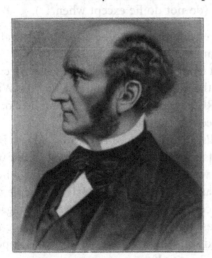

Figure 4.6 John Stuart Mill.
© Photolibrary.com.

Mill argued that there are 'higher' and 'lower' pleasures. An example of the former would be the feeling you get from successfully completing a philosophy essay, an example of the latter would be the feeling you get after enjoying a nice meal. Mill believed that in deciding how to act we must take into account the quality as well as the quantity of pleasure.

Mill was scathing about many of the objections made to utilitarianism, not least when it was suggested that utilitarianism cannot do more than pay lip service to important moral rules. In calculating how much happiness will be produced by an action it would be quite wrong, he argued, not to take into account such things as the weakening of trust, and/or the practice of promise-keeping.[15]

Rule and act utilitarianism

Traditionally it has been argued that there are two types of utilitarianism, act utilitarianism (AU) and rule utilitarianism (RU). RU was introduced as an attempt to enable the utilitarian to recognise everyday moral rules because one of the objections to AU is that it *doesn't* do this.

The AU is characterised by the belief that he must check every single individual action directly against the greatest happiness principle (GHP) which states we should produce the GHGN. So the fact that an action is a lie will not be relevant in deciding whether or not to perform it because morally speaking the only thing that matters is whether or not the action produces the GHGN.

The RU is characterised by the belief that we should check every *type* of action against the GHP. This generates rules to guide us in our daily decision-making. Then, in making decisions about particular actions, we must look to these rules. So the RU will first look at lying, as a type of action, asking whether lying usually produces the GHGN. Seeing that generally speaking lying doesn't produce the GHGN, the RU will form the rule 'don't lie'. In deciding whether or not to perform a *particular* action, he will then look to his rules. Seeing that a particular act is a lie, for example, he will not perform it.

It has been argued however that RU collapses into AU. To see this, ask yourself what should happen when the RU is considering an action that would violate a rule, but that would undoubtedly, in this particular situation, produce the GHGN. For example, the particular action he is considering is a lie. His rule says 'do not lie' because lying does not usually produce the GHGN. But it is obviously the case that this particular lie *would* produce the GHGN. There are three possibilities:

(i)   the RU would break the rule (in which case he is no different from an AU);
(ii) the RU would keep the rule (in which case he is no different from a deontologist);
(iii) the RU would make a new rule (do not do lie except when. . .).

It is only the last option that would enable the RU to be a utilitarian (rather than a deontologist) *and* be different from an AU.

But the RU would only be different from an AU in the way he makes decisions – the decisions he makes would be exactly the same as those made by the AU. Whenever an AU would break the rule and lie, the RU would make a new rule and lie. So, practically speaking, there is no difference between AU and RU.

Rather than try to maintain a distinction between RU and AU it is better to recognise that there are different sorts of rules, and different contexts in which rules must be considered. If, for example, we are legislators, considering whether to make killing people illegal, we will clearly apply directly to the GHP to decide whether or not killing, generally speaking, produces the GHGN. Arguing that a law against killing would produce the GHGN, we will pass the law. If we are a judge deciding whether or not to punish someone who has killed someone we are not entitled to appeal directly to the GHGN, we must appeal to the law itself.

The legislator, qua legislator, looks directly to the GHP. The judge, qua judge, looks only to the rule (the law). But neither can be considered an RU or an AU in the traditional sense (where *all* decisions would be referred either directly to the GHP or to rules).[16]

We have already seen in discussing deontology that the role of rules in moral thinking is hugely complex. This is another example of this complexity.

Problems for utilitarianism

There are several problems the utilitarian must grapple with, as follows:

Are there really no actions that are intrinsically wrong?
Would genocide be permissible so long as the people we killed were in the minority, and those left would be much happier without them?

Can utilitarianism recognise the existence of rights?

If anyone's rights can be over-ridden so long as the consequences are good enough, then do rights exist at all?

How do we justify the claim that we should aim to produce the greatest happiness of the greatest number?

Why is it happiness we should maximise, rather than liberty, equality or some other good?

How do we know in advance what the consequences of our actions will be?

If a company releases a drug onto the market believing that it will be hugely beneficial, but it turns out to have a side effect that leads to many deaths, has the company acted immorally?

Must we always act to produce the greatest happiness of the greatest number?

Doesn't this mean that it is immoral to relax with a drink when we could be trying to find a cure for cancer? Must we put the greatest happiness of the greatest number before the happiness of our family?

What is happiness and how do we measure it?

How can we tell what makes someone else happy? How can we balance one person's happiness against another's?

Whose happiness must be counted?

Must we count the happiness of non-human animals or not? Does the happiness of future generations count, or only the happiness of those currently alive? Might Hitler have been a good utilitarian except for the fact he didn't count Jews?

Can a utilitarian account for personal integrity?

Should someone against animal experimentation go to work in a laboratory where animals are experimented on because in doing so he could subvert the work being done?

Box 4.8 Activity: Thought experiment

Imagine that biotechnology produces a machine such that when people are attached to it they believe that they are happily living fulfilling and virtuous lives, when they are actually doing nothing but lying on a bed in a hangar-like building as these machines flood their bodies with chemicals.

The utilitarian government are considering whether or not to attach everyone to these machines.

Not everyone could be attached of course. Those on the machine must be fed, cleaned, protected. But even taking into account the unhappiness of the unattached, the greatest happiness would arguably still be produced by attaching the majority to the machines.

Should the government attach its citizens to these machines? Does conducting this thought experiment have ramifications for our acceptance of utilitarianism?[17]

Utilitarianism in this book

You will find utilitarianism discussed in:

Chapter 5 (where utilitarian arguments for therapeutic cloning are used as examples in our discussion of evaluating arguments);
Chapter 7 (in connection with the discussion about the moral status of the embryo).

Balancing the three theories against each other

The three moral theories just considered all have strengths. They also all have weaknesses. Luckily our task is not to decide which is the right moral theory, it is to decide whether the actions biotechnology makes possible are or aren't morally acceptable. We are at liberty, therefore, to use all three theories (and indeed any other consideration that seems to apply so long as we have a good argument for it).

If you are new to moral decision-making you might find it useful consciously to test a given moral dilemma against each of these theories in order to work out what each theory would say about it. Having worked out what each theory would say you will then be in a much better position to decide what *you* think.

Box 4.9 Activity: Presentations

Human therapeutic cloning involves producing a human clone in order to conduct research on it, or to harvest stem cells which may one day be used to repair human organs. Human cloning could provide huge benefits for those who are ill, their carers and their families.

For the purposes of this activity we are going to assume that human embryos have the right to life from the moment of syngamy (the point at which the sperm and the egg fuse).

Answer the following questions:

1. Would a **virtue ethicist** allow therapeutic human cloning? What reasons would he give for his view? What are the objections to his view?
2. Would a **deontologist** allow therapeutic human cloning? What reasons would he give for his view? What are the objections to his view?

3. Would a **consequentialist** allow therapeutic human cloning? What reasons would he give for his view? What are the objections to his view?

The class should be divided into three groups. Each group should take one question and prepare a presentation for the rest of the class.

We shall be discussing therapeutic cloning in Chapter 7. This activity is best completed before reading that discussion. It might be re-visited after reading that discussion.

This completes our discussion of ethical theories. Throughout this book we shall be applying all three theories to the various moral and social dilemmas we discuss.

Summary

In this section we have considered:

- three ethical theories, virtue ethics, deontology and consequentialism (in particular utilitarianism);
- the main reasons for embracing each of these theories;
- a major ramification of each theory (epistemology in the case of virtue ethics, absolutism in the case of deontology and the use of rules in the case of utilitarianism);
- a major proponent of each theory (Aristotle, Kant and Mill);
- the problems facing each of these theories;
- the fact that all three theories have strengths and weaknesses;
- the fact that we shall be applying all these theories to moral dilemmas throughout the book.

Questions to stimulate reflection

What is it that makes a person *virtuous*? Can a person be born virtuous? Is virtue a necessary condition of human happiness? How do we acquire virtue?

Is there such a thing as 'the moral law'? Where does it come from? How do we know what it requires of us? Don't rules always end up conflicting with each other? Isn't a morality of duty a heartless morality?

Is the right action the one that produces the greatest happiness of the greatest number? What is happiness? How do we measure happiness? Doesn't this claim justify violating the rights of minorities?

Additional activities

Choose a favourite moral problem and ask how each type of theorist would deal with it.

Put 'virtue ethics' 'consequentialism' and/or 'deontology' into a search engine and see what comes up.

Can you make a list of the *virtues*? Are there different categories of virtue?

What other sorts of consequentialism might there be? Consider what, other than happiness, might be deemed intrinsically valuable.

Choose a moral dilemma (for example the 'train problem' described in Box 4.6) and conduct an opinion poll amongst your family, friends and fellow students asking what people would do and why. Sort their answers by which moral theory they seem to be appealing to.

Read Dostoevsky's *Crime and Punishment* (there is a free copy here: http://www.online-literature.com/dostoevsky/crimeandpunishment/). Which theory of ethics is relied upon by Raskolnikov?

Notes

1 http://www.bbc.co.uk/ethics/introduction/virtue.shtml. A BBC website on virtue ethics.
2 http://www.youtube.com/watch?v=uNIPAwZVqb4&feature=related. Philosopher Martha Nussbaum talks to Bryan McGee about Aristotle.
3 http://www.philosophybites.libsyn.com/category/Miles%20Burnyeat. Philosopher Miles Burnyeat on Aristotle's notion of happiness for Philosophy Bites.
4 http://www.philosophybites.libsyn.com/roger_crisp_on_virtue. Philosopher Roger Crisp on Virtue for Philosophy Bites.
5 http://www.nuffieldbioethics.org/. The website for the Nuffield Council for bioethics, which often puts together committees to think about specific bioethical issues. http://www.bioethics.gov/. The website for the Presidential Commission for the Study of Bioethical Issues in the United States.
6 http://www.hfea.gov.uk/2068.html. The website of the Human Embryo and Fertilisation Authority. http://www.bionews.org.uk/page_68168.asp?dinfo=Y7N4PAmZl5Sorwq27ejPeY3Y. An article about the possibility of the HFEA being scrapped.
7 http://www.bbc.co.uk/ethics/introduction/duty_1.shtml. The BBC on deontology.
8 http://www.youtube.com/watch?v=kN5XzaWumV0. Philosopher Geoffrey Warnock talking to Bryan McGee about Kant.
9 In less formal language this could read 'act only on that maxim you could rationally wish to hold universally true'.
10 http://www.philosophybites.libsyn.com/simon_blackburn_on_moral_relativism. Philosopher Simon Blackburn being interviewed on moral relativism on Philosophy Bites.
11 http://www.bbc.co.uk/ethics/euthanasia/overview/activepassive_1.shtml The BBC gives a good account of the act–omission doctrine on this page.
12 http://www.bbc.co.uk/ethics/euthanasia/overview/doubleeffect.shtml. An explanation of the doctrine of double effect from the BBC.

13 http://www.bbc.co.uk/ethics/introduction/consequentialism_1.shtml. Consequentialism from the BBC.
14 http://ethics.sandiego.edu/theories/Utilitarianism/index.asp. Information on utilitarianism from Lawrence Hinman's site at the University of San Diego.
15 http://www.philosophybites.libsyn.com/roger_crisp_on_utilitarianism. An interview with philosopher Roger Crisp on Utilitarianism for Philosophy Bites). See also http://www.philosophybites.libsyn.com/category/Brad%20Hooker. Brad Hooker on the same topic.
16 http://www.dif.unige.it/dot/filosofiaXXI/rawls.pdf. In this philosophy paper – a bit difficult for non-philosophers – John Rawls, a famous political philosopher, discusses these ideas.
17 A version of this thought experiment was described by philosopher Robert Nozick in his book *Anarchy, State and Utopia*.

Further reading and useful websites

Fieser, J. (1999) *Metaethics, Normative Ethics, and Applied Ethics: Contemporary and Historical Readings*. Stamford, Connecticut: Wadsworth Publishing.
Graham, G. (2011) *Theories of Ethics: An Introduction to Moral Philosophy with a Selection of Classic Readings*. London: Routledge.
Timmons, M. (2002) *Moral Theory*. Lanham, Maryland: Rowman & Littlefield Publishers, Inc.

http://www.bbc.co.uk/ethics/introduction/. The BBC's Introduction to Ethics course.
http://caae.phil.cmu.edu/cavalier/80130/. An online guide to ethics posted by Dr Robert Cavalier of Carnegie Mellon University.
http://www.mariannetalbot.co.uk. Lectures discussing each of these ethical theories.

5

Identifying and evaluating arguments: logic and morality

Objectives

In reading this chapter you will:

- acquire some logical terminology;
- learn about deduction and induction;
- consider the difference between deductive validity and inductive strength;
- learn how to evaluate arguments;
- discover how to analyse arguments and set them out 'logic-book style';
- learn about a few important fallacies;
- reflect on the importance of the principle of charity.

Argument is the philosophical method. This is why philosophers study **logic**, the discipline that tells us how to distinguish good arguments from bad. There are many problems that can be approached only by using logic. Consider, for example, the following sentence:

(1) Therapeutic cloning is morally acceptable.

Therapeutic cloning (as we'll see in Chapter 7) is cloning for the purposes of conducting research on, or harvesting stem cells from, the resulting embryo. Some of us will believe sentence (1) is true. Others will believe it is false. We can't both be right. Which of us is right is not the sort of question the truth of which can be determined by observation or experiment. This can be decided only by engaging in argument.

The nature of argument

Box 5.1 Definition: Argument

When we construct an **argument** we put forward a claim and one or more reasons for believing the claim. The claim we put forward is called the **conclusion**. The reasons for believing the claim are called the **premises**.

Example: 'We have a duty not to exploit non-human animals, but when we engineer their genes this is what we are doing. Therefore we shouldn't genetically engineer non-human animals.'

Premise one: We have a duty not to exploit non-human animals.
Premise two: We exploit non-human animals when we engineer their genes.
Conclusion: We shouldn't genetically engineer non-human animals.

When we set out an argument like this we set it out 'logic-book style'.

In an argument a position is taken (the **conclusion**) together with at least one reason, possibly more, for holding that position (the **premises**). There are different types of argument, but all fall into one of two categories; they are either deductive or inductive.

Deduction and induction

Here are two arguments:

Argument one	Argument two
If the patient is in a permanent vegetative state (PVS) then he will not be conscious. The patient is in PVS. Therefore the patient will not be conscious.	People with Huntington's disease have always been observed to have the HD gene on chromosome 4. Therefore, the next person who develops Huntington's disease will be observed to have the HD gene on chromosome 4.

Argument one is a **deductively valid** argument. If the premises of this argument are true, the conclusion *must* be true. Argument two is an **inductively strong** argument. If the premise of this argument is true, the conclusion is extremely likely to be true. A deductive argument is either valid or invalid: it is an either/or matter. Inductive arguments can be strong or weak: inductive strength is a matter of degree.

Inductive arguments, even at their strongest, do not deliver cast iron guarantees because all such arguments tacitly rely on what the philosopher Hume called the 'principle of the uniformity of nature'. This belief underlies all our empirical reasoning. But it cannot be justified without circularity (see Box 5.2).

Box 5.2 Philosophical background: The principle of the uniformity of nature

Induction[1] is central to the scientific method. It extrapolates from something observed to something unobserved. Such extrapolation assumes that future observations will be like past observations.

But how do we know that we are not in the position of Bertrand Russell's chicken[2] who assumes that because the farmer has fed him every day of his life he will feed him again this morning? This morning, however, the farmer is coming to wring his neck so he can be eaten for Sunday lunch.

In expecting the sun to rise tomorrow because it has always risen before might we not be like the chicken?

The philosopher David Hume noted that every time we try to justify our use of the principle of the uniformity of nature, our reasoning goes in a circle.

We might try claiming that the future will be like the past because the future always has been like the past. But immediately the circle appears. Just because the future always has been like the past *in the past* why should we assume that the future will be like the past *in the future*?

The fact that the conclusions of deductively valid arguments are certain, and those of inductively strong arguments only *almost* certain does not make induction inferior. Science would be impossible without deduction or induction, but induction is central to the scientific method.[3]

Box 5.3 Activity: Conceptual analysis

Can you say which arguments are deductive and which inductive?

1. The sun is coming out so the rain should stop soon.
2. If Jane is at the party John won't be. Jane is at the party, therefore John won't be.
3. The house is a mess therefore Lucy must be home.
4. Either he's in the bathroom or the bedroom. He's not in the bathroom, so he must be in the bedroom.
5. The dog would have barked if it saw a stranger. It didn't bark, so it didn't see a stranger.
6. No-one in Paris understands me, so my French must be rotten, or the Parisians are stupid.

Answers:
1. inductive, 2. deductive, 3. inductive, 4. deductive, 5.deductive, 6. inductive.

Arguments one and two are both good arguments in virtue of the fact their conclusions **follow from** their premises. This is not true of the following two arguments:

Argument three	Argument four
If the patient is in a permanent vegetative state (PVS) then he will not be conscious. The patient is not conscious. Therefore the patient is in PVS.	When I passed that exam I wore my red shirt. Therefore, if I wear my red shirt next time I take an exam I will pass that exam too.

Argument three is an **invalid** argument: the premises of this argument, even if they are true, give us no reason whatsoever to believe the conclusion. Even if we are certain of the truth of these premises this tells us *nothing* about the truth of the conclusion.

Argument four is an **inductively weak** argument: even if the premise is true the likelihood of the conclusion is hardly raised at all. Even if we are certain of its truth, this tells us nothing about the likelihood of the conclusion being true.

Make sure you can see why neither conclusion **follows from** its premises before you move on.

Evaluating arguments

A bad argument tells us nothing. But it can lead us astray if we don't recognise it as bad. It is important, therefore, to learn how to evaluate arguments. In evaluating an argument we must ask two questions:

(i)   Is/are its premise(s) all true?
(ii) Does the conclusion 'follow from' the premises?

The relation of 'following from' covers two different sorts of relation between a (set of) premise(s) and a conclusion. The conclusion of a deductive argument follows from its premise(s) if the argument is **valid**. The conclusion of an inductive argument follows from its premise(s) if the argument is **inductively strong**. We shall consider how these differ below. For now we are considering what they have in common: the fact that when an argument is valid *or* inductively strong then its conclusion **follows from** its premises.

Looking at our two questions there are four possible answers to these questions taken together:

1. The answer to both questions is 'yes'
This argument is such that *all* its premises are true *and* its conclusion follows from its premises. In this situation the argument is said to be **sound**. A sound argument gives us excellent reason to believe the conclusion. A sound argument is very definitely a good argument.

2. The answer to (i) is 'yes', but the answer to (ii) is 'no'
This argument is such that although all its premises are true, the conclusion does not follow from them. In this situation the truth of the premises gives us no reason at

all to believe in the truth of the conclusion: the premises and the conclusion are not related in the right way to convince us of anything. Imagine, for example, that the premises of arguments three and four are true, this would not give us any reason to believe the conclusions would it? These arguments can't be considered 'good' in any sense.

3. The answer to (i) is 'no', but the answer to (ii) is 'yes'

This argument is such that although its conclusion follows from its premises, at least one of its premises is false. In this situation the fact that a premise is false means we have no reason to believe the conclusion despite its following from the premises. The fact that the conclusion follows from the premises, however, means that the argument can be considered a '**good**' argument. As an *argument* it is good and given that we often don't know whether the premises of an argument are true or false, this is often the best we'll get.

4. The answer to both questions is 'no'

In fact, we needn't bother with this situation because we have just seen that if the answer to *either* of these questions is 'no' then the argument gives us no reason to believe the conclusion. A fortiori, therefore, if the answer to *both* questions is 'no' the argument gives us no reason to believe the conclusion ('a fortiori' just means 'it is even more certain'). This is a very bad argument.

> ### Box 5.4 **Activity: Quiz**
>
> 1. What is an argument?
> 2. Can an argument have a single premise?
> 3. How does deduction differ from induction?
> 4. The relation of 'following from' includes two different relations, what are they?
> 5. Why doesn't induction deliver certainty?
> 6. What are the two questions we must ask in order to evaluate an argument?
> 7. What is the difference between an argument that is **sound** and one that is merely **good**?
> 8. In order for an argument to be sound must *all* its premises be true?
>
> Answers:
>
> 1. When we construct an argument we put forward a claim (a conclusion) and one or more reasons for believing the claim (the premise(s)). The argument is the set consisting in the premises plus the conclusion.
> 2. Yes.
> 3. A deductive argument, when sound, offers certainty. An inductive argument, even when sound, makes its conclusion more or less likely (possibly *much* more likely).
> 4. Validity (in the case of deduction). Inductive strength (in the case of induction).
> 5. All inductive arguments rely on the assumption that nature is uniform; that the future will be like the past. As this assumption isn't certainly true, no inductive argument can deliver certainty.
> 6. (i) Are the premises true? (ii) Does the conclusion follow from the premises?

7. A sound argument is such that all its premises are true *and* its conclusion follows from these premises. A good argument is such that its conclusion follows from the premises (we may not know whether the premises are true or not).
8. Yes.

Truth and soundness: getting the terminology right

You may have noticed that when we talked about premises and conclusions we called them *true* or *false*. But when we talked about arguments we called them *good* or *bad* or *sound* or *unsound* (or *cogent* and *uncogent*). This is important.

If you were to tell someone sincerely and non-metaphorically that a table is loud the person you're talking to would be bemused. Tables are not the sort of thing that *can* be loud. In saying a table is loud, you are demonstrating you don't understand the word 'table' or the word 'loud'. Similarly if you talk of arguments as 'true' or 'false' you demonstrate to any philosopher that you do not understand the word 'argument' or the words 'true' and 'false'. Premises and conclusions can be true or false. But arguments can't be.

Premises and conclusions are all *sentences* and it is only sentences (or the beliefs they express) that can be true or false. There are lots of philosophical theories about what makes sentences (and beliefs) true and false, but probably the most accepted one is some form of the theory that says a sentence is true when it corresponds with a fact.

Box 5.5 Philosophical background: Theories of truth

What makes a sentence (or the belief that the sentences expresses) true? One answer might be that it corresponds with some fact. So the sentence 'the litmus paper turned red' is true if the litmus paper we're referring to turned red, and it is false if it didn't.

There are many other theories of truth.[4] All fall under the sub-discipline of *philosophical logic*.

Find out more about theories of truth by putting 'theories of truth' into the search facility of the *Stanford Encyclopedia of Philosophy*: http://plato.stanford.edu/.

Arguments are not sentences. They are constituted of sentences, but in order to be an argument there must be at least two sentences, one to act as premise, the other as a conclusion, and the sentences have to be related to each other in a certain way. One of them must be being said to follow from the other(s). In evaluating an argument we must evaluate each of the sentences that constitute the argument as true or false.

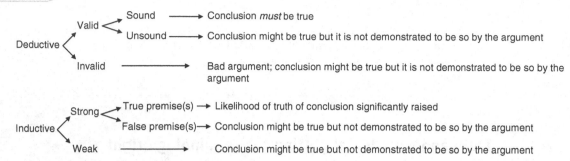

Figure 5.1 Deductive and inductive arguments.

But we must also evaluate the argument itself: the claim that the conclusion follows from the premises. If it does the argument is good (and if the premises are also true the argument is sound or cogent). If it doesn't the argument is bad (irrespective of the truth of the premises). The argument itself is neither true nor false (just as a table is neither loud nor not-loud).

Good arguments

Distinguishing good arguments from bad arguments is easier than distinguishing true sentences from false sentences. Sometimes distinguishing good arguments from bad is the only way to distinguish true sentences from false ones. This is the case with respect to the sentence with which we started this chapter:

(1) Therapeutic cloning is morally acceptable.

To know about argument is to know that if you believe this sentence is true and you want to convince others of this, you must find a (set of) premise(s) from which you can deduce, or inductively infer, it. If you want to convince others that the sentence is false you also need an argument, one from which its *falsehood* can be deduced or inductively inferred.

We have seen that an argument is **good** if its conclusion **follows from** its premises, and that there are two sorts of 'following from': **deductive validity** and **inductive strength**. Let's consider how both of these can help us decide whether sentence (1) is true or false. We'll start by looking at deduction.

Deductive validity

Here are two deductive arguments either of which would be a good starting point for an examination of the truth of sentence (1):

Argument five	Argument six
It is wrong to kill an innocent one of us. An embryo is an innocent one of us. In therapeutic cloning an embryo is killed. Therefore therapeutic cloning is wrong.	The right action is the action that produces the greatest happiness of the greatest number. Therapeutic cloning produces the greatest happiness of the greatest number. Therefore therapeutic cloning is right.

These arguments are both deductively valid. If their premises are true their conclusions *must* be true. Assuming you think the premises are at least plausible either of these arguments would be a good place to start convincing someone else of your view of sentence (1).

Box 5.6 **Activity: Evaluating deductive arguments**

An argument is deductively valid if and only if there is no possible situation in which its premises are true and its conclusion false. A counterexample is just such a situation. The existence of a counterexample, therefore, demonstrates the invalidity of the argument.

We know that argument three is invalid, so we also know there must be at least one counterexample, one situation in which the premises are true but the conclusion false.

Here is argument three. See if you can find a counterexample:

> If the patient is in a permanent vegetative state (PVS) then he will not be conscious.
>
> The patient is not conscious.
>
> Therefore the patient is in PVS.

Answer:
There are lots of counterexamples to this argument: any situation in which the patient is unconscious for reasons *other* than his being in PVS. If the patient is unconscious because he has taken a knock on the head, this would be a counterexample to argument three. Only one counterexample is needed to demonstrate invalidity.

Validity and truth

But clearly there must be something wrong. Therapeutic cloning can't be both right and wrong. That is a contradiction. At least one of these valid arguments, therefore, must have something wrong with it. But surely if an argument is valid it is a good argument?

If we understand the notion of validity we know immediately what is wrong. We know that at least one of these arguments must be *unsound*, such that at least one of its premises is false. It cannot be the case that the premises of both arguments are all true because, given the validity of both arguments, both conclusions would then have to be true, and this is impossible because they contradict each other.

Consideration of this should make it clear that a valid argument can have a false conclusion. People often find this surprising. This is usually because they have confused the notion of validity with the notion of truth and/or perhaps with the notion of soundness. Sometimes people think that because in everyday life we think of validity as good, truth as good and soundness as good, this means that validity, truth and soundness must all be the same thing. This is a bad piece of reasoning.

Box 5.7 Activity: Conceptual analysis

To make sure you are not confusing validity, truth and/or soundness look at the definition of validity then answer the questions below:

Definition: validity

An argument is valid if and only if there is no possible situation in which the premises are true and the conclusion false.

Now answer the following questions:

1. Could all the premises of a valid argument be false?
2. Should we always reject the conclusion of an invalid argument?
3. Could the set of sentences consisting of the premises of a valid argument and the negation of its conclusion be consistent (such that they could all be true together)?
4. Could an invalid argument have a true conclusion?

Answers:
1. Yes (if this is the case the argument might be good but it isn't sound).
2. No, an invalid argument tells us nothing about the truth of its conclusion and the conclusion might reasonably be believed to be true on grounds other than the argument.
3. No. Because a valid argument with true premises *must* have a true conclusion, the set consisting of the true premises plus the *negation* of the conclusion (i.e. the conclusion with 'it is not the case that' tacked on the front) must be inconsistent (such that they can't all be true together).
4. Yes. It could also have a false conclusion. The invalidity of an argument tells us nothing about the truth of its conclusion.

So we have two valid arguments, the conclusions of which contradict each other. This tells us that at least one of these arguments must be unsound, such that at least one of its premises is false.

Naturally we will all believe that the error will be found in the argument the conclusion of which we reject. If we believe that therapeutic cloning is morally *acceptable* we will think that at least one of the premises of argument five is false. If we believe that therapeutic cloning is morally *unacceptable* then we will think at least one of the premises of argument six is false. But if, on examination, we cannot show that one or other of the premises of the argument we want to reject is false we cannot rationally reject the conclusion of that argument.

The fact that an argument is deductively valid, therefore, gives us two pieces of information:

(i)   if the premises of this argument are true, the conclusion *must* be true;
(ii) if the conclusion of this argument is false, then at least one of the premises *must* be false.

Armed with a valid argument, and a proper understanding of the nature of validity, our arguments will not – or should not – go round in circles. If we accept the premises then we have to accept the conclusion. If we reject the conclusion, we know we must examine the premises to find the error.

Valid arguments and persuasiveness

A valid argument can have a false conclusion. We should never, therefore, believe a conclusion *simply* because it is the conclusion of a valid argument. We need to be especially aware of this if we are inclined to accept the conclusion on its own terms. In fact whenever we are antecedently prepared to accept the conclusion of an argument we should be *extra* vigilant both in checking that the argument really is a good one and that its premises are true.

Here is what the famous philosopher of science Karl Popper had to say about this:

'If we are uncritical we shall always find what we want: we shall look for and find confirmations, and we shall turn away from and not see, whatever might be dangerous to our pet theories.'[5]

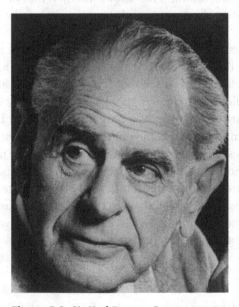

Figure 5.2 Sir Karl Popper. Image courtesy of The Library of the London School of Economics and Political Science, LSE ACHIVES/IMAGELIBRARY/5.

There are occasions other than when its premises are false, however, that the validity of an argument should not persuade us of the truth of its conclusion. We should not be persuaded, for example, of the truth of the conclusion of any argument that is circular, or that begs the question.[6] Here are examples of arguments of both kinds:

Argument seven	Argument eight
Embryos have the right to life. Therefore, embryos have the right to life.	It is always wrong to kill human babies. Therapeutic cloning involves killing human babies. Therefore, therapeutic cloning is wrong.

Argument seven is a circular argument. It is called 'circular' because its conclusion is amongst its premises (in this case the conclusion *is* the premise). Argument eight is a question-begging argument. This is because its use of the phrase 'human babies' in the second premise assumes the conclusion of the argument. If you are prepared unreflectively to call the very early embryos killed in therapeutic cloning 'human babies', this is almost certainly because you already accept the conclusion of this argument.

If you look again at the definition of validity in Box 5.7, you will see that arguments seven and eight both satisfy the conditions an argument has to satisfy to be valid: there is no possible situation in which the premises of these arguments are all true, and their conclusions false. In the first case this is obvious: how could the premise be true and the conclusion false when the conclusion *is* the premise? In the second case it is less obvious. But no one is going to accept the second premise of this argument unless they already accept the conclusion. This shows us that the validity of an argument is *necessary* for us rationally to accept the conclusion of the argument, but it isn't *sufficient*.

Of course no one would be persuaded of the conclusion of an argument as blatantly circular as argument seven. But the trouble with circular arguments is that it is not always easy to tell they are circular. Can you see that if we were to add another ten premises to this argument it would *still* be circular, though not as blatantly so? So long as a conclusion appears amongst the premises of an argument it *cannot* be the case that *all* the premises of the argument are true and yet the conclusion false.

That an argument begs the question is also something that can easily be missed. But a question-begging argument should no more persuade us of its conclusion than a circular argument should. It is especially important, when we evaluate deductive arguments, to be alert to the possibility that they are valid only because they are circular or because they beg the question. This is especially true if we have an antecedent inclination to believe the conclusion.

Fallacies

Circularity and begging the question are both examples of fallacies. A fallacy is a bad argument that can easily be mistaken for a good argument. Some fallacies, like the two

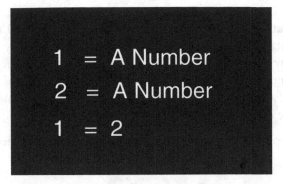

Figure 5.3 An example of a fallacy.

we've examined here, are persuasive because they are valid. Other fallacies are persuasive because they are easily mistaken for valid arguments.

For example, argument three, if you don't look at it carefully, can easily be mistaken for an argument of the same form as argument one. But argument three is an example of the fallacy of 'affirming the consequent'. Its 'logical form' (or logical structure) is:

'If P then Q, Q, therefore P.'

Any argument of this form is invalid. The logical form of argument one, on the other hand is:

'If P then Q, P, therefore Q.'

All arguments of this form are valid. This argument form is called Modus Ponens. The study of the form of arguments is called *formal logic*.[7]

Box 5.8 Philosophical background: Common fallacies[8]

Ad hominem: attacking the person instead of the argument. 'Von Daniken's books are worthless because he is a convicted forger and embezzler.' (This is true, but not why the books are worthless.)

Straw man: attacking a caricatured version of your opponent's argument. For example: 'Senator Jones argues against funding the submarine programme. Does he want to leave us defenceless?'

Fallacy of origin: if an argument or arguer has some particular origin (is poor perhaps, or black), the argument *must* be valid (or invalid).

Psychological fallacy: if there is a psychological reason why your opponent likes an argument, then he's biased, and his argument must be wrong. 'Oh, but of course you are a feminist.'

Argument of the heap: assuming that two ends of a spectrum are the same, since one can travel along the spectrum in very small steps. For example: all piles of stones are small, since if you add one stone to a small pile of stones it remains small.

False cause: assuming that because two things happened, the first one caused the second one. For example, 'Before women got the vote, there were no nuclear weapons.'

Argument by generalisation: drawing a broad conclusion from a small number of perhaps unrepresentative cases. For example, 'They say 1 out of every 5 people is Chinese. But I know hundreds of people, and none of them is Chinese.'

Non sequitur: something that just does not follow. For example, 'Tens of thousands of Americans have seen lights in the night sky which they could not identify. The existence of life on other planets is fast becoming certainty!'

Selected from a much longer list at http://www.nizkor.org/features/fallacies/.

Inductive strength

There are different sorts of inductive argument. Arguments from authority ('Einstein says P, therefore P is true') are inductive arguments, as are analogies ('The universe is like a clock, so it must have a designer') and generalisations ('He's a businessman, so he must be rich') including causal generalisations ('All As cause Bs, so that B must have been caused by an A').

We know that before they can be good, arguments must have conclusions that *follow from* their premises. The conclusion of a deductive argument follows from its premises when the argument is valid. But when does the conclusion of an inductive argument follow from its premise(s)? The two arguments in the box below are both inductive arguments:

Argument nine	Argument ten
Drug addicts often do not make good parents. Therefore, we should not allow drug addicts to become parents.	It is wrong to kill a healthy adult. A healthy embryo is similar to a healthy adult. Therefore, it is wrong to kill a healthy embryo.

Because these are inductive arguments the truth of their premises does not guarantee the truth of their conclusions. Finding a counterexample to these arguments, therefore, will not demonstrate that they are not good arguments.

Inductive strength is not an either/or matter as validity is. An inductive argument is good to the extent that the truth of its premises raises the likelihood of the truth of its conclusion (as they do in argument two), and bad to the extent that the truth of its premises does not raise the likelihood of the truth of its conclusion (as in argument four). Evaluating inductive arguments is a more subtle procedure than evaluating deductive arguments.

The best way to evaluate whether the conclusion of an inductive argument follows from its premises is to answer a set of questions. Here are the questions you might ask:

(i) **From a sample of which population is the argument extrapolating to the rest of that population? Is this extrapolation reasonable?**

Argument nine extrapolates from *some* drug addicts to *all* drug addicts. Is there reason to think all drug addicts are alike? In what respect must all drug addicts be alike for this extrapolation to work?

Argument ten extrapolates from the wrongness of killing *healthy adults* to the wrongness of killing things *similar to healthy adults*. Why is it wrong to kill a healthy adult? Does this extend to things similar to healthy adults? In what way must something be similar to a healthy adult for this extrapolation to work?

(ii) Can we question the premises of the argument?

What evidence is there for the claim that some drug addicts are bad parents? Can this evidence be questioned?

Is it always wrong to kill healthy adults? Can we think of a counterexample to this claim, a situation in which it wouldn't be wrong?

(iii) Can we undermine the similarity claim underlying the extrapolation?

Could anything be done to help drug addicts become good parents?

Are there disanalogies between healthy adults and healthy embryos that would ensure it isn't wrong to kill the latter?

In answering such questions you will get a feel for how inductively strong the argument is.

Box 5.9 Philosophical background: Causal generalisations

Arguments about causation are a sub-set of inductive arguments. The claim that As cause Bs is the claim that the occurrence of an A is sufficient for the occurrence of a B. The claim that a particular A caused a particular B is the claim that had that A not occurred that B would not have occurred.

The only evidence we can have for a causal claim is evidence that As and Bs are correlated. Correlations, however, do not always indicate causes. Nor do they always enable us to distinguish cause from effect.

If we observe that whenever a person claims to feel pain, for example, a certain type of neural event is activated, this could mean that:

- the neural event *is* the pain;
- the neural event *causes* the pain;
- the pain *causes* the neural event;
- both pain and neural event are caused by some other event C;
- nothing: the correlation could be a coincidence.

In evaluating inductive arguments you should be aware that different people have different levels of 'inductive boldness'. Some people are prepared to extrapolate from a very small sample, and/or on the ground of a very tenuous similarity. Others require a large sample and a very significant similarity. The larger the sample from which we extrapolate, the stronger the similarity on the basis of which we extrapolate, and the more reasonable the extrapolation, the stronger our argument.

> ### Box 5.10 Activity: Evaluating inductive arguments
>
> What do you think of the following arguments?
>
> 1. Einstein supports pacifism. Therefore it is right to support pacifism.
> 2. The universe, like a clock, has a designer. Therefore the universe has a designer.
> 3. All daffodils we have ever seen have been yellow. Therefore all daffodils are yellow.
>
> **Q1 From a sample of which population is the argument extrapolating to the rest of that population? Is the extrapolation reasonable?**
>
> 1. This extrapolates from the fact that Einstein is right about many things, to the claim that Einstein is right about everything. Is this reasonable?
> 2. This extrapolates from the fact that some clock-like things (clocks) have a designer to the claim that other clock-like things (universes) will have a designer.
> 3. This extrapolates from all the daffodils we have ever seen, to all daffodils (which might be grounded on the belief they share a genome).
>
> **Q2 Can we question the premises?**
>
> 1. Does Einstein support pacifism?
> 2. Are there any clock-like things that don't have designers?
> 3. Is it true that all the daffodils we have seen have been yellow? Could we have seen them all, or some of them, under a yellow light or when we had our yellow-tinted glasses on?
>
> **Q3 Can we undermine the similarity claim underlying the extrapolation?**
>
> 1. Why should we think Einstein is a good politician because he is a good physicist?
> 2. Are there any disanalogies between clocks and the universe that might undermine the analogy?
> 3. Could the daffodils we have seen be the same as each other, and yet different from daffodils we haven't seen?

Identifying and analysing arguments

The arguments above have all been presented **logic-book style**. This makes it easy to evaluate them by answering our two questions (p. 53). Most of the arguments we read in books, or hear in the classroom, the lecture theatre or the pub are more like this:

'The post is going to be late *again*! I'm fed up with it. It's pouring and the mail is *always* late when it's raining. Maybe I'll sue the post office.'

Here is this argument set out logic-book style:

Whenever it is raining the mail is late.
It is raining.
Therefore the mail will be late.

Let's see how this logic-book style argument is yielded by this informal 'pub' argument. Here is a set of steps for analysing arguments:

1. identify the conclusion of the argument;
2. identify each of the premises;
3. add suppressed premises;
4. remove irrelevancies;
5. remove inconsistent terms.

Identifying the conclusion

We start analysing an argument by identifying the conclusion, the claim for which reasons are being offered. The conclusion can often (but not always, and not in the mail argument) be identified by the fact it is preceded by a word like 'therefore', 'so', 'hence' or some other concluding word. The conclusion is not always at the end of an argument as you will see if you do the next activity.

Box 5.11 Activity: Analysing arguments

Find the conclusion

1. Since all men are mortal, Socrates is mortal, for Socrates is a man.
2. Socialism was doomed to failure because socialism did not provide the incentives needed for a prosperous economy.
3. Since many newly emerging nations do not have the capital resources necessary for sustained growth they will continue to need help from industrial nations.

Answers:
1. Socrates is mortal. 2. Socialism was doomed to failure. 3. Newly emerging nations will continue to need help from industrial nations.
See Robert J. Fogelin (1978) *Understanding Arguments: An Introduction to Formal Logic*. San Diego, CA: Harcourt, Brace and Jovanovitch, p. 34.

Identifying premises

The next step is to identify the premises, the reasons being offered for believing the conclusion. Sometimes you might think that an argument would be acceptable if it had another premise but that as it stands its premises do not provide a good reason to believe the conclusion. The following argument is such a one:

Premise one: Pupils in this school fail all their exams.
Conclusion: This school should be shut down.

As it stands, the premise is not a good reason for the conclusion, but we can easily see that it would be if we added:

Premise two: Any school whose pupils fail all their exams should be shut down.

Premise 2 is a *suppressed premise* for this argument, and it is fine to add it in setting out an argument logic-book style.

Box 5.12 Activity: Analysing arguments

Identify the premises of this argument (don't forget there might be a suppressed premise):

Socialism did not provide the incentives needed for a prosperous economy. Socialism was doomed to failure.

Answer:
Premise one: Incentives are needed for a prosperous economy.
Premise two: Socialism did not provide incentives.
Premise three: Governments fail when they do not provide what is needed to succeed.
Conclusion: Socialism was doomed to failure.
Premise three is a suppressed premise.
Taken from Robert J. Fogelin (1987) *Understanding Arguments*. San Diego, CA: Harcourt, Brace, Jovanovich, p. 34.

Remove irrelevancies

Arguing is only one of the things we do when we communicate with each other. In the mail argument for example the person is offering an argument but also communicating their frustration, and reflecting on a possible remedy. In setting out the argument logic-book style we need to disentangle the argument from the other contributions to the communication. Having done this we can then remove everything that is irrelevant to the argument.

In the mail argument the words 'Maybe I'll sue the post office' and 'I'm fed up with it' are not statements for which reasons are given, nor reasons given for a statement. The latter words express the anger that the person is feeling, the former a reflection on a possible remedy for the frustration. The words 'again' and 'always' are also used for emphasis. Once we strip out these words as irrelevant to the argument being offered the structure of the argument is revealed: we can see more clearly the statement made, and the reasons offered for it.

Remove inconsistent terms

It is fine, in setting out an argument logic-book style to paraphrase the premises and the conclusion so that the relationship between them is more obvious. What you *mustn't* do is change the meaning of the words of the argument. You will see that in this argument the wording 'the mail is always late when it is raining' has been altered to read 'whenever it is raining the mail will be late', 'it's pouring' has been changed to 'it is raining', and 'the post is going to be late' has been changed to 'the mail will be late'.

None of these alterations changes the meaning of the statements made. But they do reveal that the sentence 'it is raining' appears in both premises, and that the sentence 'the mail is/will be late' appears in the first premise and the conclusion (the change of verb from present to future is irrelevant). By such means the argument can be seen more clearly.

Box 5.13 Activity: Identifying premises and conclusions

Set out these arguments logic-book style removing irrelevancies and inconsistent terms and adding suppressed premises (if any):

1. Women's brains are on average smaller than men's. Therefore women are less intelligent than men.
2. The butler was in the pantry; therefore he couldn't have shot the master, who was in the study.
3. The green movement is wrong to think we should recycle paper and glass. Paper comes from trees, an easily renewable source, and glass is made from sand which is plentiful and cheap. Furthermore, in some American cities recycling schemes have been abandoned because they are too expensive.

Answers:
Premise one: Women's brains are on average smaller than men's.
Premise two: *The smaller the brain the less intelligent the person.*
Conclusion: Therefore women are less intelligent than men.

Premise two is a suppressed premise.

Premise one: The butler was in the pantry.
Premise two: The master was in the study.
Premise three: No one can be in two places at once.
Premise four: It is necessary to be in the same place to shoot someone.
Conclusion: Therefore the butler couldn't have shot the master.

It might be considered that premises three and four are too obvious to need to be added.

Premise one: Paper comes from trees, an easily renewable source.
Premise two: Glass is made from sand which is plentiful and cheap.
Premise three: In America some recycling schemes have been abandoned as too expensive.
Premise four: *We should only recycle if doing so saves money.*
Conclusion: Therefore the green movement is wrong to think we should recycle paper and glass.

Premise four is a suppressed premise.

Taken from Fisher, A. (2001) *Critical Thinking: An Introduction.* Cambridge: Cambridge University Press, p. 23.

Ethics, argument and charity

Whenever a philosopher hears or reads an argument his job is to subject it to criticism. He will question its conclusion by questioning the premise(s) of the argument, and asking whether the conclusion follows from the premises. By such means philosophers try to falsify hypotheses logically just as scientists try to falsify hypotheses empirically.

As bioethics is a philosophical discipline, this is what you should do as you read through the arguments in this book. You will also construct your own arguments as you form your own opinions about the issues you will read about. It is important to subject your own arguments to criticism too: it is here people often fall into Popper's trap (see p. 59). If you are working with others one of the best ways to learn is by arguing with each other, and by criticising each other's arguments.

It isn't always nice, though, to have your carefully constructed arguments criticised. Many people, afraid of this, refuse to argue. They'd rather stay silent than make themselves vulnerable to being questioned on their reasons for believing whatever it is they believe. This is particularly common when people are learning how to construct and evaluate arguments. However confident you are, however keen on offering your opinions, you might find that you become oddly shy when you are expected to argue for your opinions knowing that your arguments will not be taken at face value.

Clearly, it is a bad thing if, in asking people to explain why they believe whatever they believe, we frighten them, and possibly prevent them from putting forward their opinions. In collaborative pursuits of truth, such as science and philosophy, the more opinions we can get on the table the better. In the hope of guaranteeing this, most philosophers are scrupulous to observe the ethical principle that governs the activity of argument: the principle of charity.

The principle of charity exhorts us always to treat the appearance of falsehood, irrationality or stupidity on the part of others as evidence of *our own* misunderstanding of their argument, and for the need to try harder to understand what it is they are saying and/or why they are saying it. This was put rather neatly by the American philosopher W. V. Quine, who said 'your interlocutor's silliness is less likely than your bad interpretation'.[9]

It is amazing how often, when we check our understanding of what someone else said, we find that the other person *isn't* saying something false, irrational or stupid. Sometimes indeed, embarrassingly, we discover *we* were saying something false, irrational or stupid.

There is another important reason for using charity in argument. The only thing we learn for sure when we learn that someone else believes something opposed to something we believe is that *one of us* is wrong. We do not learn *which of us* is wrong. Unless you can be certain that you are *never* wrong the scrupulous observance of charity is the only rational way to approach argument. It is by invoking charity in argument that you will test *your own* beliefs and arguments, and it is only by properly testing these that you will be justified in thinking your beliefs are true and your arguments good.[10]

The use of charity is not only a courtesy to those with whom we are co-operating in the search for truth, it also prevents us falling victim to our own prejudices.

> ### Box 5.14 **Activity: Group discussion**
>
> Once everyone understands the principle of charity, use the following questions to stimulate discussion:
>
> - Can anyone describe a situation in which they were arguing with someone who didn't observe the principle of charity (so the person treated them as stupid and irrational or their beliefs as obviously false)? How did it make them feel?
> - Can anyone describe a situation in which, as they were arguing with someone, they discovered they were themselves wrong about something?
> - Is it possible *respectfully* to suggest that someone might be wrong? How?
> - Check out the fallacy of the 'straw man' in Box 5.8. Why should we not set up 'straw men' when we argue with someone else?

In reading this chapter you will have learned the rudiments of argument. In this book you will find many arguments on which to practise these skills.

Summary

In this chapter we have considered:

- the concepts: *argument, premise, conclusion, validity* and *counterexample*;
- the distinction between induction and deduction;
- how to evaluate both deductive and inductive arguments;
- the nature of validity and its relation to truth and soundness;
- circular arguments and question-begging arguments and how to avoid them;
- how to analyse arguments and set them out logic-book style;
- the nature of fallacies;
- the principle of charity and the role it plays in argument.

Questions to stimulate reflection

Deduction delivers certainty, induction doesn't. Does this make deduction better than induction?

Why doesn't induction deliver certainty?

What is the definition of validity? Why is validity useful if valid arguments can have false conclusions?

What is a 'counterexample'? How does a counterexample demonstrate the invalidity of an argument?

Can you name three different types of inductive argument?

What are the five steps to take in setting out an argument logic-book style?

Additional activities

Read one of the introductory books listed under further reading, doing all the exercises you find there.

Listen to the podcasts on critical reasoning given by the author of this book, and do the exercises.[11]

Reflect on how you have (or haven't) used the principle of charity in your everyday life.

The BEEP website has a discussion site designed to help students practise the skills of argument: http://www.beep.ac.uk/discuss/index.php?c=6.

Access this website and see what you can find out about critical reasoning for the Graduate Management Admission Exam for the MBA in the United States: http://www.west.net/~stewart/gmat/qmcriti.htm.

Notes

1 http://www.philosophyofscience.info/problemofinduction.html. An account of the 'problem of induction' from the website of Philosophy of Science.

2 See Bertrand Russell (1912) *The Problems of Philosophy*, Chapter VI, 'On Induction'. There are many editions of this book including one from Oxford Paperbacks, with an introduction by philosopher John Skorupski (2001).

3 It is by inductive means that science sets up testable hypotheses. It will then attempt both to confirm and falsify these hypotheses. See Chalmers, A. F. (2000) *What is this Thing Called Science?* Maidenhead, UK: Open University Press.

4 http://instruct.westvalley.edu/lafave/Truth_theories.html. A useful summary of the various theories of truth on this useful site, http://www.westvalley.edu/ph/resourc.html from West Valley College, in California.

5 Popper, K. (1991) *The Poverty of Historicism*. New York: Routledge, p. 133.

6 An argument that 'begs the question' is one that 'makes a beggar of' (or avoids) the question rather than one that begs for the question to be asked.

7 http://tellerprimer.ucdavis.edu/. A primer for modern formal logic.

8 http://www.nizkor.org/features/fallacies/. A useful list of fallacies from the Nizkor site.

9 W. V. Quine (1964) *Word and Object*. Cambridge, MA: MIT Press, p. 59.

10 Baggini, J. (2002) 'Begging Belief: To give or not to give?' *The New Humanist*, 1 September. An article on the principle of charity.

11 www.mariannetalbot.co.uk. The author's official website, look under 'podcasts'.

Further reading and useful websites

Fisher, A. (2001) *Critical Thinking: An Introduction*. Cambridge: Cambridge University Press
Priest, G. (2000) *A Very Short Introduction to Logic*. Oxford: Oxford University Press.
Walton, D. (2008) *Informal Logic: A Pragmatic Approach*. Cambridge: Cambridge University Press.

http://www.nizkor.org/features/fallacies/. A list of fallacies complied by Dr Michael Labossiere, from the Nizkor site.
http://www.philosophy.ox.ac.uk/podcasts/critical_reasoning_for_beginners. A series of podcasts on critical reasoning by the author of this book.
http://tellerprimer.ucdavis.edu/. A primer for modern formal logic (the logic we have been looking at here is *informal* logic, so this primer is only for those who would like to learn about formal logic).

6

General arguments: it's unnatural, it's disgusting, it's risky, it's only opinion

Objectives

In reading this chapter you will:

- consider whether or not something that is unnatural is also immoral;
- reflect on the arguments for and against this claim;
- consider whether morality is a matter of emotion or feeling rather than reason;
- reflect on the reasons for and against thinking that our intuitions are a good guide to morality;
- consider why many people think that it is immoral to take risks;
- reflect on the extent to which it is immoral to take risks;
- reflect on the common belief that morality is all a matter of opinion;
- consider the extent to which morality *is* a matter of opinion.

In this section we shall consider those arguments that we will come across again and again as we work through this book. There are four such arguments: (i) it's not natural; (ii) it's disgusting; (iii) it's too risky; and (iv) it's a matter of opinion. These general arguments are intuitively attractive, they often underpin discussions about ethics in the media and they almost certainly feature in your own ethical thinking. In reading this part of the introduction you may find yourself questioning some of the things you believe to be obviously true. Questioning such assumptions is an important part of thinking critically.

(i) It's not natural

Louise Brown, born in 1978, was the first ever 'test-tube' baby. Her birth caused a furore. James Watson and Max Perutz, both Nobel Prize winners, expressed fears of 'deformed babies who might be the victims of infanticide' and 'another thalidomide catastrophe'. Many obstetricians wondered who would care for the babies if this 'experiment with nature' went disastrously wrong and an American bioethicist,

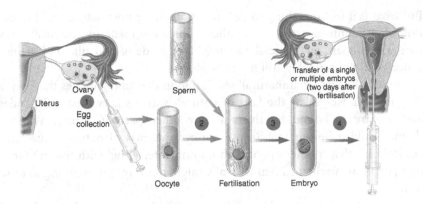

Figure 6.1 Stages of in vitro fertilisation. © Photolibrary.com.

Jeremy Rifkin, made clear his concern about babies growing up as 'specimens, sheltered not by a warm womb, but by steel and glass'.

Thousands upon thousands of IVF babies have now been born. They have no greater chance of a defect than other babies. Many IVF babies are leading productive and enjoyable lives, having given joy to parents who would otherwise be childless. It will be salutary to remember this when we look at new techniques such as cloning, artificial sperm and artificial wombs. But let's examine more closely the fears being expressed.

It is clear that people were worried about the new process causing damage. This seems reasonable. New techniques and drugs have occasionally generated disastrous side-effects. Thalidomide, hailed in the 1960s as a wonder drug for alleviating morning sickness, led to the deaths of 5,000 babies, and to 10,000 babies being born with disabilities. Worries about human intervention causing disasters are not unfounded. We shall be discussing the ethics of risk when we discuss the argument dubbed 'it's too risky'.

But there seems to be another worry behind the concerns of the people quoted: that the techniques used in IVF are not *natural*. Talk of the unnatural often grounds talk of the immoral.

Box 6.1 **Activity: Analysing arguments**

Consider the argument above about IVF being unnatural. Can you set it out logic-book style? (See pp. 64–67 for how to set out an argument in this way.) Is the result a deductive or an inductive argument?

Answer:
The 'naturalness' argument above can be analysed as follows:

> Premise one: IVF is unnatural.
> Premise two: If something is unnatural then it is immoral.
> Conclusion: IVF is immoral.

This is a deductive argument.

But what is it for something to be 'unnatural' or 'against nature'? Is it to be artificial? But what counts as artificial? Synthetic fibres are made by chemically synthesising natural materials, an artificial rose might be made of real silk, and artificial intelligence would presumably still be intelligence?

Could it be that by 'unnatural' we should understand 'violates the laws of nature'? But how can we violate the laws of nature? Nature's laws exist independently of us and we are as bound by them as any other part of nature. We *can't* violate them. Could it be our inability to control the laws of nature – the fact that *they* control *us* – that frightens people about our 'interfering' with nature? Or could it be that people are frightened that we really might one day do something to upset the laws of nature?

But on this interpretation of 'unnatural' the worry collapses into the worry with which we started: that our interference might have unpredictable consequences. This is a worry that must be borne in mind. In our discussion of the argument 'it's too risky' we shall discuss it in detail. But it is not immediately obvious that, given our previous successes, it should stop us attempting to improve on nature.

Perhaps a better understanding of 'unnatural' would be 'man-made'? This would explain why 'natural' (i.e. not man-made) goods such as natural fibres, foodstuffs and cosmetics attract a premium.

> ### Box 6.2 **Activity: Analysing arguments**
>
> The word 'unnatural' is clearly ambiguous. This means that there are different ways of interpreting the argument we analysed in Box 6.1. Each of these different arguments has to be evaluated separately.
>
> Can you identify at least two meanings of the word 'unnatural' from the discussion above, and set out logic-book style each of these arguments so the difference between them is clear?
>
> Answer:
> 1. Premise one: IVF is artificial.
>   Premise two: If something is artificial then it is immoral.
>   Conclusion: IVF is immoral.
> 2. Premise one: IVF violates the laws of nature.
>   Premise two: If something violates the laws of nature then it is immoral.
>   Conclusion: IVF is immoral.
> 3. Premise one: IVF is man-made.
>   Premise two: If something is man-made then it is immoral.
>   Conclusion: IVF is immoral.

But aren't humans natural? Very few things are free of human influence. Does this mean very few things are natural? Doesn't this strip 'natural' of any meaning?

It's not natural

As we influence virtually everything does this make virtually *everything* morally questionable? Anyway, why should human influence make something *immoral*?

It is probably true, as we saw in our discussion of ethics in general (see Chapter 2, p. 16) that only adult humans can act immorally. If so, human influence is certainly the influence of the only thing that can be immoral. But it is also probably true (for the same reasons) that only human beings can act *morally*. If so, why the emphasis on immorality? Many man-made things do not seem to be at all immoral. Are vaccinations or anaesthetic immoral? Are television and synthetic fibres *morally* abhorrent? What is immoral about watching a documentary about bioethics or even a soap opera after a hard day's work?

It is also the case that many natural things are rather obviously bad in virtue of causing much human (and non-human) suffering. Earthquakes and tsunami are natural, as are volcanic eruptions. Nature's key mechanism – often unhappily described as 'survival of the fittest' – is not obviously one to imitate. Cannibalism, infanticide and genocide are all found in nature independently of human beings. Why, therefore, should we see the natural, the non-man-made, as automatically good, the man-made as bad?

Scientists are often described disparagingly as 'interfering' with nature, as if this could only be bad. But there's no reason to accept that those who 'interfere' with nature are bad unless we accept it *is* bad to 'interfere' with nature.

But so far we have seen no reason to accept this. Science has given huge benefits to the world; mistakes such as thalidomide are hugely outweighed by these benefits. Human influence seems to be neither necessary nor sufficient for making something bad: not necessary because natural things can be bad, and not sufficient because man-made things can be good.

The argument from the unnatural to the immoral is not looking good. Nothing has been said that rules out the possibility of our one day producing something so catastrophic as to outweigh all the good science has done throughout the centuries. But, so far, the facts seem to be on the side of science.

Box 6.3 Philosophical background: Evaluating arguments

If you read Chapter 5 you will know that there are two questions we must ask to evaluate an argument (see p. 53):

(i) are all its premises true?

and

(ii) does its conclusion follow from its premises?

Answer these two questions with respect to the third argument set out logic-book style in Box 6.2. You might want to start with the second question.

Answers:
Does the conclusion follow?
The argument is a deductive argument, so it is valid unless we can find a counterexample to it, a situation in which the premises are both true and the conclusion false. But if the premises of this argument are true, surely the conclusion *must* be true. If so, this argument is valid.

Are the premises true?

Premise one seems true: IVF *is* a man-made process.

Premise two is not so obviously true. It might be grounded on man's being the only thing able to act immorally. But as man is also the only thing able to act morally this isn't very secure. We then used examples to suggest that there are many man-made things that are morally acceptable or morally neutral. This demonstrated that we do not have obvious reason to believe that being man-made suffices for a thing's being morally bad.

Our discussion does not demonstrate the falsehood of premise two, but it does give us reason to question its truth which is enough to show that the argument is not conclusive *despite* its validity.

Where this argument could be used in this book

It is unnatural:

> to clone human beings (Chapters 7 and 8);
> for older women to have babies (Chapter 9);
> to use artificial sperm, eggs or wombs for IVF (Chapter 10);
> to extend lifespan significantly (Chapter 12);
> to genetically engineer human beings (Chapter 14);
> to create life forms that don't exist in nature (Chapter 16);
> to use anything but organic farming methods (Chapter 17);
> to genetically engineer crops (Chapter 17);
> to grow human organs or to transplant pig organs into humans (Chapter 19).

(ii) It's disgusting

Most people would agree that our intuitions play a large role in our decisions about whether something is or isn't morally acceptable. It is because we *feel* that something is wrong, that we decide it is indeed wrong. Or perhaps it is because we do *not* feel that something is wrong, that we decide it must be morally acceptable.

A whole theory of ethics has been built on such intuitive reactions. It is called the 'Boo!/Hooray!' theory.[1] It says that our moral judgements are not guided by reason but by emotion, in particular by our feelings of 'approbation' or 'disapprobation'. This theory says that when consideration of a situation yields a feeling of disapprobation (a 'Boo!') this tells us that whatever we are considering is wrong, and if our feeling is that of approbation (a 'Hooray!') this tells us that whatever we are considering is right.[2]

Box 6.4 **Philosophical background: The 'Boo/Hooray' theory of ethics**

The 'Boo/Hooray' theory was propounded by A.J. Ayer in *Language, Truth and Logic* (2002, New York: Dover Publications). It is based on a theory of ethics, now known as 'emotivism', propounded by David Hume in Book 3 of the *Treatise of Human Nature* and in *An Enquiry Concerning the Principles of Morals* (both published by Oxford University Press in editions introduced by Peter Millican). The key claim of both theories is that moral judgements are not judgements of reason – as, say, Aristotle would claim – but of emotion.

The theory is much more convincing than this short description of it suggests.[3]

The American ethicists Leon Kass[4] and Alto Charo[5] have argued in the same tradition. In their contribution to the findings of an ethics committee on cloning set up by President Clinton they argued against making recommendations on the basis of reason and logic. Emotional responses, they argued, are more important in discussing political questions. This has been called the 'Yuk!' theory of morality, where the feeling that indicates immorality is a feeling of disgust, rather than simply disapprobation.

Box 6.5 **Activity: Setting out arguments logic-book style**

In the context of xenotransplantation (the transplantation of, say, a pig's liver into a human being, see Chapter 19), set out logic-book style (see Chapter 5, pp. 64–67) the argument that someone who believes the boo/hooray theory might make (which will be to do with a claim to the effect that xenotransplantation is disgusting).

Answer:
Premise one: If something is disgusting it is morally wrong.
Premise two: Xenotransplantation is disgusting.
Conclusion: Xenotransplantation is morally wrong.

But consider reading, in a tourist guide, that you shouldn't take photographs of certain people because they believe that in recreating their image you are stealing their soul. Once informed about such a belief most decent people would considerately refrain from taking photographs. But this doesn't mean they'd accept the possibility that in taking photographs they would risk stealing the soul of those they photograph. It is entirely possible to respect someone's belief without accepting that the belief is true.

Most of us would believe that the fears of these people are based on ignorance. This is the problem with intuitions: they are often grounded on ignorance.

It is understandable for people to recoil from things they know nothing about because the unknown is often frightening. But such intuitive recoils are not well-grounded.

The only way to discover whether our intuitive fears *are* well-grounded is to subject them to rational scrutiny. We shall be doing this a lot in this book.

To 'subject our intuitions to rational scrutiny' is to try to pin them down. We need to be able to recognise an intuition, find out *why* we hold it (if we can), and then ask ourselves whether our reason for holding it is, or isn't, a good one.

Box 6.6 Activity: Evaluating arguments

Once you have set out logic-book style the 'it's disgusting' argument against xenotransplantation (see Box 6.5):

(i) decide whether the argument is valid or not (such that if its premises are true its conclusion *must* be true);
(ii) decide whether its premises are true.

Answer: The argument is again valid. The truth of premise two is a matter of opinion and not obviously a matter of *truth* at all. Arguments can be given for or against the truth of premise one, which could form the basis of an interesting class discussion. The fact that one of the premises is questionable means we can rationally reject this argument even though it is valid.

Often, when we try to pin down an intuition we will find that we *are* able to back it up with good reasons. But now we have an *argument* for whatever it is we were saying, we are not relying simply on our intuitions. On other occasions we will find ourselves unable to pin down our intuitions. Sometimes this will mean that our intuitions dissolve: we will see that they had no real grounding at all. On other occasions we will be left with the disturbing feeling that *something* is wrong (or right), though we remain unable, despite our best efforts, to say why it is wrong (or right).

In such a situation the rational thing to do is to keep an open mind, to keep trying to pin our intuitions down, and to listen hard to those who believe themselves to have arguments, both for and against.

Box 6.7 Philosophical background: Intuitions

Intuition is important to both philosophy and science. We rely on intuition when we 'sense' that an argument is good or bad, a claim true or false, or a hypothesis reasonable. It is our intuition at work when, as we read something, we think 'Rubbish!', 'That's true' or 'I see that'.

To be capable of exercising reason is partly to be equipped with such intuitions. But it is one thing to say:

(i) intuitions should be taken seriously as the starting point of investigation;

and quite another to say:

(ii) intuitions should be taken seriously as the final word.

It is reasonable to take intuitions seriously in the first sense, but not the second. If we want our arguments to be well-grounded we will try to explain *why* we hold the beliefs we hold.

Where this argument could be used in this book

It is disgusting:

> to think of cloning human beings (Chapter 8);
> to use eggs from aborted foetuses for IVF (Chapter 9);
> insert genes from one species into another species (Chapter 17);
> to think of eating in vitro meat (Chapter 17);
> to transplant organs from non-humans into humans (Chapter 19);
> to experiment on non-human animals (Chapter 20).

(iii) It's too risky

Imagine we discover a drug that cures the common cold. Should it be licensed? If we think of the misery prevented and the working days saved, we will surely say 'yes'? But we must temper our excitement with caution. Are there any risks associated with the new drug? Would taking it turn us a bilious green for 6 days or give us acne?

Relatively recently the international community has been changing its attitude towards risk assessment. We have been moving from:

> **traditional risk assessment**: licensing an innovation unless there is evidence of unacceptable risk;

to

> **precautionary risk assessment**: *not* licensing an innovation unless there is evidence of *no* unacceptable risk.

The traditional model of risk assessment came under scrutiny when Germany's famous forests started dying in the 1970s. At first no-one knew why. Then the finger was pointed at 'acid rain', rain containing toxins belched out by power stations.

Despite the lack of scientifically respectable evidence for this the German government imposed strict regulations on power-plant emissions on the basis of 'Vorsorgeprinzip', the 'principle of forecaring'. This was the predecessor of the 'Precautionary Principle'.

There are many formulations of the precautionary principle. A popular formulation is the 'Wingspread Statement':

'when an activity raises threats of harm to the environment or human health, precautionary measures should be taken even if some cause and effect relationships are not fully established scientifically.'[6]

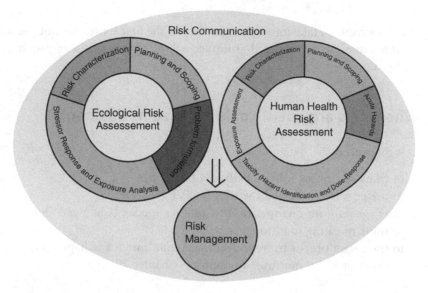

Figure 6.2 Chart showing the components of risk as understood by the US Environmental Protection Agency (http://www.epa.gov/oswer/riskassessment/risk_superfund.htm). Courtesy of US Environmental Protection Agency.

The question we shall consider is whether morality requires that we replace the traditional approach to risk with the precautionary approach.[7]

The shift to the precautionary approach is sometimes characterised as a shift in the burden of proof:

Before: the burden of proof fell on those who *didn't* want the innovation licensed. They had to demonstrate positive reason to believe in an unacceptable risk.

Now: the burden of proof falls on those who *do* want the innovation licensed. They have to demonstrate positive reason to believe there *isn't* an unacceptable risk.

This difference prompts many to believe we *should* adopt the precautionary approach on moral grounds. Isn't it wrong, they say, to leave the burden of proof on the opposers, usually members of the public or pressure groups with little backing, rather than on the proposers, usually rich pharmaceuticals or multi-national corporations who stand to make huge profits?

Also, they argue, it is simply sensible to be safe than sorry, to look before we leap: far better to insist on evidence of no risk, rather than no evidence of risk. Better to screen everyone for breast cancer, for example, even the asymptomatic. By the time symptoms show it might be too late. Screening will undoubtedly generate some false positives, but better falsely to believe there is a tumour when there isn't, than not to believe there is a tumour when there is. By the same token better to assume a risk unless we can demonstrate there isn't.

Such claims have undeniable force. If Chemie Grunenthal had been required to demonstrate that thalidomide carried no risk much suffering would have been avoided. Doesn't this show conclusively that a precautionary approach is best?

> ### Box 6.8 Activity: Small group discussion
>
> Ask participants to read this section of this chapter, then conduct some research into the thalidomide disaster. Divide them into groups and ask each group to discuss the following questions:
>
> Q1: Would the precautionary approach have prevented the thalidomide tragedy?
>
> Q2: Could the tragedy have been prevented by traditional means?
>
> Ask each group to present their findings to the rest of the group before holding a whole-group discussion.

Such considerations *are* reason for considering the precautionary approach best. But they are not conclusive. We could also have avoided the thalidomide tragedy by refining the traditional approach.

It is wrong to think the traditional model requires *no* proof from those supporting an innovation. Before our putative cure for the common cold would even become *eligible* for licensing its effectiveness would have had to be demonstrated by testing on non-human animals and by clinical trials. It is assumed evidence of risks associated with the drugs will emerge during these trials. The traditional requirement that there be no evidence of risk does not mean that nothing should be done to identify risks. It means that no evidence of risk should emerge during a process of very stringent – and very costly – testing.

The trials to which thalidomide was subjected were not rigorous enough. If thalidomide had been tested on pregnant mammals it would quickly have become clear that thalidomide was teratogenic (such that it causes birth defects). These days such tests *are* required, largely thanks to thalidomide. These days pre-clinical tests and clinical trials are extremely stringent. It is likely – though not certain – that if there is a risk associated with a new drug it would emerge during the process. The requirement that we be safe rather than sorry is met by the traditional as well as the precautionary model.

Box 6.9 Factual information: TGN1412

In 2006 the American pharmaceutical Paraxel paid six healthy young men to test TG1412, a possible wonder drug for treating arthritis, MS and leukaemia.

The trial went badly wrong when all the men suffered catastrophic organ failure and nearly died. All lived but with varying degrees of injury.

Ryan Wilson, aged 22, the worst affected, had to have some toes and several finger tips amputated, can't walk unaided and, because his skin won't heal, he can't use prosthetics. He is likely to suffer long term effects, such as cancer. He was a plumber but will probably never work again.

Paraxel admitted liability, acknowledging they should have staggered the injections and offered immediate assistance.[8]

But 'no evidence of risk' still does not amount to 'evidence of no risk'. Surely if we want to be *really* safe we should adopt the precautionary, rather than the traditional approach? But should concerns for safety *always* be paramount.[9]

Imagine if those who discovered fire or invented the wheel had had to demonstrate that fire posed no risk. They would certainly have failed. But the risks taken in adopting these innovations paid off in huge benefits for humankind.

It has been argued though that modern risks are of a different order. Jeremy Rifkin believes the risks we run now are:

'global in scale, open-ended in duration, incalculable in their consequences, and not compensational. Acid rain, the tear in the Earth's ozone layer, and the spread of virtual and biological viruses, are among the new genre of man-made threats. No-one can escape their potential effects. When everyone is vulnerable and all can be lost, then traditional notions of calculating and pooling risks become virtually meaningless.'[10]

But even if modern risks are more serious this does not mandate our acceptance of the precautionary approach. If, after all, we fail to introduce something that would be of benefit to millions, we do not *risk* loss of that benefit, we *ensure* it. If, because they cannot demonstrate there is *no* risk, a pharmaceutical company does not bring to market an effective cure for cancer, we avoid taking a risk, but at the price of continuing to die of cancer.

If proving there is no unacceptable risk is too costly, the pharmaceuticals might even go out of business. As we'll see in Chapter 19, the cost of bringing a new drug to the market in 2008 was $802 million, only 1 out of 5,000 candidate drugs ever makes it to clinical trials, and of those only 1 in 5 will make it to market. In weighing risk, even modern risk – the risk of stifling innovation – must be counted. To the extent a precautionary approach would significantly raise costs this argues against such an approach, especially if, as was suggested above, a traditional approach would enable us to rule out most risks.

Even so there are those who insist that we really must rule out evidence of *all* risks. But there is a serious question about how – and whether – we could do this. How is it possible to provide evidence of no risk in the absence of some understanding of which risks you are trying to rule out?

It is often said that it is not possible to 'prove a negative'. Even if a scientist could prove beyond doubt, for example, that he has excluded every known risk, this would not mean that there isn't another risk – an unknown one – that he hasn't excluded. But how does one go about excluding a risk that is unknown? What sort

THE FACTS

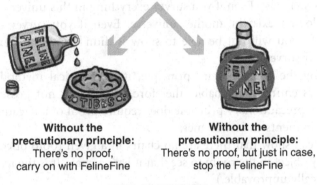

Tibbs the cat is feeling poorly.
Could it be anything to do with her
'FelineFine' vitamin supplement?

THE ACTION

**Without the
precautionary principle:**
There's no proof,
carry on with FelineFine

**Without the
precautionary principle:**
There's no proof, but just in case,
stop the FelineFine

THE OUTCOME

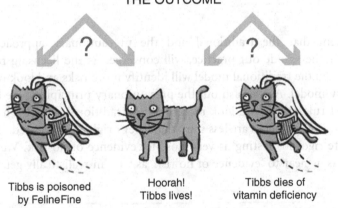

Tibbs is poisoned
by FelineFine

Hoorah!
Tibbs lives!

Tibbs dies of
vitamin deficiency

Figure 6.3 Tibbs the cat and the precautionary principle. © The Wellcome Trust
(http://www.wellcome.ac.uk).

of empirical test would enable us to rule out the possibility of a risk that no one
has anticipated?

Such considerations suggest that it is simply not possible to prove by empirical
means that something *doesn't* exist. In particular, therefore, it is not possible to prove

that an innovation carries no risk. The requirements imposed by the precautionary approach to risk assessment cannot be met.

Box 6.10 Philosophical background: Proving negatives

It is often said that we *cannot* show that something doesn't exist. But the truth of this depends on how you are trying to show that something doesn't exist.

It is possible to show by *logical* means that something doesn't exist. You do this by showing that assuming it exists generates a contradiction. For example, we can be certain that there are no square circles because anything that is a square cannot, on pain of contradiction, be circular.

If your methodology is empirical, however, then it is true you cannot show that something doesn't exist. Even if you survey everything in this universe you cannot be sure that it doesn't exist in another universe. Even if you survey everything that currently exists, you will not be able to show it didn't come into existence as you completed your survey.

In discussing the precautionary principle, it is empirical methodologies we are discussing. It is entirely reasonable, therefore, to say it is not possible to 'prove a negative'. If the precautionary principle does require proof of a negative then it is too strict: its requirements *cannot* be met.

(Note: you can show that there are no chairs in a given room of course simply by checking every object in the room to see that it isn't a chair. It is the *universal* negative that is empirically unprovable.)

It would seem that the traditional and the precautionary approaches to risk assessment, as they guide our practice, will converge. As the licensing requirements are strengthened the traditional model will identify more risks and look more like the precautionary model. As we cash out the precautionary principle so we know which risks we must rule out, it will look more like the traditional model. The differences between the two approaches are less stark than they originally appeared. 'No evidence of risk despite rigorous testing' is very close to 'evidence of no risk'. We might even think that it is as near to 'evidence of no risk' as we can realistically get.

Box 6.11 Activity: Playing devil's advocate

'The risks we run in the twenty-first century are of a quite different kind to the risks run by prehistoric human beings. The precautionary response is the only sensible response to such risks.'

Divide into two groups. One group should argue *for* this claim irrespective of the actual positions of its members. The other should argue *against* again irrespective of the actual positions of members.

Questions to help prepare:

Q: Are modern risks more worrying? Why?

Q: Is the precautionary approach the only way to manage such risks? If not how else might they be managed?

Q: Are there any drawbacks to adopting the precautionary approach?

Where this argument could be used in this book

It is too risky:

to clone human beings (Chapter 8);
to allow children to be born to drug addicts (Chapter 9);
to engineer the genes of humans (Chapter 14);
to allow the government to set up a universal DNA database (Chapter 15);
to allow free publication of security sensitive experiments (Chapter 16);
to create organisms unknown in nature (Chapter 16);
to genetically engineer crops for food (Chapter 17);
to grow crops that have been genetically engineered (Chapter 17).

(iv) It's a matter of opinion

It is common in discussions of ethics for someone to object that there is no point in discussing a given issue because it's a matter of personal opinion. 'You believe abortion is morally unacceptable,' someone might say, 'I don't. You've got no right to impose your opinion on me: even if abortion is wrong for you, it's not wrong for me, and there's an end to it.'

If this were true there would be no more to making a moral judgement than there is to making a judgement of personal preference such as 'sardines are tasty' or 'red is the nicest colour'. A warning: non-philosophers might find this argument difficult to follow. If this is true for you, you will not be alone.

Statements of personal preference (like 'sardines are tasty') are usually thought to be:

(i)   made true (or false) by some fact about the individual who makes them;
(ii) made true (or false) by some fact about which the individual is an authority;
(iii) infallible – such that the person who makes them cannot get them wrong (because that person is an authority on the fact that makes them true or false).

If Tom sincerely tells Sam that sardines are tasty, for example, Sam will conclude that Tom likes the taste of sardines, and that as Tom could hardly be wrong about liking sardines, Tom really *does* think sardines are tasty. It is Tom's liking of sardines – a fact of which Tom could hardly be unaware – that makes 'sardines are tasty' true for Tom.

To think that moral statements are comparable to statements of personal preference is to think that Sam's belief 'it is OK to rob elderly ladies' is:

(i)   made true or false by some fact about Sam;
(ii) made true or false by some fact about which Sam is an authority;
(iii) infallible, so Sam *can't* be wrong about it.

Surely, though, this is simply wrong?

It is not a fact about Sam that makes 'it is OK to rob elderly ladies' true or false, it is a fact about *robbing elderly ladies*. Why should we accept that Sam is any sort of authority on morality? And far from it being the case that Sam is infallible about this, he seems to be simply *wrong*: it is *not* morally acceptable to rob elderly ladies, Sam's belief is *false*. Statements of moral belief are *not*, therefore, comparable to statements of personal preference.

But this makes it look as if it is stupid to compare moral statements with statements of personal preference. Yet we started this section by noting that many people do just this. Doesn't this violate our commitment to the principle of charity (see Chapter 5, pages 67–69)?

It would if it wasn't relatively easy to explain why intelligent people so often make this mistake. The explanation lies in an understandable confusion between beliefs about the world (first order beliefs) and beliefs about beliefs (second order beliefs).

This is a logical distinction that often goes unnoticed even by the highly intelligent. Consider the following sentence:

Sam believes the earth is round.

This sentence embeds one sentence 'The earth is round' within another sentence 'Sam believes the earth is round':

(Sam believes [the earth is round])

The embedding sentence (in curved brackets) is about *Sam*. The embedded sentence (in square brackets) is about the earth. The truth and falsehood of the embedding sentence is quite independent of the embedded sentence as you will see if you answer the following four questions:

1. Could Sam believe the earth is round without it being the case the earth is round?
    (If so then the embedding sentence could be true whilst the embedded sentence is false.)
2. Could Sam believe the earth is round and it be true that the earth is round?
    (If so then the embedding and embedded sentence can both be true.)
3. Could it be false that Sam believes the earth is round, and yet the earth be round?
    (If so then the embedding sentence could be false whilst the embedded sentence is true.)
4. Could it be false that Sam believes the earth is round and indeed it be false the earth is round?
    (If so then embedding and embedded sentence could both be false.)

If you answer these questions you will see that the truth and falsehood of the two sentences varies independently. This is because the two sentences are made true or false by quite different facts. The embedding sentence is made true or false by some fact about *Sam*. The embedded sentence is made true or false by some fact about *the earth*.

With this in mind we can entertain the same questions with respect to Sam's belief that it is OK to rob elderly ladies:

(Sam believes [robbing elderly ladies is morally acceptable])

We will find that again the truth and falsehood of the two sentences vary quite independently: the facts that make true 'Sam believes that robbing elderly ladies is morally acceptable' and 'Robbing elderly ladies is morally acceptable' are quite different and independent of each other. The embedding sentence ('Sam believes that robbing elderly ladies is morally acceptable') is made true by a fact about *Sam*, the embedded sentence ('robbing elderly ladies is morally acceptable') is made true by a fact about *robbing elderly ladies*.

Sam may be an authority about his own beliefs, about the sort of fact that makes the *embedding* sentence true or false. But there is no reason to think he is an authority on morality, on the sort of fact that makes the *embedded* sentence true or false. To the extent we think Sam is an authority on whether or not he has a certain belief, furthermore, we might accept that his beliefs about his own beliefs are infallible. But this does not mean that his beliefs about the moral acceptability of robbing elderly ladies are infallible. About robbing elderly ladies Sam might be – indeed is – quite wrong.

It is simply not the case that a belief to the effect that robbing elderly ladies is morally acceptable is made true by a fact about a given individual, far less a fact about this individual on which he has authority. In our section on ethical theories we saw that there are many ideas about what makes a moral belief true or false (see Chapter 4). Any ethical theory stating that simply having a moral belief is sufficient to make it true would not be a very good moral theory. It would make moral error impossible.

The common and understandable confusion between first and second order beliefs can be exacerbated by a misleading ambiguity. The ambiguity lies in the sentence:

'"Robbing elderly ladies is morally acceptable" is true for Sam.'

The two meanings of this sentence that constitute the ambiguity are:

(i) Sam *believes* that robbing elderly ladies is morally acceptable
(ii) Robbing elderly ladies *is* morally acceptable *for Sam*.

We have reason to believe (i) whenever we have reason to believe that Sam believes that robbing elderly ladies is morally acceptable. It is an unfortunate fact about the way some human beings are brought up that they do form such beliefs. We will have reason to believe (ii) only when we have reason to believe that Sam's robbing elderly ladies is morally acceptable. It is difficult to imagine a situation in which we would have reason to hold the second belief. To believe this would be to have no reason to interfere with Sam's robbing an elderly lady, no reason to stop him from doing it.

To reject the claim that moral beliefs, and the sentences that express them, are comparable to beliefs and statements about personal preferences, is to reject the claim that morality is a matter of personal opinion.

> **Box 6.12 Activity: Analysing arguments**
>
> Jane and Troy are having an argument and getting very frustrated with each other.
>
> **Jane:** I would never have an abortion, I think abortion is wrong
>
> **Troy:** Abortion may be wrong for you but that doesn't mean it's wrong for anyone else.
>
> **Jane:** But I don't believe abortion is right for *anyone*.
>
> **Troy:** Who are you to say that someone else is wrong?
>
> **Jane:** If you believe that it is wrong to kill a human being, and you believe that abortion involves killing a human being, then how could you not believe that abortion is wrong quite generally?
>
> **Troy:** But other people do not believe that abortion involves killing a human being, and why should you impose *your* beliefs on them?
>
> Can you find a way of suggesting to Jane and Troy that they are not arguing about the same thing?
>
> **Hint:** Could Jane agree that Troy is right without agreeing that she is wrong? How? Could Troy agree that Jane is right to believe that if abortion is wrong it *is* wrong for everyone, without agreeing that abortion is wrong? How?

Where this argument could be used in this book

It is a matter of opinion whether:

human cloning is morally acceptable (Chapters 7 and 8);
there is a right to have a child (Chapter 9);
we should allow gamete donors anonymity (Chapter 10);
we should select against embryos with diseases and disabilities (Chapter 11);
we should pursue immortality (Chapter 12);
assisted suicide should be decriminalised (Chapter 13);
we should permit designer babies (Chapter 14);
the DNA of innocent people should be kept on the National DNA Database (Chapter 15);
it is morally permissible to synthesise the smallpox genome (Chapter 16);
to permit trials of genetically engineered crops on open land (Chapter 17);
the commercial use of human tissue is morally acceptable (Chapter 18);
clinical trials should be conducted in the developing world (Chapter 19);
animals should be used for research purposes (Chapter 20);
the non-living environment is intrinsically valuable (Chapter 21).

This completes our consideration of arguments that are common to all parts of this book. It also completes Part I.

Summary

In this chapter we have considered four common arguments that we will meet often in this book:

(i) *It's not natural*: it doesn't seem to be either necessary or sufficient for something's being immoral that it should be unnatural. There are natural things (earthquakes) that might be deemed immoral. There are things that might be deemed unnatural (anaesthetics) that are morally acceptable.

(ii) *It's disgusting*: although we rely on our intuitions to alert us to arguments and to problems with arguments, these intuitions should be pinned down by rational argument. We should not think of them as the final word.

(iii) *It's too risky*: although it is extremely important to rule out risks, this requirement does not amount to a requirement that we rule out *all* risks. Doing so would make innovation impossible.

(iv) *It's all a matter of opinion*: there is more to a moral judgement than a judgement of personal preference. We must beware of confusing first and second order beliefs, and of the ambiguity inherent in the claim 'x is right is true for Sam'.

Questions to stimulate reflection

Do you think a natural product is necessarily better than one that isn't natural? Why?

Can you think of any advantages to 'man-made' fibres or foods over natural ones?

To what extent are feelings of delight and disgust involved in moral judgements?

Can you think of something that is disgusting but not morally wrong?

Is the fact that something is risky a good reason to avoid doing it?

Can you think of three useful inventions that would have been banned had the precautionary principle been applied to them?

What makes the claim 'it is right to tell the truth' true (if it *is* true)?

Jenner injected himself with pus from a cowpox sore in order to test his idea that this would immunise him against cowpox. In doing so he took a risk. Did he act immorally? What if he had used someone else?

If Troy believes abortion is morally acceptable, and Jane believes abortion is morally unacceptable could they both be right?

Additional activities

Be alert to instances of these four arguments whenever you read a newspaper or listen to the radio or the television.

Can you find a good example of one of these arguments in a book or newspaper?

With a partner construct a role-play in which one of you makes one of these arguments and the other refutes it.

Conduct an informal opinion poll amongst your friends and family on reproductive cloning (see Chapter 8), identifying how many people cite one or other of these arguments in rejecting it (do *not* accuse them of being stupid if they do… lots of intelligent people have failed to see these arguments do not work!)

Put 'The Precautionary Principle' into a search engine and see if you can find two organisations that would have it imposed. Identify and evaluate their reasons for believing this.

Hold a debate about the precautionary principle using the motion 'This house believes it is better to be safe than to be sorry'.

Notes

1 Or more formally: 'Non-Cognitivism'. See *Ruling Passions* by Simon Blackburn (1998, Oxford: Clarendon).
2 http://www.philosophybites.libsyn.com/category/Julian%20Savulescu. Philosopher Julian Savulescu being interviewed on the 'yuk' factor for Philosophy Bites.
3 http://www.bbc.co.uk/ethics/introduction/emotivism_1.shtml. The BBC website on 'emotivism'.
4 http://www.aei.org/scholar/67. Leon Kass.
5 http://www.law.wisc.edu/profiles/racharo@wisc.edu. R. Alto Charo.
6 http://www.gdrc.org/u-gov/precaution-3.html. Information on the Wingspread Statement.
7 http://www.practicalethics.ox.ac.uk/audio/clarke_precautionary_120209.mp3. Podcast of Dr Steve Clarke, a researcher on the AHRC Project 'Cognitive Science and Religious Conflict', discussing Cass Sunstein's attack on the precautionary principle.
8 http://www.timesonline.co.uk/tol/news/uk/health/article741405.ece. A *Times* newspaper report on the TGN1412 drug trial and on why such disasters are rare.
9 http://lifeboat.com/ex/about. The Lifeboat Foundation, an organisation devoted to 'helping humanity survive existential risks'.
10 http://www.guardian.co.uk/education/2004/may/12/research.highereducation. *Guardian* newspaper, 12 May 2004.

Further reading and useful websites

Kass, L. R. (1997) The Wisdom of Repugnance. *New Republic*, **216**, Issue 22.
Levy, N. (2002) *Moral Relativism: A Short Introduction*. London: One World Publications.
Morris, J. (2000) *Rethinking Risk and the Precautionary Principle*. Burlington, MA: Butterworth-Heinemann.

http://www.independent.co.uk/opinion/a-wrinkled-saggy-woman-carrying-a-foetus-yuk-1584766.html. Journalist Polly Toynbee arguing that deep prejudice (the 'yuk' factor) is behind a familiar argument.
http://instruct.westvalley.edu/lafave/relativ.htm. A discussion of moral relativism by Sandra LaFave of West Valley College.
http://newhumanist.org.uk/2016/moral-dilemmas. An interesting article from the New Humanist by Stephen Lukes, professor of sociology at New York University.

Part II

At the Beginning and End of Life

Questions

Do you think it is morally acceptable to kill embryos for the purposes of research and organ provision?

Do you think the infertile who want genetically related children should be able to clone themselves?

Should the state ban some people – drug addicts? older women? – from reproducing? Does the state have a duty to help the infertile have a child?

Do you think it is permissible to use eggs taken from aborted foetuses for IVF so the infertile can have children?

Do you think that it is morally acceptable to use pre-implantation genetic diagnosis to identify and discard embryos that will develop diseases and disabilities?

Do you think the state should permit those who'd like to live forever to do so were it to become possible?

If there is a way of defining death that facilitates the use of organs for transplant should we favour that definition?

Should assisted suicide and/or voluntary euthanasia be legalised?

Introduction

In Part II we shall consider biotechnology as it impacts on the beginning and end of human life.

For some decades biotechnological advances in reproduction have been revolutionising the decisions we make, individually and socially, as and for potential parents and the children they may have. Decisions about whether to have children, how many and how to provide for them are amongst the most important we make: reproduction is central to our nature as biological organisms and to our understanding of our lives as having meaning. These biotechnological advances will therefore have a huge impact on our lives, introducing decisions no human has ever had to think about, or act on, before.

The end of life is ideally a time for reflection, a time to look back and see that one has loved and been loved, achieved and helped others to achieve, and been happy. But for many, if not most, the reality falls sadly short: dying can be anything but gentle. Advances in biotechnology are again holding out promise of change. Death might become easier than it has been. There is even the possibility that we might 'cure' death. But such advances will again bring with them dilemmas that are utterly new.

Part II consists in three sections, in Section 1: Cloning, Chapter 7 deals with therapeutic cloning whilst Chapter 8 looks at reproductive cloning. In Section 2: Reproduction, in Chapter 9 we consider issues generated by the technologies of assisted reproduction, whilst Chapter 10 looks at issues thrown up by the shortage of 'resources' for IVF. In Chapter 11 we shall consider pre-implantation genetic diagnosis (PGD), embryo selection and negative eugenics. Section 3: Aging And Death starts in Chapter 12 with a consideration of the issues generated by significantly increasing longevity. Finally, in Chapter 13, we shall reflect on the nature of death, and whether killing, in order to alleviate suffering at the end of life, might be morally permissible.

Section 1
Cloning

7 Therapeutic cloning: the moral status of embryos

Objectives

In reading this chapter you will:

- distinguish reproductive and therapeutic cloning;
- consider arguments for and against therapeutic cloning;
- learn more about validity and the analysis of argument;
- start to apply the moral theories outlined in Chapter 4;
- consider whether it is always wrong to kill one of us;
- reflect on the moral status of the embryo;
- reflect on the difference between therapeutic cloning and abortion.

Clones get bad press. From the re-creation of Hitler in *The Boys from Brazil* to the 'spare part' clones of Kazuo Ishiguru's *Never Let Me Go*, no one has a good word to say for them. The idea of cloning triggers, for most people, a visceral recoil (a version of the 'boo' or 'yuk' response discussed in Chapter 6).

In somatic cell nuclear transfer (SCNT) the nucleus from a somatic cell (an ordinary body cell) of an organism is inserted into the de-nucleated egg of another (female) member of the same species (or even that of another species as with chimera), and triggered into developing as an embryo. Clones can also be produced by 'twinning', by splitting apart an embryo. If done early enough each clump of cells will develop into a separate individual. This happens naturally to produce identical twins. In this chapter and the next we shall be discussing only clones produced by SCNT.[1]

The possibility of using this process on mammals generates the possibility of creating, from every cell of a human adult, a baby genetically identical to that adult. From the hair follicle you left in your hairbrush this morning it would be possible, in principle, to create many babies, each genetically identical to you.

But why would anyone want hundreds of copies of someone?[2] Could there be a benign reason? Such shiver-making thoughts might explain why, when Americans were asked what they thought of cloning after the announcement of the birth of Dolly the sheep (the first mammal ever cloned) they were against it. This might make a ban on human cloning seem a reasonable reaction to the new technology.

But as we saw when discussing the argument 'It's disgusting' (Chapter 6), before we act on the basis of intuition we should subject these intuitions to rational scrutiny. In this chapter and the next we shall do precisely this with our intuitions about cloning.

Box 7.1 Activity: Evaluating arguments

In this chapter we shall be subjecting the following argument to logical analysis.

Argument one
Premise one: It is wrong to kill one of us.
Premise two: The early embryo is one of us.
Premise three: In therapeutic cloning the early embryo is killed.
Conclusion: Therefore therapeutic cloning is wrong.

Participants might like to discuss this argument informally before we start to evaluate it more formally.

There are two purposes to which the technology of cloning can be put:

Reproductive cloning: the use of SCNT to produce human embryos to implant into the wombs of women. This will produce human babies with genomes identical to the nucleus donors.

Therapeutic cloning: the use of SCNT to produce human embryos genetically identical to the nucleus donor. These embryos are then used for research, or for the harvesting of stem cells, then destroyed.

The 'visceral recoil' noted above is usually a response to reproductive cloning. Nevertheless, we shall start, in this chapter, with therapeutic cloning because it enables us to deal immediately with the important topic of the moral status of the embryo.

Box 7.2 Philosophical background: Moral status

It was once believed that our moral status, whether we *mattered* morally, was determined by our skin colour. White people had moral status. Black people didn't. Gender counted too. Men had moral status. Women didn't. In other places and times, religion, class or income has been the deciding factor.

We now think that all human beings matter because, whatever our differences, we share a common humanity. In this chapter, however, we shall be discussing whether being human *is* sufficient for mattering morally.

In Chapter 20 we shall be considering whether we should accord moral status to non-human, as well as human, animals.

The moral status of embryos

In this section we shall be applying the skills of identifying and evaluating arguments that we learned in Chapter 5. You will therefore find this section much easier if you read it after reading Chapter 5.

The clone of someone with Parkinson's disease will have the same genes as that person. By examining this clone, we might learn how our genes contribute to Parkinson's. We might even find a cure.[3] At an early stage, furthermore, the cells of the clone have the potential to become a whole organism, or a heart, liver or some other organ. Organs grown from these 'stem' cells could be used as transplants for the original nucleus donor with a very low chance of rejection.[4]

Therapeutic cloning could provide huge benefits. A cure for Parkinson's or Alzheimer's would bring relief to thousands of sufferers, their carers and families, as would harvesting stem cells in the hope of repairing human organs (see Chapter 19). To secure these benefits we must produce clones, then conduct research on or harvest stem cells from them. Then destroy them. But are these activities ethically acceptable?

Many have thought not. Here, set out logic-book style (see Chapter 5 pages 64–67), is an argument against therapeutic cloning:

Argument one
Premise one: It is wrong to kill one of us.
Premise two: The early embryo is one of us.
Premise three: In therapeutic cloning the early embryo is killed.
Conclusion: Therefore therapeutic cloning is wrong.

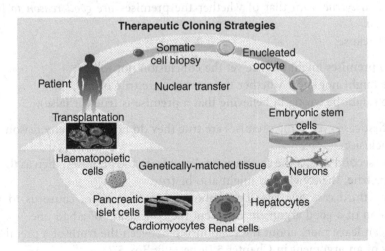

Figure 7.1 Strategy for therapeutic cloning and tissue engineering. From J. Hipp and A. Atala (2004) Tissue engineering, stem cells, cloning, and parthenogenesis: new paradigms for therapy. *Journal of Experimental & Clinical Assisted Reproduction*, **1**:3.

If this is a sound argument, then therapeutic cloning is wrong and we shouldn't do it (for the definition of 'soundness' see Chapter 5, pages 55–56).

We shall be using the phrase 'one of us' to indicate moral status (see Box 7.2.) because anything sufficiently like us in the right way to be 'one of us' will have moral status. Premise two therefore claims – possibly falsely – that the early embryo has the same moral status we have. In particular premise two implies – possibly falsely – that the early embryo has the right to life.

You might have strong intuitions about whether argument one is sound. But our task is to subject the argument to objective analysis, not to rely on intuition. In order to evaluate an argument we must ask two questions (see Chapter 5, pages 53):

(1) Does the conclusion follow from the premises?
(2) Are the premises true?

Let's ask these questions with respect to argument one.

Does the conclusion of argument one follow from its premises?

In asking this question we must put aside our actual beliefs about whether the premises are true. The question we have to ask is: *if the premises were true* would we have good reason to believe the conclusion?

Box 7.3 Philosophical background: Evaluating arguments

In evaluating an argument it is crucial to distinguish the question of whether the premises *are true* from that of whether the premises *are good reason to believe the conclusion.*
This is because:

(i)   the premises might be true yet the conclusion not follow;
(ii) we might not know whether the premises are true or not;
(iii) we might be wrong in believing that a premise is true (or false).

In the first case even if the premises are true they do not give us any reason to believe the conclusion.

In the second case, if the conclusion follows from the premises, then as the premises *might* be true, the conclusion might also be true.

In the third case our false belief about a premise might cause us to reject the conclusion of a good argument or accept the conclusion of a bad one.

You can learn more about the relationship between the truth of a premise and the validity of an argument in Chapter 5 (especially Box 5.7).

In this case, therefore, the question is: assuming it *is* wrong to kill one of us, that the early embryo *is* one of us and that in therapeutic cloning the early embryo *is* killed, would therapeutic cloning be wrong? Or can we think of a counterexample to this argument? (For counterexamples, see Box 5.6).

The answer is inescapable: if all these premises are true, the conclusion *must* be true, therapeutic cloning *has to be* wrong. Argument one is deductively valid: if its premises *are* true there is no possibility whatsoever of its conclusion being false. (See Chapter 5, Box 5.7.) This means that the only way we can rationally reject the conclusion of argument one – the claim that therapeutic cloning is wrong – is to reject at least one of the premises.

The next thing we must do, therefore, is to examine the premises to see whether one or more of them could be false.

Box 7.4 Factual information: Chimera

To produce human clones for the purpose of research, it is necessary to use human eggs. But, as we'll see in Chapter 10, these are in short supply.

It has been suggested therefore that we make clones using the eggs of another species, for example cows. SCNT would proceed as usual except that the nucleus from the cell of the donor would be inserted into a denucleated cow's egg.

The resulting embryo would be 99.9% human, with the cow providing its mitochondrial DNA to make up the remaining 0.1%. As a hybrid between two species the embryo would be a *chimera*.

It has been suggested that producing chimera, even those that will be destroyed at 14 days, is morally wrong.[5] We will discuss this in Chapter 10.

Are the premises of argument one true?

In evaluating the premises of an argument each premise must be examined separately, whilst we assume the other premises are true. As we test premise one, for example, we must assume premises two and three are true. As we test premise two, we must assume that premises one and three are true and so on. This has nothing to do with whether or not we believe any given premise *is* true: our aim is to evaluate the argument as objectively as possible.

Premise three: in therapeutic cloning the early embryo is killed

Premise three is all but unquestionable. Even if a clone survives the research procedures it has probably been so damaged many would think it wrong to let it live. In the UK, where therapeutic cloning is permitted under licence, it is required that the clone be destroyed by the 14th day. It seems safe, therefore, to accept that the third premise of our argument is true.

If we are questioning the conclusion of argument one, therefore, we must question premise one or premise two. The falsehood of either one or both would undermine the conclusion. Both these premises, however, make *huge* claims. In evaluating them we will apply all the moral theories introduced in Chapter 4. Let's start immediately, therefore, with premise one.

Premise one: is it wrong to kill one of us?

The Bible is unequivocal. The sixth commandment states: 'Thou shalt not kill'.[6] It doesn't specify *what* we shouldn't kill, but the implication is clear: we shouldn't kill each other. To the extent we accept this sort of commandment – and all the major monotheistic religions do – we accept it is wrong to kill each other.

But even the sixth commandment allows for exceptions. We are allowed to kill those who have forfeited their right to life. We are also allowed, in the context of a just war, to kill others in our pursuit of justice. The activity that is morally impermissible is not killing per se but the killing of an innocent when not in pursuit of the aims of a just war. This suggests we need to modify the first premise to: 'it is wrong to kill an innocent when not in pursuit of justice'. We can shorten this to 'it is wrong to kill an innocent'.

It is not just religion that inveighs against killing innocents, of course. It is difficult to imagine any decent legal system that does not have a law against murder, against 'illegal killing'. Some legal systems allow judicial killing in punishment for a criminal act. But such killings do not count as murder.

It would seem that whether or not we are religious we have reason to accept the truth of premise one, the claim 'it is wrong to kill one of us' perhaps modified to make it clear that it is innocents we mustn't kill.

If the clones we use in therapeutic cloning are *not* innocents, of course, this would immediately give us a counterexample to argument one. That embryonic clones *are* innocents, however, seems uncontroversial so the modification we need to make to premise one merely tightens our argument.

If you read Chapter 4 you may immediately see that premise one would be accepted by supporters of one of the theories discusses the deontologists. Deontologists believe there are absolute moral rules, binding on all of us, whether we accept them or not. Even if we *do* kill an innocent, in other words, it remains true that we *shouldn't* because the moral law (on this version of deontology) forbids it.

The price we pay for accepting a deontological approach to morality is that we have to accept there are moral absolutes, rules that bind us always, everywhere, and for all times, whether we believe them or not.

A common reason for rejecting a deontological approach to morality is the belief that there are no moral rules that do not have exceptions. It may usually be wrong to lie, for example, but it sometimes seems to be our moral *duty*. When the Nazi is at the door asking whether there are any Jews here, it would surely be wrong *not* to lie?

If we are swayed by the thought that there are exceptions even to moral rules like 'do not kill' then we will want to question premise one even if we acknowledge that religion and the law both give us reason to believe it is true. Maybe, we might say, it is *usually* wrong to kill innocents, but not always.

Here's a story that might prompt us to think we should reject premise one considered as a deontological moral absolute:

A ship is at sea, miles from land. Hundreds of sailors are on board. A fire is reported in the engine-room. The only way to save the ship (and the sailors) is to switch off the oxygen in the engine-room. The captain knows this would kill the four sailors in the engine-room.

Should the captain switch off the oxygen? Should he kill the four sailors?

Most people seem to think he should. Killing the four would save hundreds of other sailors. Also the four will die anyway if the fire isn't extinguished. Such people are expressing the intuition that 'do not kill innocents' is not an absolute rule, as (some) deontologists would have it, but a 'rule of thumb'.

Box 7.5 Philosophical background: Rules of thumb

Rules can be thought of as absolute, as unbreakable. Or they can be thought of as 'rules of thumb'. Rules of the latter sort can be broken whenever the situation is reasonably believed to demand it.

For more about the complexity of moral rules see Chapter 4, especially pages 38 and 42–44.

If you read Chapter 4 you will see that utilitarianism accounts very well for the intuition that rules like 'don't lie' and 'don't kill' are not moral absolutes. Utilitarianism is a theory according to which actions are right or wrong only in virtue of their consequences for happiness. According to a utilitarian if an action produces the greatest happiness of the greatest number (GHGN) then it is morally acceptable *whatever* it is.

Box 7.6 Activity: Conceptual analysis

Utilitarians reject the idea that rules like 'do not lie' and 'do not kill' are moral absolutes. Does this mean that utilitarians are not moral absolutists?

Answer: No. Utilitarians believe that 'produce the greatest happiness of the greatest number' (the greatest happiness principle) is true everywhere, for everyone, whether or not they believe it. This means that utilitarians believe that the GHP is true absolutely.

Embracing utilitarianism would mean that although we wouldn't want to *reject* premise one – because it is clear that killing innocents wouldn't usually promote the GHGN – we would want to modify it to demonstrate that it is not a moral absolute. We would want it to read: 'it is wrong to kill innocents unless doing so promotes the GHGN.'

This is a significant modification of our argument, however, which now reads:

Argument two (argument one with a utilitarian modification of premise one)
Premise one: It is wrong to kill an innocent unless doing so promotes the GHGN.
Premise two: The early embryo is an innocent.
Premise three: In therapeutic cloning the early embryo is killed.
Conclusion: Therefore therapeutic cloning is wrong.

This modification renders the argument invalid. There is a situation in which its premises are true and the conclusion false.

> **Box 7.7 Activity: Finding counterexamples**
>
> If argument two is invalid there must be a counterexample. Can you find one?
>
> Answer: The counterexample that proves conclusively that this argument is invalid is the situation in which therapeutic cloning promotes the GHGN.

The utilitarian can reject argument one, therefore, on the grounds that its first premise, without modification, is false. He can reject argument two because it is invalid, its conclusion does not follow from its premises. The utilitarian, therefore, has no reason that we have seen so far to accept that therapeutic cloning is wrong. If therapeutic cloning produces the GHGN it is morally unproblematic to the utilitarian.

A problem

If we reject the idea that 'do not kill' is absolutely true, and if we have a tendency to think that therapeutic cloning is a good thing, then utilitarianism, in enabling us to justify both beliefs, becomes tempting.

In adopting utilitarianism, however, we are accepting that it is morally acceptable to kill an innocent just so long as it promotes the GHGN. But do we really want to accept this? Consider the following questions:

- Would it be right to kill you in order to use your organs to save the lives of seven others?
- Would it be right to execute someone for a crime they didn't commit in order to avoid riots?
- Would it be right to slaughter all the members of a small and unpopular group because everyone else would prefer life without them?

In each of these situations killing innocents seems to produce the GHGN. If so, the utilitarian has to accept that they are morally acceptable.

But what do your intuitions say? Many people find the idea of killing innocents in these situations morally abhorrent. Could it really be right to kill in these situations? Unless it can be shown this wouldn't promote the GHGN (as perhaps it can?) the utilitarian has to say 'yes'. For many people this is a step too far.

> **Box 7.8 Activity: Small group discussion**
>
> Divide participants into three smaller groups. Each group should take one of the situations described above, and try to construct a case *against* the claim that the action described would promote the GHGN.
>
> The groups will need to consider the effect on the utilitarian calculus of:
>
> - how many people's happiness will be affected by the killing;
> - the chances of the killings being carried out in secret so the happiness of those not involved needn't be counted;
> - claiming that action is right only when no one knows about it.

Whilst there are undoubtedly occasions when many of us *do* think the right to life can be over-ridden for the sake of the GHGN – as with the ship example perhaps – there are other occasions when we would insist that the right to life trumps the GHGN. Many people reject utilitarianism because they think it doesn't take rights seriously enough.

> ### Box 7.9 Activity: Essay writing
>
> *We should reject utilitarianism because it doesn't take rights seriously enough.*
>
> *We should reject deontology because no moral claim is absolutely true.*
>
> Participants should choose one of these claims and examine it in a maximum of 2,000 words. In the essay they should:
>
> - briefly describe the theory they're considering;
> - explain the problem posed for that theory, in particular explaining why it is a problem for the theory;
> - consider at least one objection to the claim that this is a problem;
> - come to their own considered opinion, giving reasons for it.
>
> It is not necessary to come down on one side or another but it is necessary to defend the position embraced even if this is the fence-sitting position.

The third of the ethical theories we discussed in Chapter 4, virtue theory, would reject both the claim that 'do not kill' is a moral absolute *and* the claim that the promotion of the GHGN will always justify the killing of an innocent. The virtue ethicist would argue that the killing of a given innocent would be morally acceptable only if that killing accorded with the virtues: if it was wise, courageous, honest, temperate, etc.

To the extent we are troubled by the problems discussed for both deontology and utilitarianism, virtue ethics might be seen as coming to our rescue. It allows (against the deontologist) that killing could be the virtuous thing to do, but it insists (against the utilitarian) that killing for the sake of the GHGN might *not* be the virtuous thing to do. Virtue ethicists can respect both the intuition that tells us that the captain should switch off the oxygen in the engine room, *and* the intuition that genocide is wrong even if it does promote the GHGN. But what would the virtue ethicist say about therapeutic cloning?

> ### Box 7.10 Activity: Paired discussion
>
> There are many different lists of the virtues that virtue ethicists believe a virtuous person must have. Here is a list given by the BBC website on virtue ethics:[7]
>
> **The traditional list of cardinal virtues was:**
> *Prudence*
> *Justice*

Fortitude/Bravery
Temperance

The modern theologian James F. Keenan suggests:
Justice
Justice requires us to treat all human beings equally and impartially.
Fidelity
Fidelity requires that we treat people closer to us with special care.
Self-care
We each have a unique responsibility to care for ourselves, affectively, mentally, physically and spiritually.
Prudence
The prudent person must always consider justice, fidelity and self-care.
The prudent person must always look for opportunities to acquire more of the other three virtues.

In pairs, or as a whole group, participants should discuss whether a virtuous person would think therapeutic cloning accords with the virtues.

The questioning of premise one of argument one hasn't got us very far. Deontology could support it, whilst both utilitarianism and virtue ethics would reject it (at least understood as a moral absolute). But in rejecting this premise for utilitarian reasons we take on commitments many will find unacceptable. To adopt virtue ethics, however, is to be left with the question of just *when* killing an innocent would accord with the virtues.

Perhaps we would do better by questioning premise two rather than premise one? If premise two could be shown to be false, after all, the truth or falsehood of premise one would be irrelevant: argument one would have been shown to fail irrespective of the truth or falsehood of premise one.

Let us, therefore, examine premise two, the claim that the early embryo is an innocent one of us.

Premise two: the embryo is an innocent one of us

Here is our original argument:

Argument one
Premise one: It is wrong to kill an innocent one of us.
Premise two: The early embryo is an innocent one of us.
Premise three: In therapeutic cloning the early embryo is killed.
Conclusion: Therefore therapeutic cloning is wrong.

We have accepted the truth of premise three. We have found reason to question premise one, but also reason to accept it. In questioning premise two we shall, of course, assume the truth of the other premises.

If we could show that the early embryo *isn't* one of us, that it has no right to life, then our problems dissolve. If such is the case then the moral absolute 'do not kill' does not apply, nor does the embryo count in the utilitarian calculus. The way is clear for *everyone* to accept that there is no moral problem with killing the early embryo, and none, therefore, with therapeutic cloning.

Different people use the word 'embryo' in different ways. Box 7.11 below outlines the process of gestation to clarify what we will mean by the words we will use in this book.

Box 7.11 Factual information: Human gestation

Fertilisation (sometimes called 'conception') is a 24-hour process, complete at the point of 'syngamy', when the genetic materials carried by the sperm and the egg have fused.[8]

The product of fertilisation is a 'zygote' a single-celled organism. After 5 days the zygote becomes a 'blastocyst' (or 'pre-implantation embryo'), a hollow ball of about 100 cells, from some of which the embryo will develop. Other cells will become the placenta and the umbilical cord.

About 2 days later the blastocyst will implant itself into the womb, triggering biochemical signals from the mother, on which further development depends. About 75% of fertilised eggs fail to implant.

Fourteen days after fertilisation, at about the 2,000 cell stage, the cells start to differentiate, the 'primitive streak', the beginning of the nervous system, appears and individual organs start to develop.

After 7 weeks the organs are recognisable and the embryo becomes a foetus, the forerunner of the baby that will, all being well, be born 9 months after fertilisation.

We will use the word 'embryo' to cover all stages from syngamy to 7 weeks, though we will occasionally talk of the 'pre-implantation embryo' (up to 7 days).

In talking of the 'early embryo' we will mean the embryo up to the 14th day.

The question 'what is it to be one of us?' throws us into the philosophical deep end. Do we have the right to life simply in virtue of being human? Are there non-human animals with the right to life? Martians? Robots? Do we have the right to life because we are *persons*? But what is a person? Are there non-human persons or humans who are not persons?

To answer the question 'what is it to be one of us?' we should be able to answer two questions:

(i) Which conditions *must* be satisfied by a thing in order for it to be one of us?
(ii) Which conditions are such that if a thing satisfies these conditions it *is* one of us?

The first question asks for the conditions *necessary* to be one of us. The second asks for the conditions *sufficient* to be one of us.

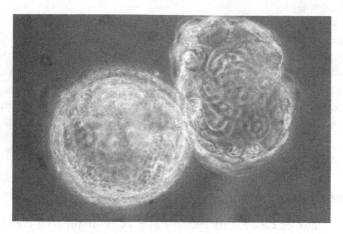

Figure 7.2 Light micrograph showing a hatching blastocyst. © Andy Walker, Midland Fertility Services/Science Photo Library.

A thing might satisfy a condition *necessary* for being one of us without satisfying the conditions *sufficient* for being one of us, or vice versa. It is arguably a necessary condition of being one of us, for example, that one be human. But is it sufficient? An early embryo is human, but is it *one of us*? It is arguably a sufficient condition for being one of us that a thing be self-conscious. But is this necessary? If so, then as the early embryo is not self-conscious it is not one of us.

It is not necessarily the case that we will be able to find conditions both necessary and sufficient to be one of us, but it will be illuminating to try.

Box 7.12 Philosophical background: Necessary and sufficient conditions

Whenever we are interested in the nature of something we can ask about the conditions necessary and sufficient for being that thing.

For example we usually recognise gold by its colour and malleability. But satisfying both these conditions is not sufficient for something to be gold, it must also have atomic number 79.

Having atomic number 79 is both necessary *and* sufficient for being gold. Anything lacking this number is not gold, however much it looks like gold. Anything that *does* have this atomic number is gold, however unlike gold it looks.

Our current interest in the question 'what is it to be one of us?' is in applying our answers to the case of the early embryo. If at any point in our discussion we find good reason to believe that the early embryo satisfies some condition *sufficient* for being one of us, therefore, or to believe it doesn't satisfy some condition *necessary* for being one of us, we will have enough for our current needs. The former finding constitutes reason to believe that premise two of argument one is true, the latter finding that it is false.

A simplifying stipulation

For the purposes of this chapter, we shall make a simplifying stipulation: that it is a necessary condition of being 'one of us' that a thing be human. We'll make this stipulation to postpone discussion of whether non-human animals could have or acquire the right to life. We shall discuss this question in Chapter 20. To assume *for the time being* that it is a necessary condition of being one of us that a thing be human does not beg this question (for the fallacy of 'begging the question' see Chapter 5, page 60).

This simplifying stipulation enables us to start by asking whether it is a sufficient condition of being one of us that a thing be human. If this is the case, then given that embryo is human from the moment of syngamy the embryo is one of us from the same moment. Here is this argument logic-book style:

> **Argument three**
> **Premise one:** It is a sufficient condition of being one of us that a thing be human.
> **Premise two:** The embryo is human from the moment of conception.
> **Conclusion:** Therefore the embryo is one of us from the moment of conception.

If this argument is sound then premise two of argument one must be true: the embryo is one of us. But is the argument sound?

Ronald Bailey, an American ethicist, denies premise two of argument three. He argues that all that comes into existence at conception is a clump of cells. In a speech denouncing President Bush's opposition to therapeutic cloning he argues:

'President Bush has declared, 'The use of embryos to clone is wrong. We should not grow life to destroy it.' In saying this Bush is confusing cellular life with human life.'[9]

It is tempting to agree that there is an important difference between a human and a bundle of cells. We might say that to claim we have a human at conception is like claiming we have a forest of oaks in our pocket when we have been collecting acorns.

But there is a problem with Bailey's argument. Is he right to say that 'cellular life' is not 'human life'? Consider scratching your finger along your arm. You will have a clump of cells under your fingernail. Now consider taking a few hairs from a mouse. You again have a clump of cells. The latter is not human. But the former is, isn't it? Something's being a bundle of cells doesn't mean it isn't human.

The cells under your fingernail are not, of course, comparable to *you*. They are not a human *being*. But you too are a bundle of cells. Bailey's argument relies on our agreeing with him that clumps of cells cannot have the right to life. But this seems, at least in some cases, to be false: the bundle of cells that is you does have the right to life.

> **Box 7.13 Activity: Analysing arguments**
>
> Read Chapter 5, pages 64–67 on how to set out an argument logic-book style, and page 60 on the fallacy of begging the question. Then set out Bailey's argument logic-book style, showing how it begs the question.

Answer: Here is Bailey's argument set out logic-book style:
Premise one: The early embryo is just a bundle of cells.
Premise two: No bundle of cells has the right to life.
Conclusion: Therefore the early embryo does not have the right to life.

Premise two is italicised because it is a *suppressed* premise: Bailey assumes it but doesn't make it explicit. This suppressed premise begs the question that we are trying to answer.

(a)   (b)

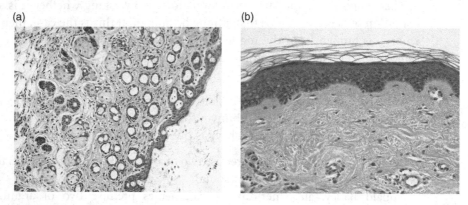

Figure 7.3 Light micrograph images showing skin cells of (a) a mouse and (b) a human. © Riccardo Cassiani-Ingoni/Science Photo Library and iStockphoto.com/Chris Dascher.

It is true that the early embryo is a bundle of cells. But is it morally equivalent to the one under your fingernail? Or is it more equivalent to the one that is *you*? It is only if it is equivalent to the former that describing the embryo as a clump of cells might ground the claim the embryo has no right to life. If the bundle of cells that is the early embryo is more equivalent to *you* then correctly describing it as a bundle of cells doesn't entail that it doesn't have the right to life.

It would seem that correctly describing the early embryo as a bundle of cells doesn't entail anything at all about the embryo's right to life, unless you tacitly assume that bundles of cells do not have the right to life. Bailey's argument begs the very question he is supposed to be answering (see Chapter 5, page 60).

Box 7.14 **Philosophical background: Redescription**

In thinking about moral issues we must avoid describing things so as to strip them of moral import. Describing a lethal injection as 'an injection' wouldn't be incorrect but it omits something of moral import.

It is not incorrect to describe an early embryo as a bundle of cells. But some bundles of cells (like you) have moral status and other bundles of cells (the one under your fingernail) don't.

So calling the early embryo a bundle of cells, even if correct, cannot say anything for or against the claim that the early embryo has moral status.

Perhaps Bailey should have argued, not that the early embryo is not human (which it is), but that it does not suffice for being one of us that a thing be human. He might claim that it is necessary also to be *a human being*. Bailey would then be rejecting the first premise of argument three rather than the second. He would be making the following argument:

Argument four
Premise one: It is a necessary condition of being one of us that a thing be a human being.
Premise two: The early embryo is not a human being.
Conclusion: Therefore the early embryo is not one of us.

This argument is valid. If its premises are true its conclusion must be true and premise two of argument one is false.

The revised argument relies on a distinction between being *human* and being *a human being*. The existence of this distinction is supported by the intuition of a moral difference between the bundle of cells that is the embryo and the one that is *you*. Both are *human*. But only you are a *human being*. This suggests that being human may be necessary for being one of us (as we have stipulated), but it *can't* be sufficient. It is also necessary to be a human being.

In making this distinction between being human and being a human being, we have both philosophy and science on our side.

Until about 14 days after syngamy, when the primitive streak forms, the embryo is capable of 'twinning', of separating into two or more embryos. This is how identical twins or triplets form. They are identical because both or all originate from *one* zygote. The zygote therefore is not obviously *a* human being: before the formation of the primitive streak it might be *one, two, three or more* human beings.

There is a logical problem, therefore, if we claim the early embryo is *a* human being. Is there *a single* human being at conception but two or more after twinning? If so what happens to this singleton? Does he or she *die* to be replaced by the other two? Does he or she *become* one or other of the two? (If so some human beings do *not* come into existence at conception, but only at twinning.) Does the singleton become *both* of the two? (But how could human being A and human being B both be human being C, when A and B are not themselves the same human being?) Identical twins might have identical genomes, but they are not identical *human beings*.[10]

Box 7.15 Philosophical background: Individuation

This logical problem is an *individuation* problem. For a concept to be coherent it is necessary for a grasp of it to enable us to tell whether the concept applies or not. If you aren't able to tell us how many cats there are in a room then we cannot attribute to you the concept 'cat'. You can't *individuate* cats.

If *none of us* can tell how many human beings exist before the 14th day, then none of us has a coherent concept of human being. An alternative is to say that the concept 'human being' does not apply to the embryo before the 14th day.

Science exacerbates this logical problem. We know that if, at the eight cell stage of development, these cells are separated, each will develop as if it was the original zygote. At this stage the cells are called 'totipotent' because they have the ability to grow into an entire human organism. This is one of the things that makes therapeutic cloning so promising.

Twinning and totipotence make it difficult to argue that *a* human being comes into existence at conception. How can we say this if we have no principled way of knowing *how many human beings* have come into existence? Is there, at conception, *a* thing with the right to life, or *eight* such things?

It might seem that the problem is merely epistemological. But the problem is metaphysical (see Chapter 2, Box 2.5). It is not just that until the formation of the primitive streak *we cannot tell* how many human beings there are, it is that until the primitive streak forms *there is no determinate number* of human beings. This makes it logically difficult to justify the claim that what has come into existence before this point is a human being.

If we accept this then whatever we have before the 14th day isn't *a human being* however human it is. If being a human being is a necessary condition of being one of us the embryo cannot be one of us until at least the 14th day after syngamy.

Box 7.16 Factual information: The Warnock Report

It was on the grounds that before the 14th day the embryo is not a human being that the Warnock Committee in the UK argued that it is morally permissible to experiment on the early embryo. (For further information about the Warnock Committee, see Box 4.2.)

This claim gives us a reason for believing that premise two of argument one is false, that the early embryo is *not* one of us. As therapeutic cloning takes place before the 14th day, if the embryo is not one of us until the 14th day, there can be no moral objection to therapeutic cloning on the basis of the claim that the embryo is one of us.

Box 7.17 Activity: Conceptual analysis

Are therapeutic cloning and abortion morally equivalent? If so, then if therapeutic cloning is morally acceptable so is abortion (and vice versa).

Can you identify a position on which we might consistently think abortion is wrong, whilst thinking therapeutic cloning is not wrong?

Answer: two beliefs are consistent if they can both be true at the same time. It is consistent to believe both that therapeutic cloning is acceptable because the embryo is killed before the 14th day, and that abortion is unacceptable because it takes place at some point after the 14th day.

To have reason to believe a claim, though, is not necessary to have *conclusive* reason to believe it. There is a problem with accepting that being a human being is a necessary condition of being one of us. To accept this is to accept that before the 14th day the embryo is morally equivalent to the bundle of skin cells under your fingernail. Both are human but *neither* is a human being, and neither, therefore, can be said to have the right to life.

But is this acceptable? An embryo, after all, has the *potential* for becoming a human being. Doesn't this have *any* moral import? Couldn't we say that the *potential for becoming* a human being suffices for being one of us, rather than requiring that the embryo *actually be* a human being? If so the embryo will once again be one of us from conception.[11] Here is the argument for this claim:

> **Argument five**
> **Premise one:** It is a sufficient condition for being one of us that a thing have the potential to become a human being.
> **Premise two:** The early embryo has the potential to become a human being.
> **Conclusion:** Therefore the early embryo is one of us.

The argument is valid and its second premise seems unassailable. To the extent we have reason to believe the first premise, therefore, we have reason to accept the conclusion which is, of course, premise two of argument one.

But there are three objections to the claim that the potential for becoming a human being is sufficient for being one of us. These are:

1. The *potential* for being something does not always confer the rights that go with actually *being* such a thing. Potential doctors do not have the rights of actual doctors.
2. Human eggs and sperm have the potential for being human beings. Conferring the right to life on gametes would have serious ramifications for daily life.
3. Every cell under your fingernail has the potential to become one of us given the technique of SCNT. Conferring the right to life on skin cells has even more serious ramifications for daily life.

These are serious objections. But perhaps we can get around them? Sometimes being a potential something does generate rights. Potential doctors have the right to proper training, for example. Could the potential for becoming human generate the right to life? In the case of the sperm and the egg, or the bundle of cells from under your fingernail, interventions would be needed to produce a human being. In the case of the early embryo no intervention is needed so long as the embryo is in a womb ripe for implantation. Could this difference generate the right to life?

> **Box 7.18 Activity: Small group discussion**
>
> Divide participants into three groups and allocate to each group one of the arguments against the claim that the potential for becoming a human being suffices for the status of a human being. Their task is to see if they can get around this argument.
>
> Each group should appoint a spokesperson to report back, the discussion can then be opened to the whole group.

Our beliefs about whether the early embryo matters morally will ground our beliefs about whether or not the early embryo can be killed with impunity (as we would discard the bundle of cells under our fingernails), or whether it must be accorded the right to life (as if it were equivalent to a human infant).

There is a profound difference between something's mattering morally and its not mattering morally. When the truth matters the principle of charity (see Chapter 5, pages 67–69) is of prime importance. If we get it wrong we could be guilty of mass murder in sacrificing thousands of early embryos in therapeutic cloning. Or we could fail to alleviate the suffering of thousands because we refuse to see that early embryos are more akin to bundles of skin cells than neonates.

> ### Box 7.19 Activity: Personal reflection
>
> *Before the 14th day it cannot reasonably be claimed that the embryo is a human being, therefore it is not one of us.*
>
> *The early embryo has the potential to become a human being from the moment of syngamy, therefore even before the 14th day it is one of us.*
>
> Identify the position towards which you tend. Then consider carefully the arguments *against* it without creating any straw men (see Chapter 5, Box 5.8).

We are not going to be able to solve this problem here. But we have enough for our purposes. We have established non-conclusive reasons for believing both:

(i) it is a necessary condition for being one of us that a thing be an actual human being and the early embryo is not an actual human being.

(ii) it is a sufficient condition for being one of us that something have the potential for being a human being and the early embryo has the potential for becoming a human being.

These claims cannot both be true.

To hold the first position is to have prima facie reason to believe that premise two of argument one is false, that the early embryo is not one of us and does not have the right to life. For you, therapeutic cloning will be morally acceptable even if you are a deontologist.

To hold the second position is to have prima facie reason to believe that premise two of argument one is true, that the early embryo *is* one of us and has the right to life. For you, therapeutic cloning will be morally unacceptable even if you are a utilitarian.

If you are a virtue ethicist, of course, you will have to take on board all these arguments in deciding whether or not therapeutic cloning accords with the virtues.

This is the point at which each of us must make a decision about the moral acceptability of therapeutic cloning. This might, of course, be the decision to keep an open mind.

Summary

In this chapter we have:

- Seen that argument one, concluding that therapeutic cloning is wrong, is valid so questioning the conclusion involves showing that a premise is false;

- considered premise one (the claim that it is wrong to kill) and seen that:
  - utilitarians and virtue ethicists could both reject it because they reject deontological moral absolutes;
  - rejecting premise one on utilitarian grounds might commit us to believing that genocide is morally acceptable;
  - rejecting premise one on the grounds of virtue ethics leaves us with the problem of deciding when killing accords with the virtues;

- considered premise two (the claim that the early embryo is one of us) and seen that:
  - if it is a necessary condition of being one of us that a thing be a human being, and before the 14th day the embryo is not a human being, it will be false;
  - if it is a sufficient condition of being one of us that a thing have the potential for being a human being, then given the early embryo has this potential, it will be true;

- seen that the moral theory you embrace does not determine whether or not you will think that moral cloning is acceptable or unacceptable.

- seen that one can believe that therapeutic cloning is morally acceptable whilst rejecting the moral acceptability of abortion.

Questions to stimulate reflection

Do you believe that it is always and everywhere wrong to kill one of us?

Do you believe that if killing one of us would produce the greatest happiness of the greatest number it is acceptable?

Do you think the fact that therapeutic cloning could save a lot of suffering means that it must be morally acceptable?

Do you think it could ever accord with virtue to kill one of us?

Do we have the right to life from conception? If not when do we acquire the right to life?

Do you think that therapeutic cloning is morally acceptable?

Additional activities

Use this website to set up a debate on therapeutic cloning:
http://www.idebate.org/debatabase/topic_details.php?topicID=142.

Find out more about why the Warnock Committee decided that therapeutic cloning is morally acceptable until the 14th day (see http://www.publications.parliament.uk/pa/cm200607/cmselect/cmsctech/272/27205.htm).

Read this debate on cloning between two scientists on Online Newshour: http://www.pbs.org/newshour/health/cloning.html.

Write a short essay about the differences between therapeutic cloning and abortion.

Access the following website at BEEP and do the thought experiment described: http://www.beep.ac.uk/content/341.0.html.

Put 'critical reasoning quiz' into a search engine, and use the results to further test your critical reasoning skills.

Notes

1 http://www.uq.edu.au/oppe/PDFS/CloningTechniques.pdf. An online factsheet from the website of the Office of Public Policy and Ethics, the Institute of Molecular Biology, University of Queensland.

2 http://www.chromosomechronicles.com/2010/01/18/genetic-identity-theft-will-you-need-to-protect-your-genome/. An article suggesting that hundreds of people might want one of the follicles from Brad Pitt's hairbrush.

3 http://news.sciencemag.org/sciencenow/2008/03/24-01.html. An article from ScienceNow on the application of therapeutic cloning techniques to Parkinson's disease.

4 http://www.telegraph.co.uk/health/healthnews/3485752/First-woman-to-have-stem-cell-organ-transplant-Exclusive-interview.html. An article from the *Telegraph* about the first woman to receive an organ grown from her own stem cells.

5 http://www.schb.org.uk/downloads/publications/ethics_of_animal-human_mixtures.pdf.

6 In the Catholic/Lutheran bibles this is the fifth commandment. It sometimes reads 'do not murder'.

7 http://www.bbc.co.uk/ethics/introduction/virtue.shtml. The BBC website on Virtue Ethics.

8 http://www.bbc.co.uk/learningzone/clips/human-fertilisation/1848.html. A video from the BBC of the moment a sperm burrows into an egg.

9 http://reason.com/archives/2001/11/28/calling-hippocrates. 'Calling Hippocrates' by Ronald Bailey Reason Online 28 November 2001.

10 http://channel.nationalgeographic.com/series/in-the-womb/4048/Overview. A video from the National Geographic on the in utero development of identical twins.

11 http://www.bbc.co.uk/ethics/abortion/child/potential.shtml The BBC Ethics website on the argument from potential.

Further reading and useful websites

Green, C. (2010) *Stem Cells (21st Century Science)*. Tunbridge Wells, UK: Tick Tock Books.

Monroe, K. R. (2007) *Fundamentals of the Stem Cell Debate: The Scientific, Religious, Ethical, and Political Issues*. Berkeley, CA: University of California Press.

Panno, J. (2006) *Stem Cell Research: Medical Applications and Ethical Controversy (New Biology)*. New York: Checkmark Books.

http://www.ornl.gov/sci/techresources/Human_Genome/elsi/cloning.shtml. Everything you
    could want to know about cloning from the Human Genome Project.
http://stemcells.nih.gov/info/ethics.asp. The website of the National Institute of Health on
    stem cells.
http://www.youtube.com/watch?v=yb8VhoVbSdk. A debate televised by the University of
    California television channel.

8 Reproductive cloning: science and science fiction

Objectives

In reading this chapter you will:

- learn about the negative public view of human cloning;
- consider the possible causes of such public disapprobation;
- reflect on the role played by the media in forming public opinion;
- note that until cloning is safe it will be wrong to clone a human child;
- reflect on whether clones would have free will;
- consider whether clones would lack human dignity;
- ask whether a clone would have confused and ambiguous relationships;
- consider whether cloning for reproductive purposes is morally acceptable.

We saw in the last chapter that embryos produced by somatic cell nuclear transfer (SCNT) can be used for therapeutic or reproductive purposes.[1] In this chapter we shall discuss reproductive cloning: SCNT (or yet-to-be-developed cloning techniques[2]) used to produce a live human baby.

The visceral recoil against cloning noted in the last chapter was particularly evident in February 1997. In this month the birth of Dolly the sheep was announced.[3] Dolly was the first mammal cloned by SCNT. The announcement triggered inflammatory headlines worldwide, and an avalanche of international legislation (see Box 8.1).

Box 8.1 Factual information: Responses to the announcement of Dolly's birth

4 March 1997: The US issued a moratorium on federal funding for human cloning and demanded an immediate report on the social and ethical issues.

18 March 1997: The House of Commons Select Committee on Science and Technology urged that existing law be tightened to ban human cloning in the UK.

14 May 1997: The World Health Assembly said: 'the use of cloning for the replication of human individuals is ethically unacceptable and contrary to human dignity and morality.'

March 1997: The European Parliament called for an explicit worldwide ban on the cloning of human beings.

Many people feel threatened by the idea of cloning human beings. In this chapter we shall consider whether this is justified or borne of media hype and science fiction.

Physical risks

Before producing Dolly, Ian Wilmut of the Roslin Institute[4] in Edinburgh failed 277 times to produce a healthy sheep. The embryos either died, or were deformed.[5] Some suspect Dolly's true age was the age of the donor of the nucleus that produced her rather than her chronological age. This would explain why she developed arthritis prematurely and died of a lung disease usually found in older sheep.[6]

This failure rate renders immoral any current attempt to produce a human clone. This technology at the moment really is too risky for the clones being produced. But the technology is improving. Our discussion will proceed on the assumption that one day the risk will be no higher than that accompanying normal reproduction. The question is whether, when we reach this point, there will still be moral barriers to cloning.

Cloning and science fiction

It is difficult to think of cloning without thinking about science fiction. Media reports of cloning (see Box 8.2) are steeped in such stories. It's likely you'll have read some of this science fiction or seen one of the hugely popular films. The enjoyable frisson we get from such stories and films are a grown-up version of that enjoyed by children when daddy jumps out at them. Children have no real reason to be frightened of dad. Do we have real reason to be frightened of human clones?

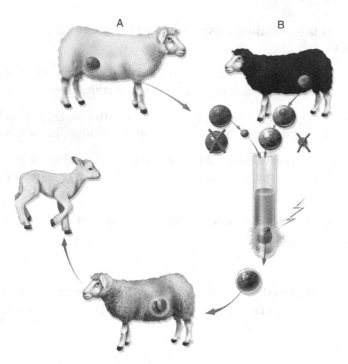

Figure 8.1 The cloning process of 'Dolly the sheep'. A cell is taken from the ewe A, of which the nucleus (genetic code) is kept. An ovum is taken from the ewe B, of which the cytoplasm is kept. In a test tube, the nucleus will merge with the cytoplasm of the other cell. The embryo is implanted into the uterus of a surrogate mother. After a few months, a ewe (Dolly) is born which is a clone of ewe A. © Jacopin/Science Photo Library.

Box 8.2 **Activity: Group discussion**

On 24 February 1997 *The Sun* (England's largest circulation tabloid newspaper – daily circulation of approximately 3 250 000) reported on Dolly's birth as follows:

SCIENTISTS have 'bred' the world's first cloned adult animal – sparking fears a woman could give birth to her father's twin.

Other horror scenarios include a dictator replacing himself, and showbiz moguls cloning dead stars. The team who made the breakthrough by cloning a sheep at Edinburgh's Roslin Institute say the idea it could be used on humans is 'repugnant'.

But expert Dr Patrick Dixon said one woman already wanted to bring back her dead father as her own baby.

The Roslin experts took a cell from a sheep called Dolly, used it to replace genetic material in another ewe's egg, then planted it in the womb of a third. The resulting lamb was Dolly's exact double.

The Sun, 24 February 1997 © News Group Newspapers Limited 2002. All rights reserved. Please contact NI Syndication at enquiries@nisyndication.com.

Discuss *The Sun*'s report of Dolly's birth. You might like to use the following questions as prompts for discussion:

1. Do you think this report is biased?
2. Has *The Sun* got the scientific facts wrong?
3. Are the 'horror scenarios' described in the report far-fetched?
4. If the horror scenarios *could* come about, however far-fetched, isn't *The Sun* right to draw readers' attention to them?
5. If you were a *Sun* reporter, would you have written this piece differently? If not, why not? If so, how would you have written it?

(Note: *The Sun* has got the facts wrong. Dolly was the product of cloning, not the sheep from whom the donor cell was taken.)

In this chapter we shall consider whether the intuitions so many people have against the cloning of human beings can be rationally justified.

Clones and free will

One argument people offer against the morality of human cloning is that human clones will lack free will.

There are numerous science fiction tales portraying clones as automata. In *The Boys From Brazil* we are asked to imagine legions of Hitler clones who have no choice but to attempt to make good Hitler's failure to rid the world of non-Aryans. In other stories we get 'armies' of clones, all identical, all obedient to some mad master, all prepared, on his command, to destroy whatever it is he wants destroyed.[7] Some stories allow clones glimmers of autonomy. This adds to the horror: these clones have some grasp of what they are missing. Could it really be morally permissible to bring such people into existence?

The first question we should ask, though, is whether we have any reason *other* than science fiction for believing clones would lack free will? There is an obvious reason for thinking the clone would *have* free will: assuming the nucleus donor has free will, why would the clone not have it? Nevertheless, here are two arguments for the belief that clones would lack autonomy:

(i)   clones are not 'ends in themselves';
(ii) clones do not have 'open futures'.

Let's look at these in turn.

(i) Clones are means to others' ends

Gilbert Meilaender, a theologian, believes that a clone would be nothing more than a 'project' of the people who produce it. It would be a means to their ends rather than an end in itself. Meilaender believes that to be born as a means to the ends of others suffices to strip you of free will.[8]

> **Box 8.3 Activity: Analysing and evaluating arguments**
>
> Can you set out Meilaender's argument logic-book style, then evaluate it in accordance with the usual procedure?
>
> Answer:
>   Premise one: Human clones will not have free will.
>   Premise two: It is wrong to bring into the world human beings who lack free will.
>   Conclusion: Human cloning is wrong.
>
> Variations on this theme are fine so long as they accurately represent this argument. The argument should be evaluated in the usual way (Does the conclusion follow from the premises? Are the premises true?).

Reflection on this, however, suggests that Meilaender cannot mean that being born as a means to the ends of others suffices *literally* to strip you of free will. If so there must be millions of human beings who lack free will.

To have a child to look after one in one's old age is to have a child as a means to one's own ends. So is having a child to carry on the family name, or inherit the family silver. Then there are those children born to satisfy their parents' desire to see how their genes would combine with those of their partner, those born to parents who 'just want someone to love', and those born to make grandparents happy. Every year millions of children are born as means to their parents' ends.

If any or all of these situations is guaranteed to result in a child who lacks free will, then millions of human beings now and throughout the ages lack, and have lacked, free will.

This is implausible. Even if there are reasons, such as those adduced for hard determinism (see pages 16–19), to suggest human beings lack free will, the idea that we lack it because we were born to care for our parents in their old age is not one of them. Charity tells us, therefore, that Meilaender can't be claiming that being born as a means to your parents' ends will *literally* deprive you of free will. (For the Principle of Charity and its importance to interpretation see Chapter 5, pages 67–69.)

It is easy to produce an alternative, and far more plausible, interpretation of Meilaender's claim. Some parents selfishly bring up a child to fulfil their own purposes rather than its own. If parents bring up a child to believe that its duty in life is to look after the family silver, the child may well grow up believing that this *is* its duty in life. These parents have succeeded in bending their child's will to their own. This child might be mistaking *their* reasons for acting for his own. When this happens, we might think of the child (metaphorically speaking) as a 'clone' of his parents, a child without a mind of his own. In this sense children born as means to their parents' ends might reasonably be said – metaphorically – to lack free will.

It would seem that, unless we can think of another interpretation of Meilaender's claim, it is either extremely implausible, or nothing more than the claim that children born as means to their parents' ends lack free will *metaphorically*.

That children brought up in the way described don't literally lack free will is obvious. The child born to care for its parents in old age may move to the other side of the world. Or refuse to help though she lives next door. The child born to inherit the family silver might make a vow to poverty. The child born to keep grandparents happy might avoid them like the plague. Many children brought up by selfish parents summon the strength of character to rebel. Such parents occasionally find themselves murdered. This is also the sort of story – in fiction at least – that gives us a little frisson of pleasure.

Even when these children do act on their parents' wishes, this does not indicate lack of free will. They are acting thus because they have chosen to do so. The mere fact that someone does something at the behest of another person does not mean that he or she is not acting freely: human beings often freely choose to act as others want them to act.

However, if the correct interpretation of Meilaender's claim is the second one, then we can see that he is right to think that a child born as a means to its parents' ends might end up without a mind of its own and in this sense lack free will. But we can also see that this wouldn't make a clone any different from any other human being. More importantly for our purposes, we might ask why anyone would go to the bother of cloning a child for such a purpose? They'd have just as much chance of success with a child born in the usual manner.

Box 8.4 Philosophical background: Equivocation

The *Fallacy* of Equivocation occurs when an ambiguous word or phrase makes an unsound argument appear sound. Consider the following example:

All banks are beside rivers.

Therefore, the financial institution where I deposit my money is beside a river.

In this argument, there are two unrelated meanings of the word 'bank':

1. *A riverside*: In this sense, the premise is true but the argument is invalid.
2. *A type of financial institution*: On this meaning, the argument is valid, but the premise is false.

In either case, the argument is unsound.[9]

(ii) Clones do not have 'open futures'

The second reason for believing that clones will lack free will derives from the fact clones are genetically identical to their donor. It is suggested that unlike the rest of us, whose futures are open to self-determination, clones are doomed to repeat the lives of their donor, to think as they think, do as they do and become whatever they became. Whereas the child of sexual reproduction will be, as philosopher Hilary Putnam puts it, 'a surprise to its parents', a clone, he says, will be anything but, its future will be mapped out, it won't have any choices to make.[10,]

This argument is distinct from the one above. Here the claim is not that the *parents* of a clone will bend it to their will, but rather that the *genetic inheritance* of a clone strips it of free will. The two arguments could be combined: imagine parents who clone someone because they want a replica of the donor, and believe that cloning will deliver this.

This argument is based on genetic determinism: the belief that identical genomes entail identical futures. Genetic determinism, however, is false. Identical genomes do not even entail that two people will be *genetically* identical. If a clone is born to a mother other than the one who carried its donor then it will differ from its donor in the mitochondrial DNA it inherits.[11]

Identical twins, however, show us that even those as close as they possibly could be in terms of nature and nurture (same genome, same mitochondria, same uterine environment, same family, at the same time) can be extremely different. There is no sense whatsoever in which even they are 'doomed' to the same future.

Box 8.5 Factual information: Conjoined twins

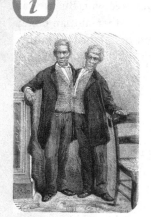

Eng and Chang Bunker were born in 1811 in Thailand (then Siam, hence 'Siamese twins'). They spent the whole of their 63 years attached to each other at the sternum. Their livers were also attached, though independently functioning.

Eng and Cheng were taken to America with a circus. Then they went into business for themselves by buying a plantation.

They married two sisters and had, respectively, 11 and 10 children. After the wives quarrelled the families lived in different houses, the twins alternating over a 3-day period.

The twins died within an hour of each other in 1874.

Figure 8.2 Chang and Eng Bunker (1811–1874). Engraving from *La Nature* (Paris, 14 March 1874). © Photolibrary.com.

The two arguments that we have considered for the claim that clones will lack autonomy have both been weak. But they have usefully drawn our attention to an equivocation (see Box 8.4). The notion of free will is ambiguous. There are three senses in which a person might be said to lack free will:

(i) Tables do not have free will in that they are not capable in any sense of choosing how to act.

Tables do not make choices at all. They are not rational or irrational. They do not act for reasons *at all*, even bad ones. Tables are *non*-rational and non-autonomous.

(ii) Animals are such that all their behaviour is determined by the laws of nature and their immediate and past environments.

Animals appear to choose how they will act. But arguably this appearance is deceptive. A woodlouse does not hide in damp places because it likes being in damp places. It rather embodies a mechanism called a 'kinesis' that ensures that the woodlouse will move whenever the air around it is dry, at a speed determined by the dryness of the air, and in a direction determined by the way it is 'pointing'. All woodlouse behaviour is explicable thus, leaving no explanatory work to be done by the notion of reason or free will.

(iii) Children might be said to lack free will if they grow up doing exactly as their parents choose.

As we are assuming that hard determinism is false (see Chapter 2) we are assuming that human beings *do* have free will. It is in the very nature of a human being to act freely.

It is easy, on first hearing the arguments of those who believe that clones won't have free will, to believe they claim that clones will lack free will in sense (i). If this were the case clones would *not* be real people, they would lack something essential to being human beings. If such were the case then it would be morally unacceptable to produce human clones.

But the two arguments we have been considering are making much weaker claims. The latter claim is arguably a claim to the effect that clones would be like non-human animals rather than humans, in that all their behaviour would be determined. But to the extent we reject genetic determinism, and identical twins show we should, we have no reason to think clones would lack free will in sense (ii).

The former claim is nothing stronger than the claim that clones would lack free will in sense (iii). Clones could be bent to the will of those who bring it up as easily as non-clones can. But this doesn't strip a clone, or any other child, of its free will except metaphorically.

We can therefore accept that *if* there is any good reason to think that clones would lack free will this would be a good reason to think that reproductive cloning is morally impermissible. But so far we have not seen any good reason to believe that clones would lack free will in any sense other than sense (iii). In this they do not differ from any other human being.

Box 8.6 Activity: Identifying and evaluating arguments

We have examined two arguments for the claim that clones will lack autonomy. Neither is convincing. But science fiction stories are often predicated on the idea that clones lack free will. Might we be missing something?

Participants should choose a science fiction book or film dealing with the issue of cloning (a couple are mentioned in the further reading section at the end of the chapter). As they read or watch it they should try to identify any argument given for *why* clones would lack free will.

These arguments should then be brought to the whole group and evaluated in the usual way. Participants might then discuss the impact of science fiction on public opinion about cloning.

This activity could also be used to stimulate discussions of other biotechnological advances where the media has greatly influenced public perception or where the 'yuk' factor (see Chapter 6 under 'it's disgusting') might arise, for example:

- GM crops (see Chapter 19)
- creating new life forms (see Chapter 16)
- xenotranplantation (see Chapter 19).

Human dignity

Gilbert Meilaender has another reason for believing that reproductive cloning is morally unacceptable: he believes that it is a necessary condition of human dignity that one be the result of an 'act of love' between a husband and wife. On the reasonable assumption that every human being has the right to dignity, this would constitute excellent reason not to produce human clones given that they are not the (immediate) result of acts of love between husbands and wives.

> ### Box 8.7 Activity: Identifying arguments
>
> Can you analyse Meilaender's argument and set it out logic-book style?
>
> Answer: Here is one analysis of the argument:
> Premise one: It is a necessary condition of human dignity that a human being be the result of an act of love between husband and wife.
> Premise two: A clone is not the result of an act of love between husband and wife.
> Conclusion: The human clone lacks human dignity.
>
> If you have something other than this you are not necessarily wrong. You should check that your conclusion really is a way of expressing the claim that Meilaender is making, and that your premises really are the reasons that he offers for his claim.

Why, though, should we accept that it is a necessary condition of human dignity that one be the result of an act of love between husband and wife? Here is Meilaender's argument:

'Our children begin with a genetic independence of us, their parents. They replicate neither their father nor their mother. This is a reminder of the independence that we must eventually grant them and for which it is our duty to prepare them. To lose, even in principle, this sense of the child as a gift entrusted to us will not be good for children.'[12]

Meilaender believes a child should spring from the act of giving and receiving love between a man and a woman committed to nurturing the child in all its independence as an equal, a replica of neither but rather 'an incarnation of their union'. Meilaender believes an act of love like this can only occur within marriage.

These acts of love, Meilaender says, free a couple from 'self-absorption', from sex as a means solely of satisfying individual needs and desires. Unless a child springs from such an act, he argues, it will be a 'personal project' of its parents: the point of its existence will not be *its own existence* but the satisfaction of its parents' desires. It will not be an end in itself.

Box 8.8 Activity: Revision

In talking of children being 'ends in themselves' Meilaender is tacitly appealing to one of the three ethical theories we considered in Chapter 4. Can you say which one?

Do you think that all those embracing this theory would have to agree with Meilaender's view?

Answer: The theory appealed to is deontology, specifically Kant's version of deontology. If cloning *does* essentially involve treating the clone as a means to the ends of others then Kantian deontologists would have to agree with Meilaender's view that human reproductive cloning is wrong.

Meilaender's description of why a child is an end in itself is moving. It is certainly the case, furthermore, that the motivations of those who want to clone a human being – especially those who want to clone themselves – should be examined very carefully. It would be morally abhorrent to allow the birth of a clone wanted only so someone can recreate and perfect *themselves*.

In fact, it is worrying to think anyone would clone a human being because they wanted a replica of another person. Given the falsehood of genetic determinism, such people are likely to be disappointed. It is not morally acceptable for anyone to bring into the world a child in whom that person is sure to be disappointed.

But there are other reasons for wanting to clone a human being. You will find three of them in Box 8.9.

Box 8.9 Activity: Small group discussion

Here are some situations in which people might want to clone a child:

1. Rob is infertile. He and Tina want to clone Rob and implant the clone into Tina's womb. Because of the contribution of Tina's mitochondrial DNA, the resulting child will be genetically related to both of them.

2. Elizabeth and David were informed after the birth of Sarah they would be unable to have more children. Sarah died in an accident aged two. Elizabeth

and David want to clone Sarah. They have had extensive counselling to make sure they are not attempting to replace Sarah.

3. The gametes of both Phil and Marti are unusable. The couple would like to clone the genome of Marti's beloved great grandmother, who lived to an old age, free from disease and sharp as a pin.

Participants should be divided into small groups and given 20 minutes to discuss the questions below before giving feedback to the group as a whole:

Would a clone produced by these couples be nothing more than a means to their ends?

If so does this mean such couples should be barred from using the technology of cloning to produce a child?

If not, is there any other reason to stop these couples from cloning (assuming the technology is now safe)?

Another problem this argument generates is that if it is sound, then in the history of mankind, very few human beings have had human dignity. The millions of human beings who, throughout the centuries, have been born outside wedlock will all have lacked human dignity. The millions born within wedlock but resulting from an act prompted by the needs of their parents, rather than the love (if any) between their parents would have lacked dignity. Anyone born of rape will have lacked dignity. It is possible that *most* human beings will lack human dignity.

Again this suggests Meilaender can't be right. Could it really be the case that only a tiny number of human beings in the history of humankind have had human dignity? Surely a human being has dignity simply in and of himself, rather than as a result of his origins? Throughout history people have believed that some people – those born outside wedlock or those of certain ethnic origins for example – have lacked human dignity. But we don't have to accept that those who believed this were right.

Box 8.10 Activity: Revision

The argument just discussed might be based on a confusion between a truth about *the beliefs someone has* with a truth about *the truth of the beliefs someone has*. We discussed this distinction in Chapter 6 (pages 86–87). Can you remember what this distinction is?

Answer: It's the distinction between first and second order beliefs. Consider the fact that there is a distinction between:

(i) Mary believes that those whose parents weren't married lack dignity.
(ii) Those whose parents weren't married lack dignity.

Claim (i) is a claim about Mary's belief about whether others have dignity.
Claim (ii) is a claim about whether others have dignity, about the *truth* of Mary's belief.

Interestingly, Ian Wilmut, the scientist who brought Dolly into the world, offered an argument against reproductive cloning that is rather like Meilaender's. Wilmut argued that reproductive cloning would be wrong because clones wouldn't be treated as real people, they would be discriminated against.[13]

But if clones would be discriminated against because they wouldn't be believed to be real people, and this belief is false then what would be wrong is the beliefs people have, and the consequent way they treat clones, not the fact that clones exist. The belief that clones are not real people would be comparable to the belief that black people or women don't deserve to be treated as real people. Such false beliefs have in the past been responsible for huge injustices.[14]

Again, the best we can say is that if we can find any good reason for the claim that clones would lack human dignity, then this would be a good reason to think that reproductive cloning is morally unacceptable. But that clones are not the result of an act of love between husband and wife does not seem to be such a reason.

Clones and family relationships

Sometimes people worry that because clones are not the result of sexual reproduction they will not, like normal babies, have a mother and a father. Nicholas Coote, for example, the Assistant General Secretary to the Roman Catholic Bishops' Conference of England argues that every child has the right to two parents.[15]

If this is an argument against reproductive cloning it appears to be based on a misunderstanding. Biologically speaking clones *do* have two parents: the parents of whoever donated the nucleus from which they were produced (see Box 8.11). They might also have two parents in the sense of having two people who, like the parents of adopted children, bring them up. The nearest a clone would get to having only one parent would be if she (and it would have to be a 'she') was the result of a woman's giving birth to her own clone and bringing her up alone. Even in this case the clone would have two biological parents (the parents of the woman who donated the nucleus and gave birth to her).[16]

Box 8.11 Factual information: The biological facts about clones

The difference between a clone and a normal human baby is that the former will only be the *mediate*, not the *immediate*, result of the coming together of a human sperm and egg.

Whilst the donated nucleus will be the result of the coming together of the sperm of the donor's father and the egg of the donor's mother, the clone itself will be the result of SCNT.

This means that the clone will be the identical twin of the nucleus donor, and the biological child of the nucleus donor's parents. The clone will also have mitochondrial genes from the woman in whose womb he or she was nurtured.

Even if we can safely put this argument to one side, there are other worries about the family relationships of a clone. Let's have a look at them.

Clones and families

The influential Cambridge philosopher Onora O'Neill claims that, for a clone, family relationships would be 'confused' (such that several individuals hold the role of one), and 'ambiguous' (such that one individual holds the roles of several).[17] She claims this means no 'responsible' parent would try to achieve a child by cloning.

It is undoubtedly true that clones *would* have confused and ambiguous family relationships on O'Neill's precise (and reasonable) definitions. If the clone's 'father' is also the nucleus-donor, then the clone would be the twin brother of the man he calls 'dad'. The clone would therefore be the 'son' of his brother. His 'grandparents', furthermore will actually be his parents. The woman he calls 'mum' won't be related to him at all except in virtue of having contributed mitochondrial DNA and a womb to gestate him. So the clone could confusedly think of at least two men as 'dad', at least two women as 'mum', and he could think of one man ambiguously as either his dad or his brother, and one woman ambiguously as either his mum or his grandmother.

If it is morally irresponsible to subject children to confused and ambiguous relations, therefore, it would seem morally irresponsible to clone a child.

The claim that it is morally irresponsible to subject children to confused and ambiguous family relationships is presumably based on the fact that children with confused and ambiguous family relationships have not flourished in the past. We need to consider whether this is true, and if so whether this means that it is morally irresponsible to bring into the world children who are likely to have such relationships.

Box 8.12 Activity: Identifying arguments

O'Neill's argument is an inductive argument. Can you identify it and set it out logic-book style.

Answer:
Premise one: Children with confused and ambiguous relationships do not flourish.
Premise two: Clones will have confused and ambiguous family relationships.
Conclusion: Clones will not flourish.

We have seen that premise two is true. If we are to question the conclusion, therefore, we must question the strength of the induction itself, or premise one, the claim from which the conclusion is inductively inferred (see Chapter 5, pages 62–64).

In order properly to evaluate the claim that children subjected to confused and ambiguous relationships do not flourish we would need to examine the empirical evidence. We can't do this here. But we can bring to bear some considerations that may tell for and against the claim.

In the days when mothers regularly died in childbirth, fathers spent years away at war, and either parent was liable to die early from disease, children were often brought up by aunts, uncles, grandparents, siblings and people totally unrelated to them. Many children must have ended up with extremely confused and ambiguous relationships. We usually think of these situations as tragic. Is this because we believe that children in these situations would have had confused and ambiguous family relationships?

Another thought is that now divorce is easier, and single parenthood morally acceptable, we often hear of children growing up in families where different men at different times play the role of 'dad'. If someone marries several times, on the other hand, their children have to get used to having several 'fathers' or 'mothers', half-siblings, step-siblings, several sets of grandparents and so on. Do we think that children will do badly in such situations? If so, is this because we believe they will have confused and ambiguous family relationships?

There are also families where the parents work such long hours that they need to employ others to care for their children. Children can hardly avoid getting confused in such ambiguous situations (is mum this woman or that?). Many people believe it is difficult for children to do well in such circumstances. Some go so far as to suggest that people shouldn't have children unless they look after them themselves. Is this a fear of children being subjected to confused and ambiguous family relationships?

To the extent we think that people who bring up their children in these ways are not doing the right thing by their children, and that this is because they are subjecting their children to confused and ambiguous family relationships, we might want to agree with O'Neill's claim that it would be morally irresponsible to bring into the world any child who will experience such relationships.

On the other hand we might reasonably ask whether children *are* invariably harmed by these situations? The stories of children who were evacuated from London, or indeed the UK, during World War II are not invariably horror stories, indeed some children seemed to have enjoyed themselves (though their parents inevitably suffered).[18] Many children of divorce would claim to have come through the experience relatively unscathed, however sad it made them. And there are now many people

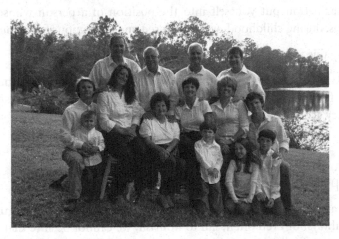

Figure 8.3 An extended family including grandparents, parents, children, siblings, grandchildren, aunts, uncles and cousins. ©iStockphoto.com/TracyHornbrook.

whose parents worked throughout their childhood, who don't seem to have been too damaged by it.

Naturally the empirical evidence would be the clincher here. But the result is not a foregone conclusion.

We might reasonably ask also whether, when children *are* harmed by such situations, they are harmed by the fact they have been exposed to confused and ambiguous relationships or by some other factor such as

(i)   the events and states of affairs that led to their having these relationships;
(ii) the way adults around them handled these events and states of affairs;
(iii) the way adults around them handled their confused and ambiguous relationships.

Naturally the empirical studies into the effect of confused and ambiguous relationships would have to allow for these other possibilities.

These studies would also need to take into account the possibility that there appear to be children who flourish despite the fact they're undoubtedly subjected to confused and ambiguous relationships.

A huge amount of confusion and ambiguity must arise in large and very close families for example. When both grannies and any one of a number of aunts play virtually the same role as mum, who should children think of as mum? All of them? There are also cultures in which extended families are the norm. In these cultures confusion and ambiguity in family relationships must be rife. Yet we have a tendency to think of extended and close families as fitting our moral ideals better than the typical nuclear families of modern Western societies.

It would seem that, pending empirical investigation, there are arguments for and against the claim that children subjected to confused and ambiguous relationships will fail to flourish.

Box 8.13 Activity: Creative writing

In your imagination put yourself into the position of a person whose family relationships, during childhood, were confused and ambiguous for some reason.

Explain why this was the case and how it affected, and affects, you.

In particular you might say or imply whether you believe that the adults responsible for putting you in that situation (if any) were morally irresponsible to act as they acted.

Morally responsible decision-making

So long as we are not sure that children subjected to confused and ambiguous family relationships always, or even often, fail to flourish, we cannot be sure that those who subject children to such relationships are being morally irresponsible. We might, however, want to say that the mere possibility that children will fail to flourish when subjected to confused and ambiguous family relationships means it would be morally irresponsible to put children into situations where they will experience such relation-ships. But would we want to say this?

Making decisions usually means choosing between two or more options. It is not always – or even often – the case that, of the options on offer, it is obvious which is the most morally responsible. Sometimes such decision-making involves choosing between two evils. The parent who is considering leaving a corrosive marriage must weigh the effects of divorce on the children against the effects of the marriage on themselves and on the children.

It is not obvious that the morally responsible choice *wouldn't* be the decision to subject children to the possibility of confused and ambiguous family relationships.

But this decision is not entirely analogous to the position of the person choosing to clone a child. The person making the difficult decision of the last paragraph is considering what to do in respect of a child who already exists. A person considering cloning a child is making a choice between bringing into the world a child who will undoubtedly experience confused and ambiguous family relationships, or not bringing such a child into the world. Such a decision is more analogous to that made by a person who, knowing they want to work full time, decides to have a child in full recognition of the fact that the child's upbringing may not be accepted by everyone as being optimal.

But the fact that not everyone would consider such an upbringing to be optimal, is not usually taken in a democracy as conclusive reason to believe that such an upbring-ing *wouldn't* be optimal. People disagree on such things as how children should be brought up. Even if everyone were to agree, furthermore, that a particular upbringing wouldn't be optimal, this wouldn't usually be taken to mean that the sub-optimality couldn't be mitigated in some way by caring parents. Many parents, for example, bring children into the world full intending to carry on working, in the belief either that working parents do not harm children at all, or that such harm is avoidable.

In the absence of clear empirical evidence for the harmfulness of a certain type of upbringing, it seems clear that this is the sort of decision that people must make for themselves. Just as there are many people who believe that parents who work full time are capable of bringing up a happy and well-adjusted child, so there will be people who believe that the confused and ambiguous family relationships of a clone could be managed so they don't result in an unhappy and badly adjusted child.

This is another point, therefore, at which you must decide for yourself whether or not you believe that the fact that clones will have confused and ambiguous family relationships means that it is morally irresponsible to clone human beings.

> ## Box 8.14 **Activity: Playing devil's advocate**
>
> *It is morally irresponsible to bring into the world a child whose family relationships will be confused and ambiguous.*
>
> Participants should be divided into two groups, one arguing for this claim the other against. If participants find themselves in a group other than that towards which they tend they should treat it as good practice in applying the principle of charity and playing devil's advocate to themselves.

Moral irresponsibility and the law

So far we have found two arguments that suggest reproductive cloning is not morally acceptable:

(i)   the argument that rests on the recognition that the technology is far from perfect;

(ii) the argument that suggests cloning is morally irresponsible because the family relationships of clones will be confused and ambiguous.

The first argument justifies the fact that reproductive cloning is currently illegal almost worldwide. But the question we set ourselves was whether, once the technology has been improved, reproductive cloning would be morally acceptable. The only argument we have currently found to suggest not is the second argument.

This makes it interesting to ask, once the technology has been sorted out, whether cloning might reasonably be legalised?

In democracies we do not usually consider the fact that something is morally irresponsible a good enough reason legally to ban it. Binge drinking might be believed to be morally irresponsible, for example, but we do not ban it. If the state were to involve itself in legislating against morally irresponsible choices it would have to interfere a great deal more in the lives of citizens than most democracies deem sensible. If we were to ban anything that resulted in children experiencing confused and ambiguous relationships, for example, we might have to ban divorce or working parents.

Legally preventing adults from making choices like this would arguably threaten things we value even more than ensuring children experience no confusion or ambiguity. It would threaten the rights of reasonable adults freely to choose the course of their own lives. During our lifetimes many if not all of us make morally irresponsible choices, especially when young. Many of these choices affect us and others adversely. But being legally prevented from making such choices would prevent us from ever making the sort of mistakes from which we might learn. Arguably such a ban would threaten the very freedom that underpins human dignity.

> ### Box 8.15 **Activity: brainstorm**
>
> *It is not good to be morally irresponsible. Therefore being morally irresponsible should be against the law.*
>
> Participants should be asked to brainstorm reactions to this claim.

Slippery slopes

There is a type of argument that we haven't yet examined. This would be a claim to the effect that to allow reproductive cloning in scenarios such as those described in Box 8.9 on page 126 would be the top of a slippery slope.[19] It is easy to see how a slippery slope might start. It would start with allowing couples like Phil and Marti (see Box 8.9) to clone Marti's grandmother, and end up with vigorous, mentally alert, elderly people supplementing their pensions by selling their genomes. Perhaps celebrities would supplement their incomes in the same way? *Hello!* magazine and the like could run special offers. Indeed, why confine ourselves to the living . . . we could grow our own J.S. Bach or Marilyn Monroe. Parents, instead of entering a genetic lottery with their own genes, would be able to choose a nucleus donor for his or her excellent genes.

It might even be that at the bottom of the slope we do not just have avaricious pensioners and celebrities, but also armies of clones, clones grown for spare parts or used as slaves or even the destruction of genetic diversity as everyone rushes to clone Elvis and Beyoncé.

It cannot be denied that to permit cloning could be the start of a slippery slope. Given this might it not be safer to ban reproductive cloning altogether?

A major problem with such an argument is that it could be used against the teaching of science in schools. It might, after all, lead to everyone making their own dirty bomb, to biological warfare between neighbours over their boundary fences or to everyone demanding their own ensuite chemistry lab.

The mere fact that a slippery slope *could* appear does not mean that it is likely. Some people who did science at school *do* make bombs. This does not incline us to ban science teaching because we don't believe it'll happen often. And how likely it is that cloning will become the preferred way of having a baby? Given how easy, cheap and enjoyable it is to make one in the traditional way it seems very unlikely.

The slippery slope argument also relies on a false dichotomy. The choice is not between banning cloning altogether or allowing cloning anywhere and everywhere. Cloning, like many other scientific advances, could clearly be used for evil purposes, and it would therefore seem sensible to regulate it. Such regulation would prevent people producing clones for frivolous or evil purposes, whilst permitting cloning whenever permitting it seems morally acceptable.

Box 8.16 Activity: Debate

This house believes that reproductive cloning, when safe, will be morally acceptable.

Participants might choose their sides freely or be allocated a side on which to argue.

We have considered several arguments against reproductive cloning. One of them – the safety argument – is currently conclusive. But if one day cloning could be made safe enough to try it on human beings this argument will no longer apply.

This is the point at which you must decide whether any of the arguments we have discussed here, or any other arguments you know of, suggest that cloning a human being would still be morally impermissible.

Summary

In this chapter we have:

- acknowledged the fact that human cloning is currently too risky to be morally acceptable;

- reflected on why people might want to produce a human baby by cloning;

- considered whether human clones would have human dignity and free will;

- reflected on whether clones would be nothing more than means to the ends of their 'parents', or such that they wouldn't have open futures;

- considered whether the fact that clones will have confused and ambiguous family relationships makes reproductive cloning morally unacceptable;

- reflected on the possibility of a slippery slope and on the possibility of regulating cloning rather than allowing a free for all.

Questions to stimulate reflection

Do you believe that there are any good reasons to bring human clones into the world?

Do you think that cloning will ever be seen as just another method of assisted reproduction?

Can you think of two reasons why someone might say that clones do not have free will?

Why will clones always have 'confused and ambiguous' family relationships?

Is the fact that clones will always have confused and ambiguous family relationships reason to believe that reproductive cloning should be banned?

Do you think that reproductive cloning will ever be morally acceptable?

To what extent do you think that the media and science fiction have contributed to popular views on cloning?

Additional activities

Access this website and take the quiz on human cloning:
http://investigation.discovery.com/investigation/quiz-central/supernatural/cloning.html.

Read *Never Let Me Go* by Kazuo Ishiguro, then write a short review of it.

Get hold of a DVD of *The Sixth Day* or *The Boys from Brazil* and use it to start a discussion of cloning.

Write a short piece of fiction imagining that you are a clone.

Conduct an opinion poll amongst family and friends on the moral acceptability of human reproductive cloning.

See if you can discover on the web how to go about cloning your pet.

Put 'cloning dinosaurs' into a search engine and see if it would be possible.

Conduct some research into claims that human babies have already been cloned. Use the results to make a presentation.

Notes

1 http://www.bioethics.ac.uk/topics/reproductive-cloning.php. A useful site for learning about reproductive cloning.

2 http://www.independent.co.uk/news/science/now-we-have-the-technology-that-can-make-a-cloned-child-808625.html. A report from the UK's *Independent* newspaper on a new cloning technique.

3 http://news.bbc.co.uk/onthisday/hi/dates/stories/february/22/newsid_4245000/4245877. stm. The BBC's report on the birth of Dolly (includes a video on how Dolly was cloned).

4 http://www.roslin.ac.uk/. The website for the Roslin Institute.

5 http://learn.genetics.utah.edu/content/tech/cloning/cloningrisks/. An article on why cloning is so risky for the clone.

6 http://news.bbc.co.uk/cbbcnews/hi/sci_tech/newsid_2764000/2764771.stm. A BBC *Newsround* announcement of Dolly's death.

7 http://www.starwars.com/databank/organization/clonetroopers/. An account of the 'Clone Troopers' from Star Wars.

8 http://www.leaderu.com/ftissues/ft9706/articles/meilaender.html. Meilaender, G., 'Begetting and Cloning' Remarks presented to the National Bioethics Advisory Commission, 13 March 1997.

9 Example taken from: http://www.fallacyfiles.org/equivoqu.html.

10 Putnam, H. (1999) Cloning People. *Genetics and Human Diversity*, ed. Justine Burley. Oxford: Oxford University Press, pp. 1–13. http://www.timeshighereducation.co.uk/story.asp?storyCode=105708&sectioncode=26. An article on human cloning from the *Times Higher Education Supplement*.

11 http://www.philosophytalk.org/pastShows/GeneticDeterminism.htm. Information on genetic determinism from PhilosophyTalk.

12 http://www.philosophytalk.org/pastShows/GeneticDeterminism.htm.

13 Ian Wilmut has been changing his views on cloning. Here is an interview with him published by *Scientific American* in 2008: http://www.scientificamerican.com/article.cfm?id=theraputic-cloning-discussion-ian-wilmut.

14 http://www.bionews.org.uk/page_37800.asp. A short article by philosopher Julian Savulescu on 'Clonism'.

15 National Bioethics Advisory Commission (1999), *Ethical Issues in Human Stem Cell Research*. Rockville, MD, p. 61.

16 Some biotechnologies would enable a person to have *three* parents. See http://www.telegraph.co.uk/science/science-news/3324321/Transplant-creates-embryos-with-three-parents.html.

17 O'Neill, O. (2002) *Autonomy and Trust in Bioethics*. Cambridge: Cambridge University Press.

18 http://www.bbc.co.uk/history/british/britain_wwtwo/evacuees_01.shtml. Stories of evacuees during World War II.

19 http://www.fallacyfiles.org/slipslop.html. An account of slippery slope arguments from the Fallacy Files.

Further reading and useful websites

Aldridge, S. (2010) *Cloning (21st Century Science)*. Tunbridge Wells, UK: TickTock Books.

Brimah, J. (2010) *The Ethics of Human Cloning: A Critical Analysis*. Saarbrücken, Germany: Lap Lambert Academic Publishing.

Wilmut, I. and Highfield, S. (2006) *After Dolly: The Uses and Misuses of Human Cloning*. New York: Little, Brown and Co.

http://bioethicsbytes.wordpress.com/2006/07/24/therapeutic-cloning-the-island/.

http://powayusd.sdcoe.k12.ca.us/projects/dolly/. A number of activities on human cloning from the 'Hello Dolly' section of the US WebQuest site.

http://science.howstuffworks.com/environmental/life/genetic/human-cloning.htm. From the 'HowStuffWorks website: how human cloning will work.

http://www.time.com/time/archive/collections/0,21428,c_cloning,00.shtml. The *Time* Magazine archive of articles on cloning.

Section 2
Reproduction

9 | Reproductive freedom: rights, responsibilities and choice

Objectives

In reading this chapter you will:

- learn about the different techniques of assisted reproduction;
- distinguish legal from moral rights;
- reflect on the 'right' to found a family;
- distinguish positive and negative duties;
- reflect on the hard financial and moral decisions governments must make;
- reflect on the differences between adoption and assisted reproductive technology (ART);
- reflect on the fairness of 'postcode' lotteries.

One of the major motivations of biotechnology has been the desire to learn how to help the sub-fertile have children. Over the 30-odd years since the birth of Louise Brown, the world's first test tube baby, huge strides have been made in the technology of assisted reproduction (ART). Many couples, thanks to biotechnology, have been able to have a family they wouldn't otherwise have had.

Box 9.1 Factual information: Technologies of assisted reproduction[1]

Artificial insemination: fertile sperm is inserted into the neck of the uterus. This permits couples to reproduce when fertilisation is not possible thanks to defective sperm. Men about to undergo fertility threatening treatment such as chemotherapy can bank their own sperm for later use.

In vitro fertilisation (IVF): a woman is treated with drugs to stimulate ovulation. Eggs are then collected and mixed with sperm in a Petri dish. Once fertilised one or more of the eggs is transferred to the uterus.

Gamete intrafallopian transfer: gametes are mixed in a Petri dish then transferred to the fallopian tubes for fertilisation to take place.

Zygote intrafallopian transfer: eggs and sperm are mixed in a Petri dish and in the hope that fertilisation has taken place, the supposed zygote is transferred to the fallopian tube.

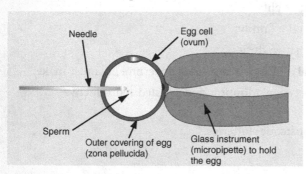

In vitro maturation (IVM): used for women who cannot take the drugs used to stimulate ovulation in IVF, IVM involves taking immature eggs and allowing them to mature in vitro before being fertilised and implanted in the uterus.

Intracytoplasmic sperm injection: used when sperm are poor, a single sperm is selected for its good quality and injected straight into the egg (see Figure 9.1).

Figure 9.1 The intracytoplasmic sperm injection technique, where a sperm is placed directly into the egg.

But our being able to help the sub-fertile have their own biological children brings many moral problems in its wake. Because it is widely (though not universally[2]) accepted that in itself assisted reproductive technology (ART) (at least in the forms described in Box 9.1) is morally permissible, many of these problems face governments rather than individuals. Once a technology is widely regarded as morally acceptable, then the moral focus shifts from the technology itself to the question of how it can be put to use and funded in such a way as to promote welfare, to be fair to everyone, and respect everyone's rights (see Chapter 3).

If ART were cheap there wouldn't be a problem. Anyone needing ART could fund their own treatment and the infertile could found families on very much the same sort of basis as the fertile always have: as and when they want to and feel they can afford it.

But ART is very costly.[3] If it had to be paid for by individuals only the rich or those prepared to cripple themselves financially for the sake of a baby would be able to afford it. Inevitably state funding is going to be needed. But given that the public purse is not bottomless this means hard decisions must be made. In this chapter we shall consider some of the questions triggered by reproductive technology and how they might be answered.

Box 9.2 Activity: Thought experiment

Many women around the age of 30 start to feel under pressure to find a partner quickly in order to reproduce.

Men, however, can reproduce naturally until late in their lives (although not necessarily without risk[4]).

The technology is now available, however, to freeze eggs so they can be used many years later to produce an embryo.[5]

If the government were to pay for all baby girls to have their eggs harvested at birth, then stored until they are needed, this would remove this inequality between men and women, enabling women too to have children at any age (so long as they had or could secure a hospitable womb).

In the light of the moral theories discussed in Chapter 4 decide whether this would be morally acceptable, and in particular whether governments should fund this service.[6]

There are also moral problems to do with the protection of people's rights versus the promotion of others' welfare. For example, should the state prevent people from using ART if it is feared they would not care properly for any resulting child? What is the state to do when the rights of different people clash in pursuit of their reproductive hopes (see Box 9.3)?

Box 9.3 Case study: Natallie Evans

In 2001 Natallie Evan was diagnosed with ovarian cancer. Her treatment involved removing her ovaries, rendering her infertile.

Natallie had always known that she wanted children. Before her treatment therefore she and her then partner, Howard Johnson, went through IVF and produced six embryos which were frozen for later use.

Natallie and Howard then split up. The six frozen embryos were Natallie's only chance of having her own children. But Howard no longer wanted to have children with Natallie and he withdrew his consent.

For 5 years Natallie took her case through every court open to her. But eventually the Grand Jury of the European Court decided that Natallie's right to found a family could not over-ride Howard's right to withhold consent. The embryos were not taken to have any independent right to life.

In April 2007 the six embryos were destroyed.[7]

These are difficult problems. Let's start thinking about them by considering the extent to which people have a *right* to found a family.

Moral and legal rights

In 1948 the United Nations Universal Declaration of Human Rights[8] laid down, in article 16, that 'men and women of full age, without limits due to race, nationality or religion, have the right to found a family'.[9]

At that time infertile people wanting a family had little option but to adopt. But people are allowed to adopt a child only if they can prove their ability to give that child a decent childhood. Nowadays the infertile can found a family by using ART. But the techniques of ART are far from perfect: most give only a 20–25% chance of pregnancy.[10] Many who embark on IVF are disappointed. The right to found a family does not entail, therefore, the *ability* to found a family.

You might think that this makes the notion of 'right' meaningless? What's the point of a right to something if it doesn't guarantee the ability to secure that something? The philosopher Jeremy Bentham[11] argued that the idea of *moral* rights is 'nonsense on stilts', they are, he said, nothing more than rights we believe we *ought* to have. David Hume (another philosopher) taught us that an 'ought' does not entail an 'is', or vice versa: even if we *ought* to have the right to found a family, therefore, this doesn't mean we *do* have this right.

Box 9.4 Philosophical background: 'Ought' and 'is'

The Scottish philosopher David Hume argued that a major source of error in moral thinking is a tendency to go from the claim something *is* the case to the claim that something *ought* to be the case.[12]

In Chapter 6 we discussed the argument 'it's not natural'. We saw there that we cannot go from the fact that something is the case to the claim that it ought to be the case (or vice versa).

This argument has been understood by many to show that facts and values are distinct and that factual judgements and value judgements are quite different.

Many philosophers now reject the claim that facts and values are distinct (because there are facts about values). But judgements of value-facts (of what *ought* to be the case) are different from judgements of non-value facts (of what *is* the case).

Even Bentham, however, believed in legal rights. These, he argued, are embedded in legal systems which make them real. Your legal right to found a family gives the state a *duty* towards you insofar as it recognises that right. John Stuart Mill (see Chapter 4, Box 4.7) would have accepted that rights entail duties, but he believed in both moral and legal rights. He argued that legal rights can be justified only on the basis of moral rights.

Most people believe there can be unfair laws, for example, but if legal rights exhaust the notion of rights, how can we have a right to anything – fair treatment for example – that is not given by the law? Conversely, we sometimes think something so unjust there should be a law against it. But again, how can we have the right to be treated justly independently of the way the law treats us if legal rights exhaust the rights there are? If this debate interests you, you might like to (re-)read the comparison of the 'moral law' and the 'law of the land' in Chapter 3, pp. 26–28.

> ### Box 9.5 Activity: Reflection and revision
>
> Are you with Bentham or Mill? Do moral rights exist? Or do legal rights exhaust the rights we have? If the former what sense can be made of a right that can't be satisfied? If the latter how to explain unjust laws, laws that *should* exist but don't?
>
> Re-read the section on utilitarianism to remind yourself why utilitarians have problems with rights.

Whatever the truth about moral rights any government recognising the UN Declaration of Human Rights confers *legal* rights on those within its jurisdiction, and a duty on itself to recognise these rights in law.

Negative and positive duties

State recognition of the right to found a family confers on the state a duty towards its citizens or subjects.[13] But is this a *negative* duty not to *prevent* adults from founding a family? Or is it a *positive* duty to *help* them found a family? Or is it both? To what extent, furthermore, are these duties entirely general (duties towards everyone), or specific (only towards particular kinds of people)?

Negative duties

Notoriously governments have been known to try to prevent adults from having children. The Nazis, for example, forcibly sterilised Jews, gypsies, homosexuals and communists.[14] Until the 1960s Sweden forcibly sterilised 60,000 people with low IQ.[15] In China people can still be forcibly sterilised if they have more than the one child allowed them by government policy.[16] It is the belief that forcible sterilisation is wrong that led to the UN Declaration of Human Rights.

This suggests that we should interpret recognition of the right to found a family as conferring on governments at least a negative duty not to *prevent* people from having children. Those who talk of 'reproductive freedom' usually mean *at least* this: that everyone should be free to have a child if that is what they want to do (and also free *not* to have a child if that is their choice: forcible child-bearing is also considered morally abhorrent).[17]

Reproductive freedom

But this immediately generates a problem. There are some people, perhaps, who *ought* to be prevented from having a child. Can a person with a very low IQ give a child a decent childhood? Should a woman of 65 be permitted to have a baby?[18] Does a drug addict or an alcoholic have the right to a child, or a woman with HIV? Do lesbians and gay men have the right to have a child? Many have thought not. In fact they have thought that given a child's right to a decent childhood, there can't be any such thing as the *right* to have a child, moral or legal. Others accept a prima facie and entirely general right to have a child, but argue that this right is negated in some cases by the right a child has to a decent childhood.

> ### Box 9.6 Activity: Test your intuitions
>
> Consider the case studies below and decide whether all these people have the right to a child.
>
> 1. Minal is 30. She has a thriving, well-paid career and wants a partner only to provide sperm. She has a brother of 32 who would play a fatherly role (not as sperm donor!).
> 2. Jane is an alcoholic. Her boyfriend, Roberto, is a drug addict. They believe that having a child would help them get clean.
> 3. Stephanie and her husband are in prison convicted of murder. By the time they get out she may be too old to have children. Conjugal visits are not allowed so they would need ART.
> 4. John (32) and David (26) are a gay couple who would like to have a child by ART and surrogacy. John is HIV positive, though he is currently fit and healthy.
> 5. Mary (65) always wanted children, but she only met the right man a year ago. Dan (69) hasn't had children either. Mary and Dan are fit, healthy and well-educated. They would be happy to adopt, but would like a child under 5 years.
> 6. Pam is a healthy 55 year old. Unexpectedly she and her husband (60) recently found themselves desperately wanting a child. They are not interested in adoption, only ART.
> 7. Ruth is a carrier of Duchenne muscular dystrophy. Any child of hers has a 50% chance of inheriting the disease. Ruth is rich enough to provide excellent child-care even for a severely disabled child.

But if the rights of a child can 'trump' the rights of a potential parent in this way, or if there isn't an entirely general right to a child,[19] then the government can't have a *general* duty not to prevent people from founding families. On the contrary, perhaps governments have a duty actively to prevent certain people from having children?

There are two big problems for the state in deciding either that it should not recognise the right to found a family, or that its recognition of this right is consistent with its taking active steps to prevent some people from exercising this right. These are:

(i)   who decides which adults should be prevented from founding a family?

(ii) how is the government to prevent fertile people from having children or rich people from getting fertility treatment?

Deciding who should be prevented from having children

These problems are worse for democratic governments because consensus on who couldn't or wouldn't give a child a decent childhood is unlikely. For every person who believes that a gay man, an older woman or a drug addict shouldn't have a baby, for example, there's bound to be someone else who insists that sexuality and age are irrelevant and that drug addicts shouldn't be penalised for what is in effect an illness. Whatever decision the government makes there'd be dissent. For a democratic government, whose very existence depends on the approval of the people, dissent is difficult.

It would be difficult, furthermore, not to think of this dissent as justified, at least in many individual cases. Governments, after all, cannot make judgements about individual cases. Instead they have to pass laws preventing certain *categories* of people from founding families.

For example, no government could prevent just Mary and Dan (see Box 9.6) from founding a family without preventing everyone over a certain age from founding a family. But what age should this be? Should it be 70? 65? Or should we play safe and make it 60, or even 55?

But is it really the case that *no* 60-year-old woman could give a child a good childhood? How would we explain the fact that grandparents often successfully rear children? How would we deal with men who have children over 60? Given that laws are blunt instruments it would be impossible to avoid injustice altogether.

It would seem that there are both moral *and* practical reasons why governments, especially democratic governments, would want to shy away from passing laws preventing certain people from having children.

Box 9.7 Activity: Role play

In 2006 Maria del Carmen Bousada de Lara, a single Spanish woman of 66, gave birth to twin sons after IVF. Two years later she died of cancer leaving Pau and Christian orphans.[20]

This has prompted much debate. Imagine that as a result of this debate your government has decided they should consider imposing an age limit on fertility treatment. To this end it has appointed a committee of the 'great and the good', otherwise known as 'the virtuous' to advise them.

Half the class will play the part of that committee. Members of this group should be appointed to play the following roles:

Chairperson: This person's job is to chair committee meetings, keep members to the agenda, make sure the committee stick to their remit and to present the final report.

Note-taker: This person's job is to keep the minutes of the meeting(s), and to produce a report of the meeting.

The other half of the class should be asked to act as witnesses called up before the committee to make arguments for or against imposing an age limit on fertility treatment. These members should represent the following organisations:

- Faith groups
- Children's rights organisations
- Organisations concerned with the rights of the aged
- Civil liberties organisations
- The social services
- The treasury

The class should be given time to conduct some research and prepare their arguments, then a meeting of the committee should be held. Witnesses should be called one by one until all have been heard. The debate should then be opened to the committee.

Preventing people from having children

Then we come to the second difficulty: it would be easy for the government to prevent certain types of people having a child if these people were both infertile and poor: they would simply refuse to fund fertility treatment. But this wouldn't prevent wealthy infertile people in these categories using ART to have children. Even if the government were to ban people from having fertility treatment, such people could simply travel abroad for treatment. Must the government ban this too? Would it be acceptable, though, for a government, especially a democratic government, to stop people travelling abroad?[21]

And how would the government stop childbearing in the naturally fertile? Would the government find itself forcibly sterilising Minal or Ruth (see Box 9.6) or locking them up? Such actions are even less in the spirit of the liberal zeitgeist than banning people from travelling abroad.

Box 9.8 **Factual information: The welfare of the child in the UK**

The Human Fertilisation and Embryology Act passed in Britain in 1990 stated that before fertility treatment could be provided doctors must 'take account of the welfare of the child who may be born as a result of that treatment, including the need of that child for a father'. Many clinics interpreted this as intending to bar single women from fertility treatment.

This clause of the Act was unpopular because:

- it discriminated against the infertile because only those needing fertility treatment were prevented from having a child without a partner;

- it forced doctors into the role of making decisions about patients' suitability to become parents;
- implementing this clause took time and effort, adding to the already exorbitant costs of ART;
- there was little evidence that it protected children (the British Fertility Society estimated it prevented about 10 births a year);
- it greatly added to the pain of a diagnosis of infertility.

In 2008 the law was reviewed and the 'good parenting test' revoked. Clinics must still take into account the welfare of the child, but they needn't consider the 'need for a father'.[22]

Acts can be against the liberal zeitgeist without being wrong, but the huge practical and moral difficulties associated with making and implementing laws of this kind are almost certainly behind the decision, of most western governments, both to recognise the right to have a child, and to interpret that right as conferring on them an entirely general negative duty, a duty not to prevent *anyone* from founding a family, even in the face of strong intuitions to the effect that some people shouldn't have children.

Adoption and rights

But we might still insist that there is a precedent for preventing some people from founding a family on the grounds that they will not care properly for that family. No decent government, after all, would allow a child to be adopted by people who wouldn't care properly for that child.[23] Why then, should a government be prepared to allow a child to be born to those who might not care for it?

There is an important disanalogy, however, between adopting a child and having a child naturally or by means of ART. A child up for adoption already *exists* and has rights in its own person. The rights of this child to a decent childhood, furthermore, have already been compromised: it wouldn't be up for adoption unless it had undergone some trauma leading to separation from its parent(s). To allow such a child to be adopted by an adult incapable of giving it a decent childhood would constitute a further violation of its rights.

In the case of someone who isn't yet pregnant, there is no child whose rights must be taken into account. The only rights in this case are the rights of the adult. There can be no weighing of the rights of a child against the rights of an adult, because there is no child whose rights can be put in the balance. We have excellent reasons for withholding rights from *possible* or *potential* people as we saw when we considered therapeutic cloning in Chapter 7 (see Box 7.15).

The fact that governments are morally required to prevent certain people from adopting, therefore, does not mean that they are morally required to prevent certain people from having their own child.

But if a state sees itself as having a duty not to prevent *anyone* from having a child then what about the rights of children to a decent childhood? Are we really saying these don't matter, or that they don't matter as much as an adult's rights to found a family?

However unfair this might seem there are three good reasons to say this:

1. There are good reasons not to accord rights to people who don't (yet) exist. Imagine having duties to all the children you might have had but didn't.
2. Offered the choice of not being born at all, and of taking one's chances on the likelihood of a decent childhood, most people would choose the latter. Can we wrong a child by allowing it to be born?
3. The right of a child to a decent childhood can always be secured after birth (once the child actually exists) by forcibly removing it from its parents.[24] By such means the rights of the parents *and* of the child can be recognised.

Box 9.9 Activity: Group discussion

No-one has the right to a child. Governments should intervene to stop children being born into families that can't or won't care for them.

Participants should be divided into two groups. One group should argue for this claim, the other against.

The group arguing against this claim might consider:

- the emotional cost to the child of being brought up badly;
- the extreme difficulty of protecting a child from its parents;
- the likelihood of the cost being passed onto the child's children;
- the cost (financial and emotional) to society of children born to dysfunctional families.

The group arguing for this claim might consider:

- the inevitable injustices of making it illegal for anyone in a whole category of people to have a child;
- the practical and moral difficulties of actively preventing fertile people from having children;
- the practical and moral difficulties of actively preventing people from travelling abroad for fertility treatment;
- the social disruption of passing laws that many would find abhorrent.

In marshalling their arguments, both groups should see if they can classify these arguments as arguments from virtue, from deontology or from utility.

For all sorts of reasons, therefore, democratic governments are likely not only to recognise the right to have children, but also to interpret this in terms of an entirely general duty not to prevent any adult from at least trying to have children, however unsuitable that adult would be as a parent.

Positive duties

But is this where the government's duty stops? Or do governments who sign up to this right also have a *positive* duty – a duty actively to *help* people have children? Such a positive duty could range from little more than adding folic acid to bread[25] to offering substantial funding for IVF and/or adoption services.

Some governments, of course, lack the resources to do anything positive to help people have a family. If a government must choose between feeding and protecting its people and giving them access to ART, morality probably requires it to do the former. This might again cause us to question the notion of a right. Must poor governments refuse to recognise the right to found a family? Or must we instead refuse to interpret this right as conferring a positive duty so we can allow for states who can't afford to help people have children?

We could, instead, simply refuse to see rights as absolute. We have already suggested this, in fact, in suggesting that a child's right to a decent childhood might 'trump' an adult's right to found a family. The possibility of 'trumping' enables us to interpret the right to found a family as conferring on governments a duty to make helping people to found a family a *goal*, to be achieved when resources permit.[26] Until the government can afford to feed, educate and protect its people, in other words, it need only see their right to found a family as conferring on it a negative duty.

This suggests we should see a government's positive duties in relation to the rights it recognises as essentially related to its resources. As a nation becomes richer, the government's positive obligations to its people increase. The question we need to address, therefore, is: do *wealthy* countries have a positive duty to help adults found families?

Box 9.10 **Philosophical background: moral versus legal rights revisited**

It is only legal rights that must be seen as relative to resources. Moral rights (if they exist) are absolute. *All* adults have the *moral* right to found a family, perhaps, but their *legal* right to do so will be relative to:

(i)   their government's recognising that right, and
(ii) their government's having the resources to help achieve it (to whatever extent).

Infertility as disease or disability

It has been suggested that infertility is a disease or a disability, and that as governments have a positive duty to provide healthcare, they also have a positive duty to provide infertility treatment. This argument suggests an argument for seeing governments as having a positive duty to help the infertile that does not depend on a government's recognition of the right to found a family. It depends instead on its recognition of a duty to provide healthcare.

This argument seems to be a good one, at least to the extent that its conclusion follows from its premises. But it is not obvious that its premises are true. The question of whether fertility is a disease or a disability depends, for example, on what we count as a disease or a disability. Even if governments have a positive duty to provide healthcare, furthermore, it is not clear they have a positive duty (or the ability) to mitigate all the effects of every disease or disability. As we shall be discussing the nature of disease and disability in Chapter 10 we shan't pursue this argument here.

> ### Box 9.11 Activity: Analysing arguments
>
> There is a deductively valid argument from the claim that infertility is a disease or disability to the claim that governments have a duty to provide fertility treatment. Can you identify this argument and set it out logic-book style?
>
> You might then like to read pages 191–194 from Chapter 11. This will enable you properly to evaluate this argument and decide whether the government has a positive duty to provide ART for the sub-fertile.
>
> Answer: The argument set out logic-book style would go:
>   Premise one: Infertility is a disease or disability.
>   Premise two: Governments have a duty to cure or mitigate the effects of disease and disabilities wherever possible.
>   Premise three: The provision of ART would mitigate the effects of infertility.
>   Conclusion: Governments have a duty to provide ART to the infertile.

Financial realities and social justice

Clearly even the wealthiest government can't make an open-ended commitment to helping people found families. ART is extremely costly: a straightforward IVF procedure costs a minimum of £3,000[27] for a single cycle and has only a 20–30% chance of success (for women under 35).[28] As new technologies are introduced, and expectations rise, costs will also rise. Countries could spend their whole GDP on fertility treatment.

Positive duties have limits, it seems, even for the wealthiest governments. Even if the right to found a family confers on governments a positive duty actively to help people found a family, therefore, this right still cannot be seen as a guarantee of the ability to found a family. No government could possibly afford financially to underpin such a guarantee. It is simply not possible for governments to avoid making hard *financial* decisions in the case of positive duties, even if they can avoid making hard *moral* decisions in the case of negative duties.

Given this, governments, even wealthy ones, could always argue that improving health and/or education or safeguarding life are more important than founding families. This could justify even the wealthiest government in refusing to allocate resources to help the sub-fertile found a family.

But in making such a decision the government must, of course, bear in mind its duty to treat people fairly. The consequences of its making *this* decision would impact far more heavily on the poor infertile than it would on anyone else. It would mean, for example, that the infertile rich would be able to fund a family, but the infertile poor wouldn't. Many people would perceive this as unfair. At the very least governments would have to take this perception into account in deciding whether or not to allocate resources for the funding of ART.

> ### Box 9.12 **Activity: Group discussion**
>
> Every government has a duty to help the poor feed and educate themselves and their children. But no government can alleviate all poverty. Helping the poor fund ART will result in the production of even more people to feed and educate.
>
> Is refusing to fund ART on these grounds:
> - an indication of the government's sensible attitude to the allocation of scarce resources?
> - an indication of the government's failure to recognise how important it is for everyone to be able to choose to have a child?

Funding ART

If a government decides it will allocate resources to funding ART it must then decide on the extent to which it will allocate resources to this end, and how they should be allocated. It is not necessarily the case, for example, that the government will use its own money – or rather the money given to it by tax payers – directly to help those in need. The modern state has many levers and instruments by which it can manipulate the resources owned by, for example, charities and privately owned companies. It also has many different ways in which it can use tax payers' money.

The government could choose directly to help its own employees *because* they are employees. It might encourage other employers to do the same by offering tax incentives (the money used by a business to fund ART for employees would be set against their tax bill). Or it might encourage donations to charities that help the infertile by offering tax incentives on such donations (so money you give to a charity for this end would be set against your tax bill). In such ways governments would be helping the subfertile poor have children, but without their own costs spiralling out of hand.

In using tax payers' money itself to fund ART, on the other hand, the state might choose to help the infertile poor on a means-tested basis: so only those on an income of less than a certain amount would be helped to fund fertility treatment or adoption. Given the administrative costs of means testing, however, it might be cheaper to guarantee a basic level of access to adoption or fertility treatment to everyone, even those who *could* pay for it themselves. This might also be deemed fairer given the huge cost of ART, and the importance to most people of having a child.

Different governments have made different decisions on whether, how and the extent to which they are prepared to allocate resources to the funding of ART in their attempts to fulfil their positive duty to help people found families.

> ### Box 9.13 **Activity: Small group discussion**
>
> *Does a wealthy government have a positive duty to help infertile people found a family?*

Participants should be divided into four groups. Each should be allocated one of the following four positions on what the government should do:

(i)   insist there are more important calls on its resources than helping the infertile have children;
(ii) provide help to its own employees, and encourage other employers and charities to do likewise by providing incentives through taxation;
(iii) provide a minimal level of help to everyone below a certain income;
(iv) provide a minimal level of help to everyone.

Participants might be expected to conduct research to support their positions (for example, those in the first group might research government expenditure).

The discussion might end with the class brainstorming ways in which governments might recognise the positive duty to help citizens found a family without breaking the bank.

In trying to solve the hard financial problems posed by the right to found a family, however, a familiar moral problem rears its head: if, for financial reasons, a government can't offer help to everyone, shouldn't it start by refusing help to those whose ability to give a child a decent childhood is in doubt?

We should note that the decision *not to help* certain types of people have children is not the same as deciding actively to *prevent* certain types of people from having children. A government's refusing financial help for ART to those believed to be unable to care properly for a child would not involve it in having forcibly to prevent anyone travelling abroad, or in it having forcibly to sterilise someone. It would merely involve it in refusing to pay for fertility treatment. Many people have thought that *omissions* (decisions *not* to act) are less morally culpable than acts themselves. We shall be discussing this in Chapter 13, see also Box 4.6 in Chapter 4.

Box 9.14 Activity: Essay writing

The argument above suggests that it might be morally acceptable to refuse funding for ART to a drug addict, yet not morally acceptable actively to prevent a drug addict having ART.

Reflect on the extent to which this distinction relies on the act–omission distinction then consider, in 1,500 words or less, how a utilitarian might respond to this.

It would still be the case, however, that someone would have to decide which groups are such that they should be refused fertility treatment. We saw above that such decisions are almost certain to be highly controversial, and also that if the government makes it illegal for certain groups to have children, injustices will almost certainly result.

But there is a way for the government to opt out of making such difficult moral decisions: it can devolve such decision-making to others. By such means it can absolve itself of any of the blame attached to the decisions made.

The government can do this either by allowing such decisions to be made by the private organisations or charities who get tax incentives to help the infertile, or by allocating budgets to lower rungs of the governmental ladder and asking those on the lower rungs to make the decisions. On the assumption that different organisations, charities and governmental bodies would make different decisions, the overall effect would not be the same as an entirely general ban on certain types of people having children. In principle this would permit an older woman who wouldn't be funded for fertility treatment by one organisation or in one region, to approach another in the hope that she might get treatment there.

Consistent with devolving the actual decision to others, the government can issue guidelines *suggesting* that certain groups be considered ineligible for funding, but without itself *stating* that such groups should be considered ineligible.

If a government devolves onto other bodies the responsibility for making decisions regarding who should and who shouldn't be eligible for funding, it avoids having to make the decision itself. But other problems will inevitably arise. For example:

- Choices might be made that some believe to be arbitrary or old-fashioned;
  If, for example, the government asks general practitioners to make such decisions some doctors might require that couples be married, or that their household income be over a certain amount.
- choices might be made that sit uncomfortably with the law of the land;
  If the Roman Catholic Church were responsible for such decisions, they might decide that gay or lesbian couples should not receive funding. Would this be permissible in a country that legally bans discrimination on the grounds of sexuality?[29]
- local government bodies might make different decisions about who to fund and on which criteria
  This will result in postcode lotteries (see Box 9.15),[30] where a couple on one street are funded, but a similar couple on the next street are not.

Box 9.15 Factual information: Postcode lotteries in the UK

In Britain the government recommends that the National Health Service (NHS) fund three full cycles of IVF for infertile couples where the woman is between 23 and 39.

The NHS, however, is funded in such a way that decisions about actual expenditure are made by the regional 'Primary Care Trusts' (PCT). PCTs are required to use their budget to fund any treatment that the government actually requires, but treatments that are merely 'recommended' often go unfunded. Recent research[31] showed that eight out of ten PCTs were failing to implement the government guidelines on fertility treatment. The recent spending cuts are likely to make it even harder to get funding.

This means that whether or not you get infertility treatment, and the amount you get, often depends on your *postcode*, on where you live (and which regional PCT is responsible for your healthcare).

Many PCTs also set their own criteria for fertility treatment, ignoring the criteria suggested by the government. Some PCTs will not treat couples if one of them already has a child. Half of PCTs require couples to have been in a relationship for at least 3 years. Some PCTs refuse to treat smokers, others the obese and some set age limits for male partners. Many PCTs will only treat women between 34 and 37. One will only treat women between 37 and 39. In 2013 PCTs are to be abolished and replaced by consortia of general practitioners. You might like to consider whether this will alleviate or exacerbate the problem of postcode lotteries.

It seems that no government will avoid having to face difficult moral and legal issues. Reflection on these arguments demonstrates the difficulties that governments have in fulfilling the remit discussed in Chapter 3: balancing public welfare, individual rights and justice between individuals.

Box 9.16 Activity: Group discussion

After the concept of 'postcode lottery' is explained, participants should be divided into groups of four and asked to discuss the following as preparation for a whole group discussion:

Postcode lotteries are unfair. The government should make a decision about the fertility treatment people should receive and require Primary Care Trusts or their successor bodies to implement that decision.

Questions to consider whilst preparing:

Why do you think the government merely 'recommends' three full cycles of IVF rather than requiring them?

Why do you think PCTs do not act on the government's recommendation, and why do they impose their own criteria for fertility treatment?

The PCTs and the government must know that postcode lotteries are perceived by the public to be unfair. Why do they not abolish them?

The government could abolish postcode lotteries by requiring PCTs to fund infertility treatment. What disadvantages might ensue from this?

What would you say to someone who says 'at least if different PCTs have different criteria, one can move'?

The interaction of practical, financial, administrative and moral decisions, together with the fact that it is very rarely the case that there will be consensus on any important issue, can make such decision-making a tight-rope-walking nightmare for any government.

Summary

In this chapter we have:

- reflected on the idea that there is a 'right' to found a family, and on whether this is a moral right as well as a legal one;

- considered whether the rights of a child to a decent childhood should trump the rights of adults to found families;

- seen that governments could interpret the right to found a family as conferring a negative or a positive duty, or both;

- seen that unless the government interprets this as conferring an entirely general negative duty, they will have to decide who should be prevented from having children, and actively take steps to prevent such people having children;

- seen that if governments do pass laws preventing certain types of people from having children, such laws are unlikely to command universal assent, and will inevitably lead to injustices;

- seen that if governments interpret this as conferring a positive right, hard financial decisions will have to be made unless the whole GDP is to be spent on fertility treatment;

- noted a disanalogy between the right to found a family by adoption and the right to found a family naturally or by means of ART;

- considered various different levers and instruments by which governments might discharge their positive duties to help people found families, consistently with the fact that its own resources are finite;

- considered whether in allocating resources for fertility treatment, it might be morally acceptable for a government to prevent certain people from having children by refusing to fund fertility treatment (by omission rather than commission).

Questions to stimulate reflection

Do you think that everyone has the right to found a family? If so, does this confer negative or positive duties (or both) on governments?

If you don't think everyone has a right to found a family, who do you think should be prevented from having children? How would you prevent fertile people in these categories from having children? How would you prevent rich infertile people in these categories travelling abroad for ART?

Do you think that there are moral as well as legal rights?

Governments do prevent certain people from adopting children. Is there a moral difference between this and preventing such people from having their own child?

Should governments help women over 60 have children? If not, isn't this unfair given that men over 60 can have children?

Given that governments could spend the whole GDP on fertility treatment how should governments allocate funding for this purpose?

Can you list the different ways in which governments might allow for the right of a child to a decent childhood consistently with recognising adults' rights to found a family?

People often say they think 'postcode lotteries' are unfair. Imagine playing devil's advocate and say how you would argue against this.

Additional activities

Write a short piece as if from the perspective of an infertile couple about the desire for a baby.

Conduct some research into infertility, its prevalence, its impact and its remedies.

Conduct an informal poll amongst your family and friends about their views on whether people should have the right to have children.

Having conducted such a poll classify people's responses according to the three moral theories discussed in Chapter 4.

Find out if you have a local IVF clinic. If so ask them what criteria they impose on prospective parents.

Access this website for a US-related quiz on reproductive rights: http://www.ipas.org/Publications/asset_upload_file642_3785.pdf.

Access this website for an interactive game on human rights: http://www.equalityhumanrights.com/wales/projects/dignity-drive/take-a-virtual-walk-down-dignity-drive/.

Access the BEEP website (see below) for further activities.

Notes

1 http://www.ehealthmd.com/library/infertility/INF_assisted.html. eHealthMD in the US: a useful summary of forms of ART.
2 Many Roman Catholics reject ART.
3 http://www.ivfcost.net/. A website comparing the cost of IVF internationally.
4 http://www.mothers35plus.co.uk/older-fathers.htm. An article on late fatherhood from the Mothers 35+ website.
5 http://www.dailymail.co.uk/health/article-28750/The-facts-egg-freezing.html. The facts about egg freezing from Mailonline.
6 http://www.bbc.co.uk/news/10419076. A BBC report on women freezing eggs to extend their fertility.

7 http://news.bbc.co.uk/1/hi/health/6530295.stm. A BBC report on Natallie Evans' final appeal.

8 http://www.un.org/en/documents/udhr/index.shtml. The Universal Declaration of Human Rights.

9 http://www.open2.net/ethicsbites/right-have-babies.html. Transcript of an interview with Baroness Mary Warnock about the right to have a baby.

10 http://www.hfea.gov.uk/fertility-clinics-success-rates.html. The HFEA on IVF success rates.

11 http://www.iep.utm.edu/bentham/. The Internet Encyclopaedia of Philosophy on Jeremy Bentham.

12 http://www.philosophy-index.com/hume/guillotine/. The 'is–ought' problem as described on the Philosophy Index.

13 http://www.publications.parliament.uk/pa/jt200809/jtselect/jtrights/47/4705.htm. An account of the distinction between negative and positive duties from the UK Parliament website.

14 http://www.jewishvirtuallibrary.org/jsource/Holocaust/disabled.html. The Jewish Virtual library on the Nazis and sterilisation.

15 http://news.bbc.co.uk/1/hi/health/background_briefings/international/290661.stm. A BBC report on Sweden's intention to compensate those who were forcibly sterilised.

16 http://www.time.com/time/world/article/0,8599,1615936,00.html. *Time* magazine on reproductive rights in China.

17 http://www.telegraph.co.uk/health/healthnews/7952231/Judge-criticises-council-for-trying-to-force-contraception-on-woman.html. A report on a judge vetoing forced contraception by social workers in the UK.

18 http://www.debatingmatters.com/topicguides/topicguide/older_mums/. A topic guide and resources on debating the moral acceptability of older mothers from Debating Matters.

19 http://www.cosmopolitan.co.uk/your-life/big-issue-IVF/v1. A discussion from *Cosmopolitan* magazine on IVF.

20 http://www.telegraph.co.uk/news/worldnews/europe/spain/5833618/Spanish-woman-who-gave-birth-at-66-dies-leaving-orphaned-twins.html. A *Daily Telegraph* report on the death of Maria del Carmen Bousada de Lara.

21 http://www.guardian.co.uk/society/2009/jun/29/women-over-40-fertility-tourism. A *Guardian* report on 'fertility tourism'.

22 http://www.opsi.gov.uk/acts/acts2008/ukpga_20080022_en_1. The HFE Act 2008.

23 http://www.baaf.org.uk/info/lpp/agencies/index.shtml. The British Agency for Adoption and Fostering lists the regulations governing adoption.

24 http://www.guardian.co.uk/uk/2009/mar/21/baby-bury-high-court-custody. A report in the UK's *Observer* newspaper about the forcible removal of a baby from its mother at birth.

25 http://news.bbc.co.uk/1/hi/health/8315836.stm. A BBC report on the folic acid debate in the UK.

26 http://plato.stanford.edu/entries/rights/#5.1. *The Stanford Encyclopedia* entry on rights, the section on 'trumping' is 5.1.

27 http://www.ivf-infertility.com/ivf/standard/procedure/costs.php. An account of the costs of IVF.

28 http://www.hfea.gov.uk/fertility-clinics-success-rates.html. The HFEA on IVF success rates.

29 http://www.guardian.co.uk/world/2010/mar/17/catholic-adoption-gay-couples. A report on a high court ruling in the UK about Catholic adoption agencies and gay applicants for adoption.

30 http://www.guardian.co.uk/society/2000/nov/09/NHS. A Q&A on postcode lotteries from the *Guardian* newspaper.
31 http://www.bionews.org.uk/page_37792.asp. A report from *Bionews* on the fact that PCTs aren't implementing government guidelines on IVF.

Further reading and useful websites

Parker, S. (2007) *In Vitro Fertilisation (Cutting Edge Medicine)*. London: Franklin Watts.

Deech, R. and Smajdor, A. (2007) *From IVF to Immortality: Controversy in the Era of Reproductive Technology*. Oxford: Oxford University Press.

Warnock, M. (2003) *Making Babies: Is There a Right to Have Children?* Oxford: Oxford Paperbacks.

http://www.beep.ac.uk/content/190.0.html. The Bioethics Education project website on assisted reproduction.

http://www.hfea.gov.uk/fertility-treatment-cost-nhs.html#1. The section on fertility treatment from the website of the Human Fertilisation and Embryology Authority.

http://www.hrea.org/index.php?doc_id=425. The Human Rights Education Associates website.

10 | The resources of reproduction: eggs, sperm and wombs for sale

Objectives

In reading this chapter you will:

- learn about a major cause of infertility;
- reflect on the reasons for the shortage of donor gametes;
- consider what it would be like to have no idea who your parents are;
- reflect on ways to alleviate the gamete shortage;
- ask whether we should use eggs from aborted foetuses to alleviate the egg shortage;
- ask whether it is right to use artificial sperm to alleviate the sperm shortage;
- consider whether paying for reproductive resources is a morally unacceptable 'commodification' of the human body;
- reflect on artificial wombs and the extent to which they will relieve women of the burden of carrying babies to term.

A major cause of infertility is the inability to produce fertile gametes.[1] Since women have been having babies later this type of fertility has increased. Many men have low sperm counts, or even no sperm at all and sperm counts quite generally seem to be decreasing.[2] Sometimes the problems are not with gametes but with difficulty in providing a womb hospitable to a developing foetus. For many sub-fertile people, therefore, their chance of a child still depends on their ability to secure fertile gametes, and/or a hospitable womb. Securing these 'resources' is not easy.

In this chapter we shall consider the ethical and social issues emerging from the demand for and supply of gametes and of hospitable wombs. We shall start by considering gamete donation then turn to surrogacy.

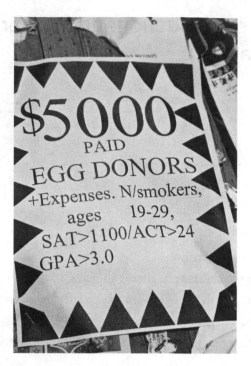

Figure 10.1 An advert posted at the University of Texas campus, offering money to egg donors with qualifications. © Photolibrary.com.

Gamete donation

The first recorded act of medical sperm donation was in 1884.[3] Many women have used artificial insemination both formally and informally as a means of securing a much-wanted child. Such a procedure depends on a man willing to donate sperm. But donating sperm is easy and many men have proven willing.[4] Now IVF is possible and infertility rates are rising (partly thanks to sexually transmitted diseases such as chlamydia), the demand for sperm is growing.

Reproductive technology has introduced a demand for eggs. Donating eggs is not easy. A woman must take drugs to stimulate egg production and undergo invasive procedures so the eggs can be harvested.[5] There have never been enough eggs donated to meet demand, especially as in recent years that demand comes, not just from infertile women, but also from researchers who study human reproduction and need a ready supply of eggs and sperm (and early embryos). Therapeutic cloning too (see Chapter 7) depends on a ready supply of eggs, though these needn't be human eggs.

The shortage of available gametes has been exacerbated recently in many countries by the passing of two laws:

(i) a law requiring the details of gamete donors be registered and made available on request to the child(ren) of any resulting pregnancy from the date of their 18th birthday;[6]

(ii) a law forbidding payment of anything but expenses to gamete donors.[7]

Box 10.1 Factual information: Fresh versus stored sperm

Until 2007 the UK laws banning anonymity and payment to sperm donors covered only sperm that will be stored. It was legal to donate fresh sperm anonymously and for payment.[8] In 2007 regulations were extended to include fresh sperm. It is, however, proving easy for the unscrupulous to evade the regulations.

The benefits of storing sperm should not be underestimated. Many sexually transmitted diseases, HIV for example, cannot be detected for some months after infection. Bona fide fertility clinics test prospective donors for STDs, and store their sperm for 6 months. They then test the sperm to make sure it is disease-free before use.

Anyone trying to circumvent the laws on anonymity by donating or using fresh sperm may be giving more than the gift of life to their donor-conceived offspring.

It is easy to see why these laws have led to a fall in the number of donors. Sperm donors, in particular, have traditionally been impecunious students in need of cash. Such students have no desire to be fathers, no yearning to take responsibility for anyone or anything, and often no thought for the future. All they want is beer money. When donations were anonymous they could pocket the cash without consequences.

Now not only can they only charge expenses (and receipts are required), they also have to sign up to be revealed as the biological father of children born as a result of their donation. Luckily, no countries have made loss of anonymity retrospective: there would be many men who could be contacted by literally hundreds of offspring. Most countries that have banned anonymity simultaneously limited the number of 'childbirth events' per donation (multiple births count as one 'childbirth event') to avoid this. But there are not many young men who would welcome the idea that they might, in their forties, be contacted by teenage offspring. Most would rightly wonder how their future wives and children would react.

The dilemma facing the countries passing the two laws is that of trying to secure sufficient gamete donations to meet demand. In the UK, after the anonymity law was passed, the number of treatment cycles using donated eggs fell by 25%, the number of women using donated sperm by 30%.[9]

You might immediately think that it was a mistake to pass one or both of these laws. Why impose laws almost guaranteed to decrease donations in the context of an increasing need for donations?

This seems such a sensible question that we'll start by considering why so many countries have passed one or both of these two laws and whether, in the light of the arguments *for* these laws we continue to think that repealing these laws is the obvious way to meet the shortage of gametes.

Gamete donor anonymity

The downside of donor anonymity, and the reason so many countries no longer offer it, is the effect on children born as a result of donation.

If you are lucky enough to have grown up with one or more biological parents, close your eyes and think about them. Do you resemble them? Do you share mannerisms with them? Do your family tease you about the traits you have in common with them? This might infuriate you. But it might also give you a warm sense of belonging. It is usually a wonderful thing to know one's parents. It confers a sense of identity, a secure sense of knowing who you are and where you came from.

As you get older further benefits might accrue. The medical history of your biological family may become important to you or to your children. Or you may become interested in the non-medical history of your biological family, perhaps when you have children of your own. Your parents, siblings, aunts and uncles, grandparents and cousins all hold part of a jigsaw that you may or may not want to construct. No one ever knows everything about their biological family, some people know very little, some people are not interested. But at least they have the choice.

In the past donor-conceived children have not had this choice. They may have loving parents and grow up in happy families, but they often know very little, if anything, about at least one of their biological parents. This is also true, of course, for most adopted children. Sometimes such children will have access to basic facts such as height and eye colour. Sometimes they may have some biographical information. But often they have nothing. For some such children, especially as they get older and have children of their own, this matters a great deal.

Box 10.2 **Case study: A donor-conceived child's experience**

Caroline Halstead is a donor-conceived child who struggles to come to terms with the fact she was conceived 'in a Petri dish by artificial insemination at a Harley Street Clinic in London.' She believes this was a 'horrible, clinical way to be conceived'. All my life' she says 'I've felt as if I'm only half a person.'[10]

Caroline describes herself as 'haunted' by the way she was conceived and by the fact she will never know or meet her father.

The Commission on Parenthood's Future conducted a study that suggests donor-conceived children often feel confusion, isolation and hurt. Half are disturbed that money was involved in their conception. And as many again admitted that when they see someone who looks like them, they wonder if they're related. Two-thirds argue that they should have the right to know their parents.[11]

It is easy to say that at least donor-conceived people have lives they wouldn't have had their biological parent(s) not chosen to donate gametes. To the extent that their biological parent(s) wouldn't have donated gametes had they not been guaranteed anonymity, this might be some consolation. But are we sure they wouldn't have donated gametes without anonymity? And why, we may want to ask, should donors want anonymity?

Perhaps they are afraid they will become responsible, legally, financially or even morally, for their donor-conceived offspring? If so their fears are unfounded. Gamete donors are never regarded as responsible in law, legally, financially or morally, for their donor-conceived offspring.[12]

The answer to the question of why donors want anonymity goes back to the moral queasiness of an earlier age. Before egg donation became possible sperm donation was often considered morally questionable. The image of a sperm donor was not that of an altruistic man prepared to give the gift of life. It was rather that of a furtive man masturbating over pornographic pictures. Sperm donation was considered by some to be tantamount to adultery.[13]

One can see why anonymity was attractive. But surely these days we're more morally robust? Why did the guarantee of anonymity not fall away with the social changes that have revealed sperm donation, never mind egg donation, to be an altruistic act, an act to be lauded? Why aren't sperm and egg donors *proud* of their willingness to donate?

It is now a legal right, in many countries, to know where you came from. Perhaps it always was a *moral* right? Either way the donor-conceived child's right to know its biological parent has been given priority over prospective donors' apparent desire for anonymity.

The fact that this is the way things *are* does not, of course, mean that this is the way things *ought to be*. If refusing to guarantee anonymity means that fewer donor-conceived children are born and that more infertile people are disappointed in their quest for children, might it not be morally required of us to repeal the laws that result in this?

> ### Box 10.3 Activity: Small group discussion
>
> *Restoring donor anonymity will probably lead to an increase in gamete donation. So donor anonymity should be restored.*
>
> Participants should be divided into small groups and asked whether or not they agree with this claim. They should be allowed 15 minutes for discussion before feeding back to the whole group to whom the discussion should then be opened.
>
> It would be interesting to ask after the whole group discussion whether anyone has changed their mind. This will involve taking a poll before starting the exercise.

Anonymity and the internet

Some have suggested that anonymity, at least for sperm donors, cannot be secured even if the law 'guarantees' it. That this is the case was proven by a 15-year-old American in 2005. The teenager sent a swab of his saliva to a company that profiled his DNA and recorded it on their database.[14] When close matches are found between profiles on their database the company sends email alerts to the people whose DNA matches. Within a few days two matches had been found with the boy's Y chromosome. The matches suggested a 50% chance that the boy and the two other men had the same father, grandfather or great-grandfather.

Exploiting the fact that it is not just Y chromosomes but surnames that are passed from father to son, the boy went to another company,[15] where he checked the shared surname of the two men he matched against the details he had about his biological father from the fertility clinic organising his conception. These details included date and place of birth, and his biological father's college degree. These details were sufficient for him to find his father.[16]

It is not recorded whether this story had a happy ending. But for our purposes what matters is that no illegal act was perpetrated by the boy. Yet within 10 days he found his biological father despite the guarantee of anonymity his father had been given when he donated the sperm that led to the boy's conception.

Given this we might reasonably ask whether there would be any point in repealing the law that forbids anonymity?

Payment for gametes

We could alleviate the shortage of gametes by allowing people to pay for them. But some people believe that this is morally unacceptable because it is a 'commodification' of the human body.

Would you happily sell your body for sex? Would you buy sex? Many people wouldn't. They believe it would be demeaning. Sex, to most people, is a move in a human relationship, not a move in a commercial transaction. If you think like this, you are likely to think that sex cannot, without moral and psychological distortion, be marketed like a pint of milk or a bag of coal.[17]

Many countries have banned payment for gametes because they believe that permitting payment is 'commodifying' something that shouldn't be commodified, in this case the 'gift of life'.[18]

Such a view is consistent with paying donors out-of-pocket expenses, even perhaps with covering loss of income, but it is not consistent with a full blown *market* for gametes or wombs.

Interestingly, even in countries like the United States, Russia, the Czech Republic and Spain, where it is legal to buy and sell gametes, the language of altruism, rather than the language of commerce, is often used. Young women are urged to 'donate' eggs, and offered 'compensation' for their time and trouble. Even where commerce is legal lip service is paid to the idea that the means of human reproduction should not be commodified. That the transactions are commercial is clear: why otherwise would a tall, blonde, Ivy Leaguer be able to command $50,000 for her eggs, whilst a short dark woman from an also-ran university gets only $5,000? Is it really so much more inconvenient for the former to donate her eggs?

'You'll want my sperm after you see pictures of my kids!'

'I am a 30-year-old white male and father of two. I am healthy, do not use drugs and have two beautiful children. Due to the economy I am thinking outside the box and have resorted to sperm donation for extra income. I WILL ONLY DO THIS ONCE so you need to seize the opportunity and get my sperm before I change my mind. I am willing to give it to you through the bank or the old-fashioned way if the price is right and you are disease-free. Please email me and we will talk. Thank you.'

Advertisement on 'spermbanker.com'

Another objection to permitting payment for gametes is that it condones the exploitation of the poor by the rich. The only reason that people would sell their gametes, it is claimed, is their need of money. The only people who could afford to pay for gametes are the rich.

Interestingly, many accepted that for male students selling sperm was a good way of making beer money, yet there has been an outcry about young women selling their eggs to pay university fees. Maybe this is because of the increased risk? Or could there be a whiff of sexism: women are supposed to be nurturers not purveyors of eggs. But of course it is not just female students with excellent life-chances who could be tempted to sell their eggs: poverty-stricken women in developing countries may well be overwhelmed by the temptation.[19]

But is it right that the ability of the infertile to have children should depend on their disposable income? And isn't the gift of life, when motivated by poverty, diminished?

Box 10.4 Activity: Creative writing

Imagine you are an impoverished student wondering whether to sell your gametes to pay off your debts. Ask yourself what your parents would think, how you will feel about yourself later on, how it would feel to know you had children you'll never know...

Banning payment for gametes may enable us to relax in the confidence that we are properly honouring the gift of life and refusing to condone the exploitation of the poor, but it might also condemn thousands to childlessness. It will also make finding the gametes needed for research harder. If so perhaps it is morally required of us to repeal the laws barring payment?

We might adduce in support of this claim the fact that passing laws banning payment for gametes only prevents the law-abiding from buying and selling gametes: everyone else can simply use the internet. To see how easy this is perform an internet search for 'sperm donor' and see how quickly and easily you would be able to get hold of some sperm.

Box 10.5 Case study: Jamie and Sarah

In 2004 a donor-conceived child was born to lesbian couple, Jamie and Sarah, from Liverpool in the UK.[20]

The couple had been together for 4 years, and had desperately wanted a child for 2 of them. Seeing they were getting nowhere with their GP, they approached a website called 'Man Not Included'.

This website was launched specifically to cater for single women and lesbians. The website currently has 5,500 prospective donors, and 3,000 prospective recipients. The basic service cost the couple £830. Customers can also ask, at the time of the original donation of fresh sperm, for another fresh sample from the same donor to be frozen to permit biological full siblings. This extra service cost £1,365.

The service includes a home ovulation kit so when Jamie knew she was at her most fertile she alerted the website, a sample was collected from their chosen donor and rushed to Jamie and Sarah's house by courier. Jamie and Sarah used the sperm to inseminate Jamie, who conceived immediately.

Before the birth Jamie said 'Everything happened when they said it would and doing everything at home meant it was private and comfortable. We know that some people will be against what we have done and they are entitled to their opinion. As long as our child is loved and wants for nothing, I can't see how it is wrong.'

Of course no law can prevent transgressions. But could it be the case that the law banning the sale and purchase of stored gametes merely generates a thriving internet black market? Could it even be forcing people to risk their health and that of their children by using fresh sperm or buying eggs through disreputable clinics? It certainly seems to be forcing more and more women into 'fertility tourism' where they travel to countries with different laws, either to buy eggs or to 'donate' them for payment. Given this, couldn't it be the case that we are morally required to legalise the market in gametes, imposing strict regulations ensuring that all gametes sold are stored for long enough to be guaranteed disease-free?

Box 10.6 Activity: Group discussion

Many people are happy that the sale and purchase of gametes is illegal. But some would like to see it:

(i) decriminalised (such that the law has no interest whatsoever in the buying and selling of gametes, rather as the law has no interest in the buying and selling of sweets).

Others would like to see it:

(ii) legalised (such that the law regulates it as it regulates the sale of alcohol, imposing conditions on its sale, such as 6 months of storage to check for disease).

> Divide the group into three. Allocate to each group one of the moral theories discussed in Chapter 4 and give them 20 minutes to discuss whether theorists of their kind would be for or against decriminalising or legalising the sale of gametes.

Securing reproductive resources without payment or anonymity

If it were possible to secure a ready supply of gametes without guaranteeing anonymity or making payment we would clearly have the best of both worlds: the infertile would get their children, those children would get their lives, donor-conceived offspring would get to know who they are *and* we would be properly honouring the gift of life.

Before we can properly answer the question, therefore, of whether we should or shouldn't repeal the laws forbidding anonymity and payment, we need to ask what alternatives there are: is there any way we could increase supply to meet demand *without* needing either to pay and/or guarantee anonymity?

There are several things we could try, other than repealing these laws, to ensure supply meets demand. We could:

- use family as donors;
- approach donors on a different basis;
- relax the restrictions on donations;
- encourage 'egg sharing';
- use eggs from aborted foetuses;
- use artificial gametes;
- accept chimera.

Let's look briefly at each of these:

Using family donors

With egg donation familial donation has long been popular: a sister, for example, distressed by her sister's inability to have a baby might provide her sister with eggs.[21] Recently, in England, a mother whose daughter has Turner syndrome, a condition that will render the daughter infertile, has frozen her eggs so her daughter, should she ever want children, has the choice of using her mother's eggs rather than the eggs of a stranger.[22]

Men also engage in familial donation. Recently a 72-year-old man gave sperm to his daughter-in-law.[23] In another case a man donated his sperm to his sister who was using a donated egg.[24]

Critics have argued that such cases will lead to the sort of confused and ambiguous family relationships we discussed in Chapter 8. Others argue there can be no greater act of family love than giving the possibility of a child.

Approach donors on a different basis

The laws against payment and anonymity are likely to deter the traditional sperm donor.[25] But would they deter everyone? Egg donors often donate because they cannot bear the thought that some people cannot have children. They want to help. They don't want anything more than expenses, and they are prepared to have their details given to their donor-conceived offspring. Mightn't there be men who would feel the same if the idea was put to them that they could give the gift of a child to another couple?

Such men would probably fit a very different profile from traditional sperm donors. They are likely to be older, have long-term stable relationships and children of their own. Such men, enjoying their own children, may be prepared to help, especially if their wives (and children?) were supportive. They would not need more than expenses. Nor, given their wives' support, would the thought of their offspring contacting them fill them with horror (understanding they have no legal, financial or moral obligations in respect of their donor-conceived offspring). A variation on this theme would be to try to encourage all men having a vasectomy to donate a few samples.

Such men would have to be treated differently from the traditional donor. The best approach would probably be a 'self-esteem' based approach rather like that used for blood donors.[26] Potential donors would have to be convinced that what they were doing was admirable and they would have to be treated with respect. But it seems at least possible that such an approach would result in as many donations as the traditional payment-based approach did.

Relax the restrictions on donations

Another way of helping supply meet demand would be to relax some of the restrictions on the use of donated gametes.[27] At the moment in the UK men cannot donate after 45 or women after 35. Perhaps these age restrictions might be loosened slightly, especially if it is believed that altruistic donors will be older than traditional donors.

There is also an upper limit on the number of 'childbirth events' (multiple births count as one 'childbirth event') allowed for each donor. In the UK, for example, no donor is allowed more than 10. Perhaps this could be revised so each donor was allowed 15 or 20 childbirth events?

Finally there is an upper limit on the length of time donations can be frozen. Perhaps this too could be revised?

These upper limits were, of course, imposed for reasons. Human eggs start to deteriorate after 35, and there is evidence that there might be problems with older fathers. The limit on 'childbirth events' is intended to minimise the chances of half-siblings marrying in ignorance of their biological relationship. The limit on the length of time gametes can be frozen is a fear that they deteriorate over time (though recent events – the successful birth of a child from eggs frozen for over 13 years – suggest that the upper limit could safely be revised). Nevertheless we would not have to revise the upper limits significantly to increase the number and usefulness of donations.

Encourage 'egg sharing'

In many countries clinics offering IVF now ask couples undergoing IVF if they will donate gametes for others' use.[28] Often such requests are accompanied by offers of significant discounts on the cost of their treatment. As a woman who is having IVF is already undergoing the unpleasant procedures necessary to harvest her eggs, asking her to share her eggs (given that she will produce more eggs than she needs) is not asking her to do anything other than make it possible for another woman to have a child (and be prepared for the possibility that child will get in touch in 18 years' time).

It has been argued that this is simply payment for gametes in another form. In countries that ban payment but permit egg sharing charges of hypocrisy abound. A discount of £1,500 on a course of IVF is not a small inducement.[29] Perhaps it preserves at least the spirit of the law, whilst at least mitigating the shortage of gametes? But is there really a moral difference between a discount of £1,500 and a payment of £1,500?

The downside of egg sharing is of course that the fertility of the woman who is sharing her eggs is already comprised. But at least egg sharing does give the chance of a child to the infertile. It is likely, however, that this way of securing eggs for donation will dry up as ways are found of helping women to have children without their needing to produce multiple eggs.

Use eggs from aborted foetuses

A female child is born with all the oocytes she'll ever have. These develop early in foetal development and can be extracted from foetuses from about week 13. Between 16 and 20 weeks each female foetus has about 6–7 million oocytes each potentially capable of maturing into a fertile egg. In many developed countries abortion is legal well after the 13th week of pregnancy. It would be possible therefore to ask every woman undergoing abortion if she would permit the oocytes of any female foetus to be donated to the sub-fertile. By such means we need never be short of eggs ever again.[30]

At least this would be the case so long as enough women undergoing abortions were prepared, in future, to become grandmothers without having ever mothered the mother of their grandchild. The question of whether they'd even know about their grandchildren (as an actual fact) is a moot one. The legislation banning anonymity requires potential *parents* to be prepared for their details to be given to offspring, but it says nothing about *grandparents*. As no child would result from this particular pregnancy, the law seems to be silent on whether details of the woman having an abortion, but allowing her aborted daughter's oocytes to be harvested, would have to be registered.

Clearly the law would have to be re-visited if this method for alleviated the egg shortage were used. Should grandparents be allowed to retain their anonymity? Would lack of knowledge about one's grandmother be comparable, psychologically and emotionally, to lack of knowledge about a parent?

Perhaps though it would not be lack of knowledge of one grandmother that would prompt psychological and emotional problems so much as the knowledge that your mother had been aborted? How would you feel knowing that your biological mother had *never* lived except as a foetus? How would you feel knowing that it was a decision made by your grandmother that had led to your mother's extremely premature death? Consideration of this might prompt us to think that anonymity *should* be permitted to those who donate eggs in this way. Perhaps it would be best never to tell such a child of their origins? But this would involve lying to the child. Would this be morally acceptable?

Box 10.7 Activity: Creative writing

Write 500 words from the perspective of a child conceived from an egg harvested from an aborted foetus.

You might like to consider the following:

- Had it not been for your grandmother's willingness to donate her foetus' oocytes, you would not exist.
- Isn't it better that your mother should at least have had a child even if she never had a life?
- Has your life been blighted by the discovery of your origins?
- Would it have been better that you were never born?
- Would it have been better for you never to have known your origins?

Use artificial gametes

Technology is fast developing another way in which the gamete shortage could be alleviated: by producing 'artificial' gametes.[31] 'Artificial' gametes are a bit like 'artificial' intelligences: the only difference between them and the real thing is their origin. See the Box 10.8 for the different ways of producing artificial gametes.

Box 10.8 Factual information: Ways of producing artificial gametes

There are different ways of producing artificial gametes:

- Directly converting somatic cells from mitotic division to meiotic division so they carry just one set of chromosomes instead of two.
- Dedifferentiating somatic cells into embryonic stem cells and re-differentiating these stem cells into germ cells.
- Extracting adult stem cells and re-differentiating them into gametes.

The first sperm cells have now been grown in the laboratory[32] and researchers from the Women and Infants' Hospital, Brown University, Rhode Island, have created an artificial ovary from slivers of ovarian tissue, which can mature eggs.[33]

In contrast to other ways of producing gametes it is easier to produce artificial eggs than it is artificial sperm. Because all normal male mammals have one X chromosome it is even possible to produce eggs from male stem cells.

That this is the case is considered by some to demonstrate the moral unaccept-ability of artificial gametes: it could permit a single sex male couple to produce a baby genetically related to both of them by means of one providing the egg, the other the sperm. Even more controversially it could permit a man, by means of a surrogate mother, to provide both the egg *and* sperm in his quest for a baby. But could it ever be right for a man to be both father *and* mother to a child? How confused and ambiguous would this child's family relationships be?

Box 10.9 Factual information: The end of men?

When artificial sperm were first mooted the newspapers heralded the 'end of men'. They argued that if sperm could be made from the cells of women this would lead to men becoming redundant.

In fact, as women do not have a Y chromosome it would be harder, maybe even impossible, to create sperm from a female cell. It is more likely, therefore, that artificial human gametes would lead to the end of *women*.

Of course, this ignores the fact that only the infertile need to use artificial gametes. The rest can make babies the usual way which, apart from anything else, is far cheaper.

It seems unlikely that the successful production of artificial human gametes will prove the last salvo in the war between the sexes.

But there are other moral barriers in the way of artificial gametes. The only way of testing whether these gametes work is to use them, see if fertilisation proceeds and, if it does, whether the fertilised egg develops normally.

This has been done with mice. The first mouse born by such means, Eggbert, died very young having lived a very sickly life. But healthy mouse pups have since been produced from artificial mouse sperm.[34] Maybe it is only a matter of time until we can do the same for humans.

But this would involve experimentation on human embryos, and such experimen-tation would *have* to proceed beyond the 14th day. At the moment most countries forbid experimentation on embryos beyond the 14th day for all the reasons discussed in Chapter 7. Would the promise of artificial gametes to help the infertile render the arguments against such experimentation obsolete? But why should it? If it didn't how could we ever successfully demonstrate that artificial gametes work like natural ones? Many believe – with good reason – that such 'suck it and see' techniques with respect to humans are morally abhorrent.

Accept chimera

In Greek mythology the *chimera* was a fire-breathing creature constituted of several different animals. She (it was female) had the body of a lion, from whose back emerged a goat's head, and a tail that ended with the head of a snake. To biotechnolo-gists a chimera is slightly less alarming. It is an embryo that results from inserting a human nucleus into the egg of a non-human, a cow, for example.

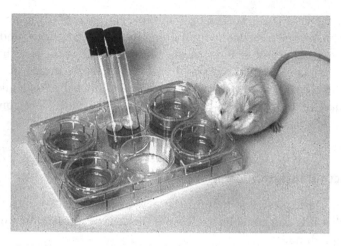

Figure 10.2 Eggbert, the first mouse born from a lab-cultured egg, suffered obesity later in life. Reprinted with permission from Macmillan Publishers Ltd: 'Developmental biology: Synthetic sex cells' *Nature*, **424**, 364–366, © 2003.

The creation of chimera was, in the UK, approved in 2007 after the HFEA conducted a public consultation.[35] It has been approved, however, only for research purposes. There is no suggestion that chimera be produced for the purposes of producing live chimera.

But would this be so bad? A human–cow chimera is 99.9% human, and only 0.1% cow. Might we, taking a very deep breath, approve of the use of chimera for reproductive purposes. . .?

> ### Box 10.10 Activity: Creative writing
>
> Write a short story about the use of chimera for reproductive purposes. Consider the feelings of the parents, the grandparents and the child itself.

It is clear that there are several means of attempting to secure a ready supply of gametes other than repealing the laws forbidding anonymity and payment. But it is not obvious that all these means are themselves morally acceptable. Let's now turn to the other resources needed for reproduction.

> ### Box 10.11 Activity: Group discussion
>
> Participants should discuss:
>
> (i) whether society has an obligation to help those whose infertility stems from the inability to produce fertile gametes.
> (ii) by which (combination of) means society should help.

Participants should remember that egg donation differs from sperm donation to such an extent that some may think they should be treated differently.

Alternatively the group could restrict the discussion to one aspect of this debate as follows:

- Should payment for eggs be permitted?
- Should anonymity for sperm donors be restored?
- Is the use of eggs from aborted foetuses morally permissible?
- Is the use of artificial gametes morally permissible?
- Would it be morally acceptable for single sex male couples to produce a child with one of them providing the egg, the other the sperm?

Surrogacy, society and morality

A woman born with 'Mayer–Rokitansky–Kuster–Hauser Syndrome'[36] (MRKH) has no womb. Women with this syndrome obviously cannot bear children for themselves; but the possibility of using a surrogate mother can be the answer to their prayers.[37] Other conditions, including endometriosis and hysterectomy, can also lead to a woman's needing a surrogacy arrangement.[38]

Surrogacy is becoming quite commonplace in the developed world. About 300 babies are born each year to surrogate mothers in the United States. In the UK, despite much stricter regulation, there will be about 30–40.[39] These figures probably grossly underestimate the true number of surrogate births because fertility tourism for the purposes of surrogacy is big business. India, for example, has been called 'the cradle of the world': estimates of the value of the surrogate industry to India vary between £250 and 500 million a year.[40] The typical Indian clinic has 40 potential surrogates on their books, 20 of whom will be pregnant at any one time, and charges about £6,000 for the whole procedure, including legal and medical fees. This compares with approximately £25,000 in the UK and $100,000 in the United States.[41]

The fear of exploitation is as much of an issue with surrogacy as it is with gamete purchase. This is especially the case when the surrogate is from the developing world.

Box 10.12 Activity: Paired discussion

Najima Vohra from near Anand in India is being paid £2,750 to carry a child for an American couple. She plans to buy a brick house, invest in her husband's business and pay for her children's education: 'My daughter wants to be a teacher', she says, 'I'll do anything to give her that opportunity.'

One thing Vohra is doing to give her daughter this opportunity is living a lie. Her extended family, friends and neighbours 'think that immoral acts take place to get pregnant. They'd shun my family if they knew'. She, her husband and children have temporarily moved to another village to hide what she is doing.[42]

Discuss with a partner whether the commissioning parents are exploiting Najima or helping her to give her children a future.

Being a surrogate mother is no sinecure. Pregnancy can be a life-threatening condition. The procedures one must undergo to become a surrogate are no walk in the park. There are two types of surrogacy: partial, where the surrogate's eggs are fertilised by the sperm of the commissioning father, and full, where an embryo created from the eggs and sperm of the commissioning parents is implanted into the surrogate's womb.

But many women enjoy pregnancy and find it easy. This partly explains why so many women are prepared to carry babies for other women for nothing more than expenses. But many who need surrogate mothers will not regard the payments they must make as 'nothing more than' anything. Surrogacy is not an option for the poor unless a friend or family member can be found who'll do it for love. (It is believed that many informal surrogacy arrangements never appear on the records.) Once again nations threaten to divide into those who can afford surrogacy to alleviate infertility and those who can't.

It might be thought that surrogacy would be a risky venture in that surrogate mother must often find themselves unable to hand over the baby: apparently the question surrogates are most often asked is *how* they can do it. In the UK surrogacy is not recognised as binding agreement: either side can pull out. In fact the surrogate's name must appear on the birth certificate and the intended parent must formally adopt the baby at 6 weeks old. Research suggests, however, that only 4% of surrogates refuse to hand over the baby, and many express themselves delighted to see the happiness it gives to the commissioning parents. When a surrogate does refuse to hand over the baby, however, it can lead to great heartache (see Box 10.13).[43]

Box 10.13 Case study: Baby M

In 1985 a wealthy American couple, Bill and Elizabeth Stern, offered Mary Beth Whitehead $10,000 to bear Bill Stern's baby. Elizabeth was physically capable of bearing a child but she believed a pregnancy might prompt a recurrence of her multiple sclerosis. Mary Beth and her husband Richard signed a contract agreeing to some stringent healthcare conditions after going through it for several hours with an independent lawyer.

Whitehead was inseminated with Bill Stern's sperm and in July, after nine attempts, she became pregnant.

The baby, a girl, was born in March 1987. The Whiteheads had not mentioned the surrogacy arrangement to the hospital in which she was born, and when the Sterns arrived they were not allowed to hold the baby. Later that day Whitehead relinquished the child, but the next day she threatened suicide unless she could keep the baby.

The Sterns' contract was upheld by the family court in Hackensack and the Whiteheads were ordered to surrender the baby. Instead they fled with their children to Florida where they remained hidden for 3 months.

When they were found the judge at Hackensack made Elizabeth Stern the legal mother of baby M and made a specific order that Mary Beth Whitehead was to have no visiting rights.

This ruling was reversed by the Supreme Court of New Jersey, who found that surrogacy contracts amounted to 'baby-selling'.

The court allowed the Sterns to keep Baby M so that she had a stable life (by that time the Whiteheads were divorcing), but they gave extensive visiting rights to Mary Beth who took full advantage of them throughout Baby M's childhood.

When Baby M, now revealed as Melissa Stern, reached 18 she voluntarily severed contact with Mary Beth Whitehead and formalised her adoption by the Sterns.[44]

Did Mary Beth Whitehead 'sell' her baby then renege on the sale? Did The Sterns exploit the Whiteheads (who were bankrupt when they signed the contract)? Should the Sterns have allowed the Whiteheads to keep baby M?

Surrogacy for social reasons

There is a suspicion, however, that not all women or couples who use surrogates do so for medical reasons.[45] It has recently been suggested that some women, in particular certain celebrities, are paying other women to have their babies for the sake of their figures or their careers. Why go through a pregnancy, suffer stretch marks, months of sleeplessness, possible weight gain and all the health risks attendant on pregnancy when you can pay someone else to do this for you, and still have your own biological child?

Some have suggested that this is immoral. Why have children, they ask, if you are not going to look after them yourself? On the other hand, why shouldn't a woman pay someone else to carry her child if she can afford it? Men have always found someone else to carry their children. In 2010 the footballer Christian Ronaldo paid a surrogate to have a child for him.[46] If, by paying a surrogate, a woman is able to help the surrogate provide for her own family isn't this a plus all round?

> ### Box 10.14 Activity: Group discussion
>
> *If a woman is capable of carrying her own child, she should do this. It would be wrong to pay a surrogate in the absence of a medical need.*
>
> Half the group should take one side of this argument, the other half the other side.

Artificial wombs

One day it will not be necessary for women even to pay surrogates.[47] Scientists have been working on producing artificial wombs for some time now. Two different avenues are being explored:

(i) Cells have been taken from the lining of a woman's womb and grown in the laboratory on scaffolds of biodegradable material moulded in the shape of the interior of a uterus. As the cells become tissue the scaffold disintegrates and oestrogen and nutrients can be added to the tissue.

(ii) The construction of tanks of amniotic fluid stabilised at body temperature, in which foetuses can be put and connected to machines that pump in nutrients and dispose of waste.

The first method is ideal for starting a pregnancy off and getting it to settle in the laboratory before the whole apparatus is put into the body of the mother or a surrogate to bring the baby to term. Embryos left over from IVF have already been placed in these 'wombs' and successfully implanted before being destroyed as required by the law.

The second method is useful part way through a pregnancy. A foetus in trouble in the womb can be removed and brought to term in the amniotic tank. So far this method has been tried only with goats.

It has been suggested that the advent of the artificial womb will be the fulfilment of the feminist dream. No longer, it is thought, will a woman be disadvantaged by the need to bear children. Just like a man she will be able to have her children without any career break, without compromising her health and without ruining her figure.

Employers too may benefit. No longer will they need to look askance at women of child-bearing age. Unless a woman is old-fashioned enough to insist on bearing her own child, she will be able to farm out the bearing of the child and the employer will not need to pay her any more maternity leave than he'd pay a man. Health insurers, too, might be delighted. Once artificial wombs are tried and tested the use of them could become a condition of certain policies.

Finally, once artificial wombs are a reality no foetus ever again need be aborted. As soon as its unwanted presence is registered it could be removed from the womb of the woman who doesn't want it and placed in an artificial womb, from whence it could be offered for adoption. No longer would adoptive parents have to reconcile themselves to adopting an older child or one with disabilities, they would be able to take their pick of hundreds of babies still in the womb.

Box 10.15 **Activity: Opinion poll**

Amongst your friends and family conduct an informal opinion poll on attitudes to artificial wombs. Prepare by constructing a list of pros and cons for people to read, then note their responses.

Classify these responses in terms of the ethical theories discussed in Chapter 4. Then use the results to stimulate group discussion.

This concludes our discussion of the shortage of reproductive resources. In the next chapter we shall consider the technologies that permit us to select for and against foetuses on the basis of their genome.

Summary

In this chapter we have:

- noted that there is a severe shortage of 'resources', especially gametes, for fertility treatment;
- considered whether laws requiring identification of donors and forbidding payment are responsible at least in part for this shortage;
- reflected on the reasons these laws were passed and on whether they should be repealed;
- considered other means of alleviating the shortage of gametes, including using eggs from aborted foetuses and artificial gametes;
- reflected on the possibility of introducing a market in gametes in the face of the fear it represents a commodification of the gift of life;
- considered the problems of surrogacy, and the possible exploitation of the poor by the rich;
- noted that artificial wombs might soon be a reality, and considered the possibility that women might one day use surrogacy or artificial wombs for social rather than medical reasons;
- reflected on the fact that artificial wombs might remove the need for abortion, and provide a steady stream of embryos for adoption.

Questions to stimulate reflection

'We should restore donor anonymity and pay donors a proper market rate to halt the decrease in the supply of donated gametes.' Do you agree?

To what extent do you think everyone has the right to know 'who they are'?

Would you be prepared to use the eggs of aborted foetuses as a supply of eggs for infertile women needing IVF?

Is the use of artificial gametes an acceptable way of responding to the gamete shortage?

Is paying a market rate to women prepared to be surrogate mothers unacceptable exploitation?

'The development of artificial wombs is an unacceptable interference with nature.' Is it?

Once we have artificial wombs women will be able to opt out of pregnancy for the sake of their careers or their figures. A welcome equality? Or a step too far?

Artificial wombs will obviate the need for abortion. This can only be a good thing. Is this right?

Additional activities

Write a short (120 word) article for a tabloid newspaper about career women who choose to use surrogate mothers so their career isn't interrupted.

Listen to Hillel Steiner on Exploitation on this website: http://itunes.apple.com/gb/podcast/philosophy-bites/id257042117 and use it to reflect on whether those who use surrogate mothers from other countries are engaged in exploitation.

Read this article http://news.scotsman.com/ivftreatment/Warnock-backs-babies-from-aborted.2440539.jp then see whether you agree with Baroness Warnock on the use of eggs from aborted foetuses.

Imagine that you are the result of the use of artificial sperm. Write a short (500 word) letter to your mother.

Find a partner, spend half an hour separately wandering the web looking at the testimony of donor-conceived children, then discuss whether you think the law against anonymity should be repealed.

Conduct an informal poll amongst your friends and family about people's views on buying and selling gametes.

Notes

1 http://www.babycentre.co.uk/preconception/suspectingaproblem/majorcauses/?_requestid=251404. Chart of the major causes of infertility.
2 http://www.ispub.com/ostia/index.php?xmlFilePath=journals/iju/vol2n1/sperm.xml. An academic paper about decreasing sperm counts.
3 http://fertilitylabinsider.com/2010/06/whos-my-daddy-the-issues-of-sperm-donation/. An account of this act of medical assisted reproduction.
4 http://www.londonspermbank.com/. How to become a sperm donor from the London Sperm Bank.
5 http://www.chiark.greenend.org.uk/~rmc28/eggs/egg_index.html. A personal account of egg donation.
6 http://news.bbc.co.uk/1/hi/health/4397249.stm. A BBC news report of the ending of donor anonymity.
7 http://www.hfea.gov.uk/784.html. A statement of the HFEA position on payment for gametes.
8 http://www.ivf.net/ivf/fresh_sperm_sales_banned_in_uk-o2227.html. An account of the change in the law in 2006 (implemented 2007).
9 http://www.timesonline.co.uk/tol/news/science/article4215440.ece. A report on the fall in gamete donors since the anonymity laws were passed.
10 http://www.dailymail.co.uk/femail/article-1289042/Caroline-fathered-sperm-donor–does-bitterly-resent-stranger-gave-life.html#ixzz0wxOmFpwK. Case study adapted from this article from Mailonline.
11 http://www.familyscholars.org/assets/Donor_FINAL.pdf.
12 http://www.ngdt.co.uk/. The legal facts about gamete donation from the National Gamete Donation Trust.

13 http://www.cartoonstock.com/directory/s/sperm_bank.asp. A series of cartoons depicting sperm donors.

14 www.familytreedna.com.

15 www.omnitrace.com.

16 http://news.bbc.co.uk/1/hi/health/4400778.stm. A BBC report of the boy's quest.

17 http://www.thestudentroom.co.uk/showthread.php?t=798614. A discussion about selling sperm in The Student Room. http://www.fertilitynation.com/females-selling-human-eggs-for-cash-stirs-controversy/. A discussion about egg donation on *Fertility Nation* in the United States, including a video from ABC News.

18 http://www.dailymail.co.uk/news/article-1257816/Human-egg-raffled-IVF-promotion. html. A report of the raffle of a human egg.

19 http://news.bbc.co.uk/1/hi/health/8401770.stm. A BBC site discussing payment for eggs.

20 http://icliverpool.icnetwork.co.uk/0100news/0100regionalnews/content_objec-tid=13126049_method=full_siteid=50061_headline=-Baby-conceived-thanks-to-internet–name_page.html. A report on icLiverpool.

21 http://www.guardian.co.uk/lifeandstyle/2003/may/14/familyandrelationships.features101. A woman donates eggs to her sister.

22 http://www.squidoo.com/ivf-pregnancies. A report from Squidoo on a mother donating eggs to her daughter.

23 http://news.bbc.co.uk/1/hi/health/7030267.stm. Report on a man donating sperm to secure a grandchild.

24 http://fertilityblog.fertilitystories.com/2006/02/donating-sperm-for-sibling-brothers.html. A letter to an agony column about a brother's donating sperm to his sister.

25 http://www.bionews.org.uk/page_59862.asp. An article on ways of approaching sperm donors from *BioNews*.

26 http://news.bbc.co.uk/1/hi/england/manchester/8567999.stm. A report on an attempt to get sports fans to donate sperm.

27 http://www.hfea.gov.uk/5605.html. HFEA's review on the restrictions governing gamete donation.

28 http://www.hfea.gov.uk/1411.html. The HFEA on egg-sharing schemes.

29 http://www.bionews.org.uk/page_57629.asp. Egg-sharing and the sale of gametes from *BioNews*.

30 http://news.bbc.co.uk/1/hi/health/3031800.stm. BBC report on the use of eggs from aborted foetuses.

31 http://www.dailymail.co.uk/sciencetech/article-1223617/No-men-OR-women-needed-artificial-sperm-eggs-created-time.html. Report on the development of artificial gametes from the *Daily Mail*.

32 http://wadhaf.com/archives/1926. *Guardian* report on the first sperm cells grown in the laboratory.

33 http://www.telegraph.co.uk/health/women_shealth/8004552/Artificial-ovary-gives-fertility-hope-to-cancer-sufferers.html. *Telegraph* report on artificial ovaries.

34 http://www.newscientist.com/article/dn3700-stem-cells-can-become-normal-sperm.html. A report on artificial sperm from the *New Scientist*.

35 http://www.hfea.gov.uk/docs/Hybrids_Report.pdf. The HFEA report on hybrids and chimera.

36 http://www.mrkh.org/. The website for the Mayer–Rokitansky–Kuster–Hauser Syndrome Organization in the United States.

37 It may, in the relatively near future, be possible for such women to have a womb transplant from living or dead donors.

38 http://www.hfea.gov.uk/fertility-treatment-options-surrogacy.html. The HFEA site on surrogacy.

39 http://www.surrogacyuk.org/. The website of the Surrogacy UK organisation.

40 http://mmabbasi.com/2010/07/30/world-centre-of-surrogacy-tourism-will-introduce-radical-legislation-to-regulate-1–5bn-industry/. A report on surrogacy tourism to India.

41 http://www.surrogacy.com/. The website of a surrogacy clinic in the United States.

42 http://www.marieclaire.com/world-reports/news/international/womb-rent-india-6. Adapted from an article on surrogacy in *Marie Claire* magazine.

43 http://www.bionews.org.uk/page_54221.asp. Information on when surrogacy goes wrong from *BioNews*.

44 http://writ.news.findlaw.com/grossman/20100119.html. An article on Baby M and recent court rulings in the United States on surrogacy.

45 http://www.timesonline.co.uk/tol/life_and_style/health/article6319240.ece. An article mentioning suspicions of the social surrogacy phenomenon.

46 http://www.dailymail.co.uk/tvshowbiz/article-1292094/Cristiano-Ronaldo-father-paying-surrogate-baby.html. A report on Ronaldo's surrogacy arrangements from the *Daily Mail*.

47 http://www.timesonline.co.uk/tol/news/uk/article560384.ece. A *Times* newspaper report on artificial wombs.

    http://www.informaworld.com/smpp/section?content=a770467448&fulltext=713240928. Landau, R. (2007) Artificial womb versus natural birth: an exploratory study of women's views. *Journal of Reproductive and Infant Psychology*, **25**:1, 4–17.

Further reading and useful websites

Day-Sclater, S., Ebtehaj, F., Jackson, E. and Richards, M. (2009) *Regulating Autonomy: Sex, Reproduction and Family.* Oxford: Hart Publishing.

Ehrensaft, D. (2005) *Mommies, Daddies, Donors, Surrogates.* New York: Guilford Press.

McWhinnie, A. M. (2006) *Who am I? Experiences of Donor Conception.* London: Idreos Education Trust.

http://corethics.org/. Comment on reproductive ethics, a website from a group who see 'absolute respect for the human embryo as a principal tenet'.

http://humupd.oxfordjournals.org/cgi/content/short/9/4/397. The website of the journal *Human Reproductive Update* from the European Society of Human Reproduction and Embryology.

http://news.bbc.co.uk/1/hi/health/3853237.stm. A BBC report on fertility tourism.

11 Screening and embryo selection: eliminating disorders or people?

Objectives

In reading this chapter you will:

- learn about pre-implantation genetic diagnosis;
- consider whether it is morally acceptable to select against embryos with diseases and disabilities;
- reflect on whether good intentions make an action morally acceptable;
- ask about the value of a life compromised by disease or disability;
- reflect on whether diseases and/or disabilities are socially constructed;
- consider the moral acceptability of 'saviour siblings' and gender selection.

In 2003 the Human Genome Project was completed.[1] It sequenced and mapped the human genome, demonstrating there are fewer genes than expected (25–26,000 instead of 80,000–140,000), and that 50% of the genome consists of 'non-coding DNA', repeated sequences of DNA that do not code for proteins. The next step – already well advanced – is to identify the functions of the genes that make up the genome, their interactions with each other and with the environment.

We shall be discussing the activities made possible by our understanding of human genetics in several parts of this book. In this chapter we shall consider only using genetic information to test embryos before implantation, and selecting for and against embryos on the basis of such tests.

Pre-natal testing, genetic diagnosis and embryo selection

In the 1980s it became possible for doctors to diagnose various genetic and chromosomal disorders in very early embryos produced in vitro. The procedure is known as pre-implantation genetic diagnosis, or PGD (sometimes PID). In this procedure a single cell is removed from an eight-cell embryo and analysed genetically. Removal of this cell does not affect the development of the embryo.[2] Recently a different technique, karyomapping, which, it is hoped, will make the process more effective, has been under development.[3]

Box 11.1 Factual information: Pre-natal testing

Before Pre-Implantation Genetic Diagnosis (PGD or PID) was developed embryos at risk could be tested by amniocentesis and chorionic villus sampling (CVS). Both techniques are invasive and carry a high risk of miscarriage.[4]

If these procedures indicate a risk the parent can go ahead or opt for an abortion.

These techniques are far from accurate. Estimates suggest that in the UK about 400 healthy babies a year are aborted after tests suggest they are at risk of some disease or disability.[5]

PGD and karyomapping allow a couple who know their embryos to be at risk to undergo IVF to produce several embryos.[6] These embryos are then tested and one or two healthy embryos selected for implantation. Other healthy embryos, if any, can be frozen for later use or donated to others (see Chapter 10). Embryo(s) with diseases and disabilities are discarded. By such means parents avoid the trauma of having a child with a disease or disability without having to have an abortion.[7]

We shall start by discussing the moral acceptability of selecting *against* embryos, then turn to that of selecting *for* embryos.

Box 11.2 Factual information: Genetic testing and screening

DNA genetic testing and genetic screening involve the same testing processes to confirm or refute a suspected DNA change. Tissues tested include blood, skin, saliva and hair follicles and, prenatally, embryo, placental tissue and amniotic fluid; DNA can be tested using blood.

Genetic screening is done for a particular condition in individuals, groups or populations *without* family history of the condition.

Genetic testing is done for a particular condition where an individual is suspected of being at increased risk due to their family history or the result of a genetic screening test.

Direct gene testing looks at the presence or absence of a known gene mutation by examining the sequence of letters in the information in the gene.

The test is very accurate and used for diagnosis and screening including prenatal, genetic carrier testing and screening, presymptomatic and predictive testing.

Limitations include:

- interpretation of the test result, e.g. finding that a person has a faulty gene does not always relate to how a person is, or will be, affected by that condition;
- the testing may be time-consuming and expensive for the health service if not for the patient;
- for some complex conditions, e.g. cancer, the testing may have to be done on a family member with the condition to identify a family-specific mutation in the gene (mutation searching) before unaffected family members can be offered predictive testing.

Indirect gene tracking (linkage) relies on comparing DNA markers from family members with the condition to markers in unaffected relatives. Used in situations where the gene itself has not been precisely located or where mutation(s) in a gene have not yet been defined, the test is not as accurate as direct gene testing but can be used in diagnosis including pre-natal and presymptomatic and predictive testing.

It may not always be possible to find DNA markers that enable the scientists to tell the difference between the faulty gene copy and the working gene copy.

Selection against

. . . .

Some people have objected to PGD and other genetic tests for fear of a slippery slope.[8] We might start by discarding embryos with nasty diseases, they think, but end by eliminating redheads because of the prejudice against 'gingers'.[9]

But the use of PGD depends on IVF. IVF is risky, unpleasant and costly. It is implausible to expect people will use it to eliminate trivial conditions, or even non-trivial conditions whose effects are far in the future or manageable in some other way. How many parents would deem it worth going through IVF to eliminate embryos who may develop Alzheimer's disease (which usually reveals itself in the 80s),[10] breast cancer[11] or heart disease (both of which develop in mid-life and can be managed in other ways)?

It is also, of course, possible to regulate PGD in such a way that use of it for trivial purposes is illegal.

If a couple are using IVF and PGD to guard against serious, unmanageable and immediately threatening genetic conditions, they *may* decide also to discard embryos with red hair (or Alzheimer's). But given they underwent IVF to produce a healthy child this seems unlikely. Given the tiny number of people at risk of serious genetic diseases, even if a few did discard red-headed embryos this would not impact significantly on the number of redheads.[12]

In a society that permits abortion it would seem particularly odd to ban PGD for fear it would lead to discarding embryos for supposedly trivial conditions: if PGD were banned, parents determined not to have a child with a given condition would simply opt for abortion.

PGD, it seems, is likely only to be used to identify and discard embryos with seriously disabling diseases and disabilities.[13] Given this, we might wonder how there could be any moral objection to it? Surely any procedure that could (in principle) rid the world of Huntington's disease[14] must be morally acceptable?

But we saw earlier (Box 7.14) that in considering the moral acceptability of an action the way we describe the action can be crucial. Some descriptions tempt us to think the argument is one-sided (see Box 11.3 if you'd like to try redescribing an act so as to strip it of its real import). But this is rarely the case. The use of PGD and embryo selection could, in principle, rid the world of Huntington's disease.[15] But so, in principle, would shooting everyone with the HD gene.

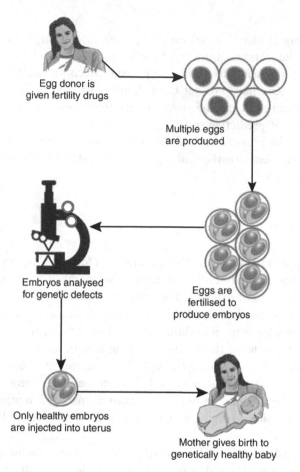

Egg donor is
given fertility drugs

Multiple eggs
are produced

Embryos analysed
for genetic defects

Eggs are
fertilised to
produce embryos

Only healthy embryos
are injected into uterus

Mother gives birth to
genetically healthy baby

Figure 11.1 Preimplantation genetic diagnosis involves screening embryos for genetic defects.
© HowStuffWorks 2001.

Some people believe that using PGD to select against embryos because they have diseases and disabilities is no different from shooting people with the HD gene.

Box 11.3 Activity: Small group work

In groups of four think of an activity you believe to be morally wrong (murdering grandmothers, robbing blind people, pushing children off bicycles. . .).

Now describe these actions so as to strip them of their moral import ('I was teaching the child how to handle the unexpected. . .').

Each group should choose two contributions to present to the rest of the class.

The class might then discuss situations in which actions have been re-described in attempts to exonerate the perpetrators. (e.g. the Nazi claim that they were 'just obeying orders'). The discussion might also consider how one person's terrorist is another person's freedom fighter.

The point is to teach participants to guard against allowing descriptions to influence their moral reasoning.

Many people miss this because they confuse:

(i) **genetic engineering** in which we transform a child who would have had a disease or disability into a child without that disease or disability;

and

(ii) **PGD and embryo selection** in which we discard – i.e. kill – an embryo who would have developed into a child with a disease or disability.

In the first case there is a given embryo who, without the intervention, would develop into a person with some disease or disability and who, with the intervention, will develop into a person who does not have any disease or disability.

In the second case there is a given embryo who, without the intervention, would develop into a person with some disease or disability and who, with the intervention, will die.

In using PGD to select against embryos with the genetic make-up that would lead to certain diseases we are not eliminating *diseases*, we are eliminating *embryos with diseases*. There is an important moral difference.

The right to life

There is a major disanalogy, of course, between shooting everyone with Huntington's disease and discarding embryos after PGD because they have some disease or disability. The first violates the undoubted right to life of those being shot. But very early embryos do not obviously *have* the right to life.

Anyone who believes that early embryos have the right to life will believe that PGD is as morally problematic as shooting those with HD. But if you believe the right to life emerges only at the 14th day or some later stage you will reject the idea that embryos destroyed at the eight-cell stage of development had the right to life.

Box 11.4 Activity: Creative writing

Imagine you are an embryo with Huntington's disease. Write a 500-word piece on how you feel about discovering your parents are trying to decide whether to use PGD and embryo selection to discard embryos like you.

There is no need to repeat our discussion of the moral status of the embryo (see Chapter 7 pages 104–113). Instead let's ask whether those who *deny* the right to life to the early embryo could themselves have reason to find PGD morally unacceptable.

Consider the fact that someone can consistently be pro-abortion yet morally outraged by the routine abortion of female embryos. In India, for example, it is estimated that ten million girls have been aborted over the last two decades.[16] To find this morally unacceptable is not necessarily to think that the females aborted had the right to life. It might be to think that being female is not a morally acceptable reason to abort a foetus.

Analogously, we might think that discarding embryos because they have diseases or disabilities is morally unacceptable because someone's being disabled or having a disease does not justify killing them.

Box 11.5 Philosophical background: Arguments from analogy

An argument from analogy identifies a similarity between two things and concludes that they are probably similar in some other respect. The most famous argument from analogy is probably that used by William Paley to argue for the existence of God.

That argument went:

Premise one: A pocket watch is so complex that it must have had an intelligent maker.
Premise two: The universe is at least as complex as a pocket watch.
Conclusion: Therefore the universe must also have had an intelligent maker.

Arguments from analogy are *inductive* arguments. As with all inductive arguments the premises of an analogy can be strong or weak reason to believe the conclusion. See Chapter 5, pages 62–64.

A revival of Nazi eugenics?

This suggests that rather than think of PGD as the alleviation of suffering we might instead, and just as accurately, think of it as the revival of Nazi eugenics. The Nazis sent many people to the gas chambers because they had diseases and disabilities. In the eyes of the Nazis the lives of such people were worthless. For this (and other things) the Nazis were vilified the world over.

But in condoning the use of PGD to identify and kill embryos because they have disease and disabilities, would we not be guilty of the very same thing?[17]

It is true that those *we* kill know nothing about being killed whereas many of the Nazis' victims were agonisingly aware of their imminent death. But would the Nazis' actions have been morally acceptable had they done what they did in such a way that their victims were oblivious to their deaths? Would it have been OK if they did it while their victims slept?

Or we might try to justify our use of PGD by claiming that we are doing it for the sake of those we kill. It might seem obvious that anyone who could choose to live without a disease or disability would choose that over living with the disease or disability.

But as we saw above in PGD this isn't the choice: the choice is between living with a disease or disability, and not living *at all.*

However, we might still think that if it were us, we *would* choose not to live rather than to live with a given disease or disability: 'I'd rather be dead' is not a thought foreign to us.

But if you ask those *without* a given disease or disability what life would be like with that disease or disability, people will usually demonstrate pessimism about whether life would be worth living. Those lucky enough to be healthy cannot imagine how it could be possible to live satisfactory lives were we less lucky.

There was a time when it was not deemed necessary to consult with those who actually had diseases or disabilities (the 'does he take sugar?' days). But just as feminists have persuaded us we should listen to the views of women as well as men, disability rights activists are trying to persuade us we should listen to those with disease and disabilities, as well as those who are able-bodied.[18]

Try asking a teenager with cystic fibrosis whether her life is worth living. If you're lucky enough to pin her down as she leaves for an evening out, she'll laugh at the thought that it isn't, even if she has spent an hour that day enduring a vigorous massage to remove mucus from her lungs, has to take pills with every meal, and has had to come to terms with the probability that she will die young.[19] Just watch a few young adults with Down's syndrome, smiling and laughing; it will be obvious that they love the lives they have, however restricted those lives are by our lights. We may express horror at the thought of becoming demented, but many people who are demented have no insight into their condition and clearly enjoy the lives they are leading.

According to the testimony of those with certain diseases and disabilities, then, their lives are far from valueless. The idea that they would choose never to have lived, rather than to live the life they do live, the only life they *could* live, is ruled out by such testimony.

Box 11.6 Case study: Christopher Nolan

Christy Nolan was deprived of oxygen at birth and suffered from cerebral palsy. Nolan couldn't walk, talk or use his hands. He spent his short life (he died aged 43 in 2008) in a wheelchair.

Until Nolan was 11 he couldn't communicate with words at all. Then a new drug Lioresal made it possible for him to use a 'unicorn stick' on a headband.

In 1987, with the help of his mother Bernadette, Nolan published his autobiography entitled *Under The Eye of the Clock.* Nolan's mother held his head whilst he picked out the letters he wanted. He managed a couple of pages a day.

The book won the Whitbread Award and was described as 'astonishing' for its extraordinary use of language, comparable, it was said, to Yeats and Joyce.

Here is Nolan's description of the process of writing:

'My mind is just like a spin-dryer at full speed; my thoughts fly around my skull while millions of beautiful words cascade into my lap. Images gunfire across my consciousness. Try then to give expression to that avalanche in efforts of one great nod after another.'

It is undeniable, of course, that there *are* diseases and disabilities that are incompatible with a worthwhile life. Tay Sachs disease leads to certain death by the age of 4 after the child has become progressively paralysed, deaf and blind. It is difficult to imagine that such a life could be deemed worthwhile even from the point of view of the one whose life it is. It also seems reasonable to think that anencephaly, the condition of being born without a functioning cerebellum, is incompatible with a worthwhile life.

But the existence of such diseases and disabilities does not detract from the fact that the vast majority of genetic diseases and disabilities are entirely consistent with a life that, *seen from the point of view of the one who will live it*, is entirely worthwhile.

Once this is accepted it might not seem so straightforwardly morally acceptable to discard or abort embryos with diseases and disabilities. At the very least the claim that in discarding them we are attempting to alleviate *their* suffering will not stand up. Indeed this claim, if it is not just confused, starts to look unbearably self-serving.

Morality and intention

We have been suggesting that we might distinguish morally between Nazi eugenics and parents' use of PGD on the grounds of their intentions. Most people who use PGD would be horrified at being compared to the Nazis.

But even if we assume the vast majority of parents who use PGD have benign intentions, we can't assume this clinches the case for the moral acceptability of PGD. If, in shooting those with Huntington's disease, we sincerely intended to eliminate suffering would this make it morally OK? If the gas chambers were sincerely intended to relieve the suffering of the Jews would this make the Nazi actions acceptable?

Box 11.7 Philosophical background: Intentions and moral evaluability

If you read Chapter 4 you will know that ethical theories differ in their attitudes towards the intentions with which actions are performed.

Utilitarians evaluate actions morally only by appeal to the consequences of that action, not by intentions.

Deontologists do evaluate actions by their intentions. Kant, for example, believes that an action is only right if it is performed out of 'reverence for the law'.

Here is an imaginary situation that might support the deontological position:

> Two friends are walking down the road towards each other. At the place where they meet sits a beggar and her child. Each friend gives the beggar a £1 coin. One of them does this because he wants to impress his friend. The other because he believes it is the right thing to do.

Question: are the actions of the two friends morally alike?

The utilitarian cannot distinguish these two actions morally unless they differ in their consequences.

The deontologist would argue that the action of the person who tried to impress his friend was self-seeking and not a moral action at all, whilst the other action was morally admirable because it was performed because the agent believed it to be right.

The virtue ethicist could also distinguish the two actions by arguing that the person who acted to impress his friend did not act virtuously.

Caring for those with diseases and disabilities

Even if we can't reasonably claim that in using PGD to select against embryos with diseases and disabilities we are trying to save *them* from suffering, perhaps we could claim that we are attempting to alleviate *our own* suffering? When parents discard an embryo with a disease or a disability they might do so because they think their marriage might not stand the strain of caring for such a child, or that they will focus on this child to the detriment of their other children. Or they might believe they would not be able to be decent parent to such a child. Or they might simply believe that their own lives would not be worth living if they had to care for such a child.[20]

It is possible to imagine any number of motivations of this sort, all of them compatible with the belief that the embryo, allowed to live, would have a worthwhile life.

In many societies the lives of people who care for those with debilitating diseases or disabilities can be almost intolerable. Carers complain of having no social life, of having to give up work, of finding themselves penniless and of having to deal with endlessly frustrating petty administrative duties. Some carers argue that being a carer can be almost as disabling as suffering from the disease itself.

Is it morally contemptible to use PGD and embryo selection to avoid having to become a carer? Can such a person be compared to the Nazis? Most people wouldn't think so. A parent who decides to go ahead with a baby who will have to be cared for throughout its life may be especially praiseworthy for performing a supererogatory act (see Box 11.8). It is surely not right to condemn the actions of those who find themselves unable to do this.[21]

Box 11.8 Philosophical background: Supererogatory actions

We can categorise actions morally as follows:

- actions that are good to do and bad not to do (required);
- actions that are neither good to do nor bad not to do (permissible);
- actions that are bad to do and good not to do (forbidden).

Some philosophers, however, would like to add another category:

- actions that are good to do but not bad not to do.

This last category is that of the *supererogatory*. You perform a supererogatory act whenever you go beyond the call of duty, you do *more* than is morally required of you.

The soldier who throws himself on an exploding hand-grenade to save others is performing a supererogatory act. His action is not morally required, because he could not be blamed for not doing it. For doing it he deserves extra praise.

It is the performance of supererogatory acts that attracts the appellation 'saint' or 'hero'.

It wouldn't only be the parents who would have to care for the child, of course. Eventually, even if only when the parents died, the state would become involved. Money that could be spent on other things would have to be spent on catering for the person who would not have been born had PGD been used to select against him at birth. There is a sense in which *all* of us will suffer if we allow that person to be born, if only because he or she will use more resources than a healthy person.

Perhaps then, an embryo's having a disease or a disability *does* give us a moral licence to kill that embryo, not to alleviate *its* suffering, but to alleviate the suffering of those who will have to care for it, and to avoid its becoming a burden on society?

Box 11.9 Activity: Research

Go to the website of an organisation such as Carers UK (http://www.carersuk.org/Home) or the Princess Royal Trust for Carers (http://www.carers.org/), log onto a 'chat zone' and read the postings from the many carers who use these sites.

You might also post a request for them to tell you something of their lives, explaining why you need the information.

Having gathered the information write a short essay (500 words) about what it is like to be a carer. Say in particular whether you think the downside of caring justifies the use of PGD to select against those with diseases and disabilities.

The social status of caring

But at this point we might ask another question: isn't there something wrong with a society in which caring for someone with a disease or a disability is so distressing that it is better for us to deprive those with diseases and disabilities of the only life they'd be able to have? Isn't there something wrong with our values if the only way we can think of to deal with the distress of caring is to eliminate those who need care?

We should remember, of course, that we are never going to be able successfully to eliminate the need to care for others. Not so long as people are helpless when young, and often also when old, and so long as people have accidents. Perhaps the better thing would be to do something to make caring less distressing? In fact we might think the only truly moral thing to do would be to rearrange things so that carers can live worthwhile lives consistently with caring for loved ones.

Were we successfully to improve the lot of carers, parents would have less incentive to undergo the discomforts of IVF and PGD to select against embryos that might need extra care. We would also, perhaps, eliminate some of the fear we have of becoming old and helpless, knowing that in doing so we will almost certainly become a burden on those we love.

> ### Box 11.10 Activity: Film review
>
> Get hold of a copy of the film 'Logan's Run' (in which people over 30 are disposed of so they don't become a burden on society). Write a 500 word review of it. Consider especially whether it is acceptable to eliminate people because they are about to become a burden.

But once we get on to this question, there is a related question that is even more pressing: to what extent is society responsible for the very existence of disabling diseases and conditions?

The social character of diseases and disabilities

Some disability rights activists would say that many conditions that are currently disabling are so only because of the way society is set up.[22] Consider this extract from a letter written to the author in the 1970s:

'When I arrived in Sweden I was astonished by the number of people in wheelchairs. They seemed to be everywhere. I speculated on why this should be so. I considered whether it was something in the water, some function of the Swedish upbringing, or whether the accident rate was just extraordinarily high. After a while the truth dawned on me: the incidence of wheelchair use is no higher in Sweden than in England, it's just that in Sweden people in wheelchairs can get out and about.'

The writer graphically illustrates the contribution the social environment can make to whether a physical impairment becomes a disability. In Sweden being in a wheelchair is less of a disability than it is elsewhere because in Sweden people in wheelchairs are catered for.[23] If a society doesn't cater well for people in wheelchairs, such people are invisible and largely excluded from many activities the rest of us consider unexceptional, such as going to the cinema or travelling by train. If a society does cater well for such people, being unable to walk is far less disabling.

Another tale further illustrates this point. In his excellent book *Choosing Children: Genes, Disability and Design* Jonathan Glover[24] describes the fact that in Martha's Vineyard in the late nineteenth century hereditary deafness meant that one person in every 155 was born deaf. So many people were deaf that even hearing people picked up sign language and, according to a report written in 1985, the two became so 'mingled' that both were used in conversation almost unconsciously. Deafness was so common, and its drawbacks so catered for, that someone was able to say in an interview 'Oh those people weren't handicapped, they were just deaf'.

Were we to adopt the view that those who differ from 'normal' people are not disabled but merely different, and were we to start catering for them, the incentive to undergo IVF in order to 'discard' those with differences would decrease. Not only will the value of the lives of those with physical impairments be more obvious, such people will need much less care because independence will be much easier.[25]

Of course even if we can minimise the disabling effects of various physical impairments, we might still insist that there is little we can do about genetic diseases.

But even here we might ask whether the appropriate response to this isn't to put more effort into curing these diseases. The fewer people who are born with these diseases, of course, the less incentive there is for pharmaceutical companies to invest money and time in searching for a cure.[26] The less likely it is that we will find a cure, the more reasonable it might seem simply to discard embryos with the disease.

Armed with PGD and other technologies that make it easy for us to eliminate those who might become a burden on the rest of us, it would be very easy for us to travel the route of seeing such elimination as the only sensible way to behave. Once we start to think like this our actions could spiral us into a situation in which suffering of any kind is deemed unacceptable. Yet throughout the ages suffering has often been seen as an essential precursor to wisdom.[27] Each of us, perhaps, will have stories about how we have, by going through hardship, emerged as better people.

There are all sorts of reasons, therefore, to stop and think about whether using PGD to identify and eliminate those with diseases and disabilities is the right response to these diseases and disabilities. Science and technology might be used just as effectively, after all, to cure, or mitigate the effects of, the diseases and disabilities. In a society in which physical impairments are not allowed to become disabilities, no one need suffer the indignity of becoming a 'burden'.

Box 11.11 Factual information: The Disability Discrimination Act

In 1995 The Disability Discrimination Act[28] came into force in the UK. This act gave disabled people the right not to be discriminated against:

- in accessing everyday goods and services provided by local councils, doctors' surgeries, shops, hotels, banks, pubs, post offices, theatres, hairdressers, places of worship, schools, courts and voluntary groups such as play groups. Non-educational services provided by schools are also included;
- in buying or renting land or property;
- in accessing or becoming a member of a private club;
- in accessing the functions of public bodies.

Under the DDA, it is illegal for service providers to treat disabled people less favourably than other people for a reason related to their disability.[29]

Under the Act service providers must make all the 'reasonable adjustments' needed to make it possible for disabled people to access their services including:

- providing induction loops for the hearing impaired;
- giving the option to book tickets by email as well as by phone;
- providing disability awareness training for staff;
- providing larger, well-defined signage for people with impaired vision;
- putting in a ramp at the entrance to a building as well as steps.

Failure or refusal to provide a service that is offered to other people to a disabled person is discrimination unless it can be justified.

Differences or disabilities?

But in the context of a worry about which conditions might be considered disabling enough to warrant elimination we might reconsider the slippery slope argument with which we started.

We noted earlier the outrage some people feel about the routine abortion of foetuses because they are female. We feel outraged by this because we reject the idea that being female is inconsistent with living a worthwhile life. We reject the idea that being female is a *disability* of any kind, we see it as nothing more than a *difference*.

But there are cultures in which being female *is* undeniably disabling. Would you have wanted to be female in the days when you had little choice but to produce children year in year out, when work outside the home was either not an option, or mandated by poverty and not in the slightest bit fulfilling? Would you want to be female in Taliban-governed Afghanistan where, in 2007, at least 184 Afghan women preferred to die by self-immolation than live the lives they were living?[30]

We also think of being homosexual as nothing more than a difference, but in some societies it is undoubtedly disabling: in Iran for example it is a hanging offence, even for people as young as 15.[31]

Naturally we want to say that these societies have it wrong. We will insist there is nothing intrinsically disabling about being female or about being homosexual; if being female or being homosexual is disabling, this is because of the way the society is set up. The cure is to change society not to accept that it is reasonable to abort foetuses because they are female or homosexual.

At this point we might start to think that our own attitudes towards the diseased and disabled might be deemed analogous to these other cultures' attitudes towards females and homosexuals. Perhaps our great-grandchildren will think that we are as bigoted in our views on those with physical impairments as we think the Nazis were in relation to their views on Jews or the Talib are in their views on women?

To assume that a condition is necessarily disabling, or that caring for someone with such a condition is necessarily catastrophic, is an assumption that we make within the context of a society in which both these things are true. But there is no obvious reason why either *must* be true. No doubt bringing about a society in which physical impairments are not disabling would incur huge expense and upheaval. But it wasn't easy or cheap to give women the vote either...

> ## Box 11.12 Activity: Group discussion
>
> Consider again the analogy we considered on page 186:
>
> > **Premise one:** Being female is not a morally acceptable reason for aborting an early embryo.
> > **Premise two:** Aborting an embryo because it has a disease or a disability is like aborting an embryo because it is female.
> > **Conclusion:** It's having a disease or disability is not a morally acceptable reason for aborting an early embryo.
>
> Discuss in class the truth of the second premise of this argument. The exercise could also be done by exchanging 'female' for 'homosexual' or another condition that would make the exercise more meaningful to participants.

Selection for

In the UK recently there has been a major debate about the extent to which deafness is a difference or a disability. The debate was triggered by the desire of a deaf couple to use PGD to select *for* a deaf baby. We shall consider this debate by considering the newspaper article reproduced in the box.

Box 11.13 Case study: 'Of course a deaf couple want a deaf child'

Adapted from the article by Dominic Lawson *The Independent* Tuesday 11 March 2008. http://www.independent.co.uk/opinion/commentators/dominic-lawson/dominic-lawson-of-course-a-deaf-couple-want-a-deaf-child-794001.html.

Few broadcasters convey outrage as skillfully as the BBC's John Humphrys. Yesterday it was not a politician who got Humphrys to hit his top note. It was a bloke called Tomato – Mr Tomato Lichy, to be precise. The programme's listeners never heard Mr Lichy speak: he answered Humphrys' questions in sign language, and someone translated his answers into spoken English for our benefit.

Tomato Lichy and his partner Paula are both deaf, as is their child Molly. Paula is in her 40s and the couple believe they might require IVF treatment to produce a second child. They very much want this child to be deaf and are prepared to undergo IVF to achieve this.

Here's where it gets political: the Government is whipping through a new Human Fertilisation and Embryology Bill. Clause 14/4/9 states that, 'Persons or embryos that are known to have a gene, chromosome or mitochondrion abnormality involving a significant risk that a person with the abnormality will have or develop a serious physical or mental disability, a serious illness or any other serious medical condition must not be preferred to those that are not known to have such an abnormality.'

This, Tomato Lichy signed to Mr Humphrys, means that he and Paula would be legally obliged to discard the very embryos they wished to implant: 'I couldn't participate in any procedure which forced me to reject a deaf embryo in favour of a hearing embryo.' Mr. Lichy argued this legislation was discrimination against deafness. He's quite right.

The explanatory notes to the clause inform legislators: 'Outside the UK, the positive selection of deaf donors in order deliberately to result in a deaf child has been reported. This provision would prevent (embryo) selection for a similar purpose.'

This stems from a case in the US when a lesbian couple, Sharon Duchesneau and Candace McCullough, both deaf, selected a sperm donor for his family history of deafness.

In an email interview in the *Lancet* Duchesneau and McCullough wrote: 'Most of the ethical issues that have been raised in regard to our story centre on the idea that being deaf is a negative thing. From there, people surmise that it is unethical to want to create deaf children, who are, in their view, disabled.

'Our view is that being deaf is a positive thing, with many wonderful aspects. We don't view being deaf along the same lines as being blind or mentally retarded; we see it as more like Jewish or black.'

This is a clear exposition of the concept of 'cultural deafness'. Adherents of this philosophy believe themselves to be members of a 'linguistic community'. Mr. Lichy said he felt 'sorry for' John Humphrys for not being able to appreciate 'deaf plays'. The proponents of cultural deafness, in virtue of their separate language, describe themselves as an ethnic minority. This makes any legislative attempt to weed them out as embryos analogous with the most insidious racism.

In the most obvious sense, the argument that deafness is not a disability is self-evidently wrong. The absence of one of our most valuable senses brings with it many practical disadvantages. A deaf boy might have fantasies about being a soldier or a fireman, but fantasies are what they will remain. Humphrys tasked Tomato Lichy with the fact he would never be able to enjoy the music of Beethoven – a low blow as Beethoven himself was tormented by increasing deafness.

But if you have never been able to hear music, then you cannot be said to miss it. I know one or two people, completely tone deaf, who are not in the least miserable about it: their only irritation lies in having to hear 'noise' rather than silence. The idea that congenitally deaf people are 'suffering' strikes me as mere presumption.

It is not as if the implantation of an embryo thought likely to be deaf is equivalent to deliberate mutilation. The choice isn't whether that embryo could be 'made deaf' or not. The choice is whether to discard an already existing embryo for another one believed to be less at risk of turning out to be deaf.

The real issue here is whether the state should be able to dictate to the Lichys which of their embryos to select, and which they should be compelled to reject. I am not surprised he can't understand why he and his partner should be legally prevented from choosing the embryo which might most turn out to resemble them.

John Humphrys argued that most people would regard his demands as profoundly selfish: Mr. Lichy and his partner might want a deaf child, but what about the views of the child itself? I suspect that the child in question would be intelligent enough to be able to understand that the only alternative deal for him or her was never to have existed at all.

It is clear that Mr Lichy and his partner believe that deafness is a difference not a disability. If so then why shouldn't they be able to select *for* rather than *against* a child who is deaf? In the same way a homosexual couple might want to select for a child who is gay. Many parents would want a child who resembles them in some way, especially perhaps in the ways that they consider to be an important part of their identity.

> ### Box 11.14 Activity: Playing devil's advocate
>
> *Tomato and Paula Lichy should be able to select for a deaf child.*
>
> Participants should be allocated to one or other side of this argument without reference to their actual beliefs. Otherwise the discussion should be a free one with all participants invited to contribute.

Saviour siblings

IVF and PGD can also be used to identify and select for embryos who are immunologically compatible with another person, and therefore able to provide stem cells to treat that person.[32] 'Saviour siblings', for example, are children who are born, as the result of IVF and PGD, to save the life of a sibling.[33]

Box 11.15 Case study: The Whitakers

Jamie Whitaker was born in 2003 so that he could save the life of Charlie, his older brother.[34]

Charlie has Diamond–Blackfan anaemia (DBA), a rare genetic condition treatable only by a stem cell transplant from a matching donor.

The boys' parents, Michelle and Jayson Whitaker, selected the embryo that became Jamie, after IVF undertaken solely in the hope of producing a genetic match for Charlie.

The Whitakers had to travel to the United States for treatment because the Human Embryo and Fertilisation Authority in the UK refused to grant the Whitakers' application because there would be no direct benefit to the unborn child.[35]

The argument against this use of PGD is based on the idea that the saviour sibling is being used as a means to others' ends. It seems undeniable, in fact, that the 'saviour' child is being used as a means to the ends of its parents and its sibling.[36] You might like to remind yourself about this Kantian requirement by re-reading Chapter 4, pp. 37–42.

In evaluating the moral acceptability of this it is important to recognise that the Kantian requirement always to treat others as ends in themselves is consistent with treating them *also* as a means to your own end. Every time you ask someone to do something for you, you treat them as a means to your own ends. What is important, from the Kantian point of view, is treating them *also* as ends in themselves. You do this by *asking* them if they will do something, by giving them the choice of saying 'no'. Anyone who responds to someone's request to lend them a pen is allowing himself to be treated as a means to someone else's end. But assuming he has chosen freely to lend the pen, he is also being treated as an end in himself.

But it is not possible to ask the saviour sibling for his consent to being used: until he is born he doesn't exist to have his consent sought.[37]

There is also a whiff of a slippery slope. If it is acceptable to use IVF and PGD to select for a child with a compatible immune system from whose umbilical cord stem cells can be taken, is it also acceptable to have a child because they have kidneys one of which could be used for a transplant into a sibling, or because it has a liver part of which could be used to provide a liver transplant? In discussing the ethical acceptability of 'saviour siblings' the chairman of the HFEA in the UK noted that such siblings might better be called 'spare-part sisters' or 'bred-to-order brothers'. Would such uses of a child be permissible?

We might say that no-one would prefer not to have been born than to have been born in order to be used as a means to someone else's end. But this claim might not be generally true: it depends on the way in which, and the extent to which, a child will be used as a means to the ends of others. If a saviour sibling, once it has served its purpose, is neglected and/or abused, or if something prevents it from serving its purpose and it is rejected, then this is morally unacceptable because the child clearly was being used *solely* as a means to the ends of others, in contravention of the Kantian maxim.

But where do we draw the line? At what stage do we call a halt to one child's being used as a means to the health of another? Does the difficulty of drawing this line suggest that saviour siblings should be banned completely?

> **Box 11.16 Activity: Writing a review**
>
> Read the book *My Sister's Keeper* by Jodi Picoult (2009) Hodder Paperbacks (or watch the film which is not so good – http://www.imdb.com/title/tt1078588/). Write a 500-word review of the book and/or use it to stimulate discussion.

Selecting for sex

We know that many embryos are selected against because they are female because in many cultures being female is considered intrinsically less valuable then being male. But not all sex selection is based on such a belief. Some parents wish to select for a sex for the purposes of balancing a family or in order to avoid a sex-linked condition such as haemophilia.[38]

There are two complications with permitting parents to select against embryos for the purposes of 'family balancing':

(i)   it is hard to distinguish those who have genuine reasons for wishing to select for a sex from those who believe one sex is intrinsically preferable;

(ii) it is socially valuable for there to be roughly equal numbers of males and females and nature is good at ensuring this.

The latter is a good reason, perhaps, for refusing to interfere with nature, especially in the light of the former. It is probably for this reason that many countries ban the use of PGD (and other methods such as sperm selection) to choose a baby's sex.[39] This does not, of course, stop people from travelling abroad to countries where they are permitted to choose the sex of their baby.

> ### Box 11.17 Activity: Group discussion
>
> In 2001 Alan and Louise Masterton applied to the HFEA in the UK to be allowed to use IVF and PGD to select the sex of a baby.[40] The Mastertons had four sons, and then 15 years later had had a much-wanted daughter, Nicole. Sadly Nicole died in a fire at 4-years-old. The Mastertons badly wanted to select for another daughter.
>
> Should the Mastertons have been granted their wish?

This concludes our discussion of the ethical and social issues attending PGD, and also of the issues that arise at the beginning of life. In the next chapter we shall turn to the issues that arise at the end of life.

Summary

In this chapter we have:

- distinguished between eliminating diseases by genetic engineering and eliminating embryos with diseases by PGD;

- noted that we can reject PGD even if we deny the right to life to embryos (because we object to eliminating embryos with the genetic make-up that will lead to diseases and disabilities);

- considered the analogy between Nazi eugenics and the use of PGD to eliminate embryos with diseases and disabilities;

- reflected on whether good intentions can make a wrong action into a right one;

- considered whether PGD is morally acceptable because it relieves the able-bodied of the burden of caring for someone, and society of the need to provide extra resources;

- wondered to what extent it is society that makes a physical impairment into a disability;

- reflected on the fact that some cultures see mere differences where others see disabilities.

Questions to stimulate reflection

Could permitting parents to use PGD to select against embryos with undesirable characteristics lead to parents using this technology to discard embryos for trivial reasons?

To what extent should intentions be counted in evaluating actions morally?

Assuming an early embryo has no right to life does it matter why we discard it?

Should a parent have the right to decide not to care for a diseased or disabled child?

To what extent are disabilities created by the social set-up? Could there ever be a society in which no physical impairment amounted to a disability?

Is it acceptable to bring a child into the world so it can save the life of a sibling?

Would it be short-sighted to permit sex selection given that nature is herself so good at balancing the sexes?

Why shouldn't a family with four sons choose the sex of their next child?

Additional activities

Listen to Women's Hour in the UK talk about karyomapping: http://www.bbc.co.uk/radio4/womanshour/04/2009_27_tue.shtml.

Conduct an opinion poll amongst your family and friends on whether selection for sex should be permitted.

Prepare a short presentation on PGD and eugenics using power point.

With a partner who disagrees with you discuss whether or not disabilities are social constructs.

Find out if there is a carers' centre near you. Ask if you might interview a carer about his or her caring responsibilities.

Conduct some web research on the disability rights movement.

Read Christy Nolan's book *Under the Eye of the Clock* (1988, Pan Books). Write a review.

Wear a blindfold for a day and with the help of a partner experience something of what it must be like to be blind. The following day help your partner experience the same thing.

Arrange a debate on whether it would be a good thing completely to eliminate suffering.

Notes

1   http://www.sanger.ac.uk/about/history/hgp/. The website of the Human Genome Project.
2   http://www.hfea.gov.uk/PGD.html. The HFEA on PGD.
3   http://www.timesonline.co.uk/tol/life_and_style/health/article5004111.ece. A *Times* report on karyomapping.
4   http://www.patient.co.uk/health/Pre-natal-Screening-and-Diagnosis-of-Down's-Syndrome.htm. A website about PGD and Down's Syndrome. http://www.down-syndrome.org/editorials/2087/. Research from Down Syndrome Education International.
5   http://www.down-syndrome.org/editorials/2087/. Research from Down Syndrome Education International.
6   The Children's Mercy Hospital in Kansas City, Missouri, have produced a low cost test which could be used to screen young people, before they become parents, for up to 600 disorders. Here is an article about this in Disabled World: http://www.disabled-world.com/editorials/genetic-screening.php.
7   http://www.beep.ac.uk/content/163.0.html. A case study from the Bioethics Education Project website.
8   http://www.independent.co.uk/life-style/health-and-families/health-news/embryo-selection-critics-fear-slippery-slope-1243030.html. An *Independent* article raising fears of a slippery slope.
9   http://news.bbc.co.uk/1/hi/england/2367917.stm. A BBC report of the discovery that an abortion had been carried out because a baby had a cleft palate. http://news.bbc.co.uk/1/hi/7918296.stm. A report on a US clinic offering PGD to choose eye colour.
10 http://www.timesonline.co.uk/tol/news/science/article1596809.ece. A couple who had PGD to avoid early onset Alzheimer's disease.
11 http://www.guardian.co.uk/science/2009/jan/10/pgd-baby-debate-breast-cancer. A *Guardian* report on the first baby born in the UK after PGD for breast cancer.
12 http://www.disabilitynow.org.uk/latest-news2/politics-1/matters-of-life-and-birth. An article on PGD from Disability Now.
13 http://scienceblog.cancerresearchuk.org/2009/01/30/brca1-free-birth-isnt-a-slippery-slope-to-designer-babies/. A Cancer Research UK article on PGD and slippery slopes.
14 http://www.hda.org.uk/. The Huntington's Disease Society website.
15 http://www.bbc.co.uk/health/physical_health/conditions/huntingtons1.shtml. The BBC health site on Huntington's disease.
16 http://news.bbc.co.uk/1/hi/world/south_asia/4592890.stm. A BBC report about the 10 million lost girls.
17 http://www.dailymail.co.uk/health/article-1249448/Eugenics-fear-British-couples-offered-online-gene-test-100-inherited-diseases.html. A *Daily Mail* article about a genetic testing kit for parents and the fear of eugenics.

18 http://www.independent.co.uk/opinion/commentators/clair-lewis-disabled-people-need-assistance-to-live-not-die-1911313.html. An *Independent* article on death and disability.

19 http://www.youth-web.org.uk/ashfield/index.html. A disability awareness site from Youth Web.

20 http://www.timesonline.co.uk/tol/life_and_style/article633433.ece. An article by the parent of a child with Down's syndrome.

21 http://www.cafamily.org.uk/index.php?section=861. A website for families of children with disabilities.

22 http://www.accessiblesociety.org/topics/demographics-identity/dkaplanpaper.htm. An essay on different models of disease and disability from the Centre for an Accessible Society.

23 http://sweden.gov.se/sb/d/2197/a/15254. Swedish Disability Policy.

24 Glover, J. (2006) *Choosing Children: Genes, Disability, and Design.* Oxford: Oxford University Press, pp. 6–7.

25 http://www.equalityhumanrights.com/scotland/projects-and-campaigns-in-scotland/capturing-the-gains-of-the-public-sector-duties-in-scotland/capturing-the-gains-case-studies/case-study-tayside-police/. A case study from Tayside Police who introduced an SMS text messaging service for deaf and hard-of-hearing people so communication would be easier.

26 http://www.wisegeek.com/what-is-an-orphan-disease.htm. A short account of 'orphan diseases' from wisegeek.com.

27 http://clarkescott.org/is-wisdom-really-necessary-in-order-to-generate-compassion/. A discussion of suffering, wisdom and compassion by a Buddhist monk.

28 http://www.inbrief.co.uk/disability-discrimination.htm. A brief description of the Disability Discrimination Act 1995.

29 http://www.direct.gov.uk/en/DisabledPeople/RightsAndObligations/DisabilityRights/DG_4001068. A description of the DDA from the UK government.

30 http://news.bbc.co.uk/1/hi/world/south_asia/7942819.stm. A BBC report on self-immolation by Afghan women.

31 http://www.ukgaynews.org.uk/archive/2005july/2101.htm. A report from *GayNews* on the hanging of two teenagers for being gay.

32 http://www.hfea.gov.uk/preimplantation-tissue-typing.html. The HFEA on saviour siblings.

33 http://news.bbc.co.uk/1/hi/health/4972142.stm. A BBC Q&A on saviour siblings.

34 http://news.bbc.co.uk/1/hi/health/3756556.stm. A BBC report of this case study.

35 http://www.independent.co.uk/opinion/leading-articles/the-law-on-designer-babies-should-be-changed--but-carefully-541244.html. An *Independent* article on the Whitakers' situation.

36 http://news.bbc.co.uk/1/hi/health/955644.stm. A BBC report on 'designer babies'.

37 http://biochem118.stanford.edu/Projects/2008/Elizabeth.pdf. A presentation on the ethical implications of PGD by Elizabeth Kersten of Stanford University.

38 http://www.fertility-docs.com/fertility_gender.phtml. A US website offering PGD for sex selection.

39 http://news.bbc.co.uk/1/hi/uk/7696698.stm. A BBC report on gender selection.

40 http://news.bbc.co.uk/1/hi/scotland/955672.stm. A BBC report on this case study.

Further reading and useful websites

Gavaghan, C. (2006) *Defending The Genetic Supermarket.* London: Routledge-Cavendish (you can find a review of this book here: http://www.bionews.org.uk/page_39410.asp).

Shakespeare, T. (2006) *Disability Rights and Wrongs.* London: Routledge.

Swain, J., French, S. and Cameron, C. (2003) *Controversial Issues in a Disabling Society (Disability, Human Rights & Society).* Maidenhead, UK: Open University Press.

Wilkinson, S. (2010) *Choosing Tomorrow's Children: The Ethics of Selective Reproduction (Issues in Biomedical Ethics).* Oxford: Oxford University Press.

http://bancroft.berkeley.edu/collections/drilm/index.html. The Disability Rights and Independent Living Movement based at Berkeley University in the United States.

http://www.debatingmatters.com/topicguides/topicguide/genetic_screening/. A 'Debating Matters' topic guide to genetic screening.

http://www.equalityhumanrights.com/. The Equality and Human Rights Commission in the UK (put 'case study' in the search facility for lots of case studies).

Section 3
Aging and death

12

Aging and immortality: the search for longevity

Objectives

In reading this chapter you will:

- reflect on the claims of those who promise a significant increase in longevity;
- consider whether you would like to live for 1000 (or even 150) years;
- examine the social consequences of everyone's having the choice of living much longer;
- examine the moral consequences of a significant increase in lifespan;
- consider whether a normal lifespan is part of what makes us human;
- ask yourself whether normal humans and 'immortal' humans could belong to the same species.

Having considered the ethical and social issues generated by biotechnology at the beginning of life, we shall now turn to the issues that arise at the end of life. In this chapter we shall consider the issues generated by the possibility of significantly extending our lives.

The possibility of 'eternal' life

If someone were to offer you the gift of eternal life, would you cry 'let me at it!' or would you be suspicious?

It wouldn't be unreasonable to be suspicious. Since the beginning of time people have sought the fountain of youth,[1] and so far all have been disappointed.[2] Quite a few scientists, however, believe the gift of all-but-eternal life is within our grasp not through magical potions but through genetic know-how.[3]

The bio-gerontologist Aubrey de Grey of Cambridge University[4] believes we are on the very verge of conquering death. He believes the first 'immortal' might already be 60.[5] Once we conquer death, according to de Grey, we will live on until, inevitably, we have an accident. He calculates (by extrapolating from teenage lifespans and accident rates generally) that the average lifespan will then be 1,000 plus.[6] Not quite immortality, but close. Perhaps if you were *very* risk-adverse you could achieve the real thing.

Many reject de Grey's claim that we could extend lifespan to this extent.[7] But most accept that it is already extending in the western world, and is likely to continue doing so for a while at least.[8]

Box 12.1 Activity: Brainstorm

Participants should imagine that someone offers them the gift of eternal life, but gives them only half an hour to decide whether or not to accept it.

In pairs participants should decide on the questions they would want answered before they accepted this gift.

The questions should then be collected and possible answers and responses to these answers brainstormed.

(This exercise will have more 'bite' if it is assumed that those to whom the gift of eternal life has been given cannot commit suicide.)

A poll on whether people would or wouldn't accept the gift might be taken before and after this exercise.

So obvious is it that we wouldn't want to live forever without being healthy that, for the sake of argument, we will stipulate that reasonable health is part of the package.[9] Imagine spending (at least) 900 of your 1,000 years (or 60 of your 150 years) in a nursing home for the demented: if health were not part of the package that's what most of us would do.[10] (Imagine the cost to the state.) The question we need to ask is whether it is morally acceptable to extend our lives in the light of this stipulation.

It seems hugely likely that given a guarantee of good health (and the option of suicide should it prove too much) most people would love to live longer. If you read about utilitarianism in Chapter 4 you will see that this gives us a prima facie utilitarian argument for claiming it is morally acceptable significantly to extend our lives: doing so would promote the greatest happiness of the greatest number.

The tragedy of the commons

To go from the claim that individuals believe they would be made happier by increasing longevity, however, to the claim that the greatest happiness of the greatest number would be served by increasing longevity, is to commit a fallacy.

Box 12.2 Philosophical background: The 'tragedy of the commons fallacy'

When people were free to graze their sheep on common land, everyone took to grazing as many sheep as they could, each believing their own happiness would be promoted by this.

Soon the land became over-grazed. The sheep started to starve and to die. People lost their livelihoods and eventually their lives.

The activity that might be chosen by each individual as contributing to his or her personal happiness does not necessarily produce the greatest happiness of the greatest number.[11]

Individuals might be happy initially to know that they are immortal, but their happiness might fade in discovering the impact of *everyone's* becoming immortal. Consider the effect on marriage of spouses living for 1,000 or even 150 years, on the economy of paying pensions for people who will live as long as this, on education of having to school such people, on the environment of all these extra people, their cars and their waste...

Box 12.3 Activity: Small group work

Every government has departments devoted to consideration of the impact of a new development on their area of remit.[12] Each of these departments will be headed by someone whose task it is to brief the head of government on this impact.

These 'areas of remit' will include: education, health, finance, social services; infrastructure (transport, towns and cities), security, international relations, culture, business...
Participants should be divided into groups, each group with one of these areas of remit. Each group should appoint one of their number as head.

The task is to discuss the possible impact of significantly increasing longevity (to an average of 150 years) on their area. The group head should report their findings to the group as a whole.

This exercise could be done over time: each group, for example, might have one week in which to prepare their report.

We might also consider the effect on political relationships between people both within and across nations. Conflict would certainly arise if only the rich were able to afford to make themselves immortal. de Grey believes that states would pretty soon be forced, through fear of political unrest, to make the intervention available to everyone. If so, this conflict would be short-lived. But there's plenty of scope for others...
Might we also see the emergence of intergenerational conflict[13] as older people take all the jobs and younger people have to wait for years (and years) to get proper jobs?[14] When older voters hugely outnumber younger voters, will the government ever be able to launch initiatives to benefit the young?[15] Won't the needs and wants of older

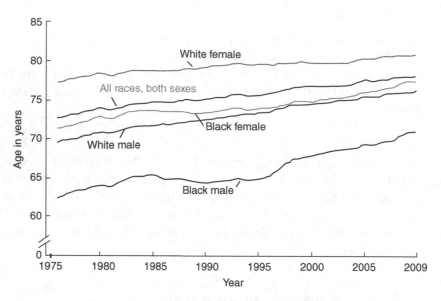

Figure 12.1 Life expectancy at birth, by race and sex: United States, 1975–2007 final and 2008–2009 preliminary results. US life expectancy at birth rose steadily between 1975 and 2007. The increase is due mainly to falling rates in almost all the leading causes of death. *Source:* Centers for Disease Control and Prevention, USA.

people always have to come first as a matter of political pragmatism?[16] Will states be able to afford *anything* much once they've paid all the pensions and provided housing for those who need it?

There would also be scope for conflict between nations. Even if rich nations were to provide life-extending treatment to all citizens, the poorer nations are unlikely to be able to do this. We would soon reach a stage where, in the developed nations, most citizens would be elderly (and, Fukuyama believes, female) and in the developing nations most citizens would be young (and Fukuyama believes, male). Fukuyama believes the developed nations would find themselves having to bring in young male labour from developing nations. This would mean that a developed country would soon have an indigenous population of rich elderly females, and an immigrant population of poor young males.[17] If Fukuyama is right do you think this would be conducive to social stability?

De Grey believes that, for fear of another 9/11, the richer nations would soon start to subsidise life-extending treatment for poorer nations. But would the richer nations also subsidise life-enhancing programmes such as food relief? If not would the poorer nations accept life-extending treatment? Would you like the idea of starving forever?

It seems clear, from reflecting on these practical problems, that there are excellent consequentialist arguments *against* embracing significant extensions to longevity. But do these arguments outweigh the consequentialist argument for extending lifespan that arose from consideration of the personal pleasure we might believe we'd get from living forever?

> ### Box 12.4 Activity: Creative writing
>
> Imagine you are the Prime Minister of the UK, the American President or the head of state of some other nation, and that you are faced with deciding what to do with a new technique that will significantly extend lifespan. Imagine the thought processes you might go through.

De Grey believes these practical problems can be resolved.[18] Housing won't be a problem, he says, because we'd all be so fit we could live in high-rise blocks, and anyway, we'll eventually have the option of living on other planets (and perhaps increasing longevity will make this sooner rather than later). He points out that people might choose to have fewer children, with the result that there won't *be* a population explosion. As for the money running out, well, he says, if HIV suddenly became transmissible in the way the common cold is, and just as infectious, you can bet your bottom dollar governments would subsidise an effective treatment whatever it cost. 'What's the difference?' asks de Grey.

> ### Box 12.5 Activity: Brainstorm
>
> Do a group brainstorm and come up with a list of:
>
> (i)   the practical problems that might be generated by increasing longevity;
> (ii) suggested solutions to these problems.
>
> Participants can be as inventive and creative as they like.

If the practical problems can be overcome, of course, this would mean that the consequentialist arguments based on these problems would also dissolve. But there would still be problems of principle.[19]

Aging and human nature

Some pundits (Kass,[20] Fukuyama[21]) argue that even if we can find solutions to the practical problems that would be triggered by increased longevity, it is morally unacceptable to halt the process of aging. To interfere with the process of aging and death, they say, is like trying to interfere with adolescence and sexual maturity, it is to interfere with the natural way of things. It is human nature, they argue, to age and eventually to die. It comes to all of us, and it is right that it should do so.

On the face of it this appears to be a version of the argument we were warned against in Chapter 6, the one that goes: if it is unnatural it is morally bad. We saw there that this argument just won't do, there are many natural things (pain in childbirth, for example, or dementia) that we are happy to interfere with, so why not old age and death?

But those who make this argument are not obviously guilty of arguing quite so egregiously. They are not afraid of immortality simply because it is unnatural. They are afraid that becoming immortal will dehumanise us. It is, they argue, part of human nature to be mortal, part of the human condition to know that we will one day age and die. On this story to embrace immortality is to turn our backs on being human. There is more to this than simply the claim that if it is natural it is good.

Some of these commentators, for example Kass, intend this claim metaphorically. Others, for example Fukuyama, mean it literally. Let's look first at Kass' argument, then at Fukuyama's.

The dehumanising effects of immortality

There is a long tradition in fiction of people who have been made immortal only to discover it is a curse rather than a blessing. Leon Kass would accept this: he identifies four benefits of mortality, all of which he believes will be lost if we make ourselves immortal. They are: (i) our interest and engagement with life, (ii) our seriousness and aspiration, (iii) beauty and love, (iv) virtue and moral excellence.[22]

Clearly it would be extremely serious to lose such things. But why should becoming immortal – or at least living for a lot longer than we currently do – threaten them?

(i) Interest and engagement

In making his case for the claim that becoming immortal would cause us to lose interest in the world and become disengaged from it, Kass quotes a poet he doesn't name (but is, I suspect, Seneca):

'We move and ever spend our lives amid the same things, and not by any length of life is any new pleasure hammered out'

and asks why we should think that the fact we enjoy something for 40 years means that we would enjoy it for another 40, never mind 400?

It's a reasonable question. But why should we accept the implication that all we would do with our extra years would be more of the same? One of the main advantages of living longer would surely be that we could do all sorts of things that we don't currently have time to do? Think of the degrees we could do, the languages we could learn, the technologies we could master, the books we could read.

de Grey believes that only those sorely lacking in education would reject the gift of immortality for fear they would be bored.[23] The remedy for boredom, he argues, is getting an education, not rejecting immortality. But is *everyone* capable of getting an education that would enable them to stay interested and engaged for many more than three-score years and ten? Will having an education protect us against getting bored however long we live?

It is important to recognise that no one will, or could, offer us leisure even for the lifespans we currently live, never mind if we lived for significantly longer. Life is costly and must be paid for however long it is.[24] There'll be no retiring at 65 in a world of immortals or even in the world of living to 150, 950 (or 130) would be more like it. This will have a huge effect on our working lives. Living longer would also have a huge effect on our family lives.

Working life

Many people long for retirement after 45 working years,[25] what would 950 years of work feel like? We might think that in all that time we could have lots of different and exciting careers. But amazingly few people change their careers, even though 45 years would seem to allow for this. Would this change if we lived much longer? Perhaps we'd still prefer to stick with the familiar, even if we were bored for 900 years?

Then it is only the lucky few who have a job that even starts off being interesting. Would you fancy attaching widget E to the wotchdyamacallit for 930 years? Would anyone? The idea of a working life of 950 years could be anything *but* attractive.

Then if we all live to 1,000 why should we think we'll advance in our careers fast enough to maintain the sense of challenge? It is unlikely we'll be promoted beyond making the tea and doing the photocopying until we're 300. Perhaps the time for submitting a PhD, for example, would be revised from the current 3 years to more like 100 years? Perhaps we'd have to stay at school until we were 200?

Family life

Perhaps the time and energy required to change careers would be released by the fact that increased longevity would mean we wouldn't have to juggle families with work: the part of the jigsaw represented by family life will drop away after 50 years, leaving us 950 years to work on our careers and other interests.

But why would family life drop away after 50 years? Any minute now artificial wombs, together with frozen or artificial gametes, will ensure that the menopause is no barrier to having children. So why should we restrict reproduction to the years from 16–40? We could postpone child-rearing until we are 250 or even 750. Perhaps this will be what keeps life interesting?

But de Grey warns that having children is one of the things, along with eating too much[26] that we might have to give up to become immortal. Child-bearing and rearing is just too physically demanding. How do you feel about giving up children so you could live for 1,000 years? (How do you feel about giving up pizza?)[27]

Anyway, even if we didn't continue reproducing ourselves we could still find ourselves juggling family responsibilities. How many progeny might you and, say three children, have produced by the time you are 900? Could having hundreds of great-great (etc.) grandchildren become boring? Or at least not as interesting as it once was? Would you be able to keep up with (and afford) the birthday presents? What on earth would Christmas be like?

Perhaps there is something in Kass' claim that it would be difficult to remain engaged and interested over 1,000 years?

> ### Box 12.6 **Activity: Paired discussion**
>
> Do you think you would remain interested and engaged in life even if you lived for 1,000 years?
>
> Having decided what you think (and why) find someone who believes the opposite.
>
> Each participant should then make the case *against* themselves.

(ii) Seriousness and aspiration

Kass believes that life's meaning is predicated on its having limits. The only way we can make our days count, he argues, is to number them. Only this spurs us to the pursuit of things that are worthwhile.

Again a quick response to this suggests that it is wrong. Learning is a worthwhile activity, as is the activity of nurturing family and friends, but it is not obvious that either depends on our being limited to 80 years' worth of the pursuit of them.

But have you ever gone to sleep on a Friday night dreaming of everything you are going to get done over the weekend, then found on Sunday afternoon that you have done nothing? It happens to most of us. The fact that we have all that time, together with the fact we're tired from our week's work, means that instead of getting on with whatever we've got to do, we do nothing. We read the paper, wander in the garden, paint our nails, watch a bit of television, chat with a friend... Could the same thing happen with a life of 1,000 years?

Most older people would agree that it is only when we are in our 40s that our mortality suddenly comes home to us. This is the reason many people cite for their 'mid-life crises'. Mid-life crises may not be pleasant. But they can be a spur to action. The sudden recognition that life really *is* short is an extraordinary motivator. Were life to be long, would we find such motivation elsewhere? Or would motivation, as Kass suggests, just go missing?

> ### Box 12.7 **Activity: group discussion**
>
> *It is because we know we will die at about 80 that we are motivated to achieve the things we achieve. A significantly increased lifespan would drain us of motivation.*
>
> Participants should be allocated a side for which to argue irrespective of their actual views.

(iii) Beauty and love

Kass believes only mortals could be moved to make things of beauty. This is because, he says, such things are made to be appreciated by those who come after us. He also suggests that many natural things, sunsets, for example, or seasons, are beautiful only because of their transience. 'Could the beauty of flowers' he asks 'depend on the fact they will soon wither?' From this thought he proceeds to wonder whether love itself could depend on our appreciation of our mortality. 'How deeply', he asks, 'could one deathless human love another?'

To this we might ask why we should find a bluebell less beautiful if it lasted for 2 months, or a year, or forever? It is certainly true that plastic or silk flowers, however realistic, do not have the same effect on us. But might this not be because they are plastic or silk rather than real?

Perhaps the beauty of Michelangelo's David depends on its 'timelessness', the fact it was made so very long ago, and that it will outlive anyone alive today (even perhaps if de Grey is right about the imminence of our immortality). But did Michelangelo make the David because he wanted to make something timeless? It's true that a David carved in butter or ice doesn't have the same impact on us, but might this not again be because we find marble intrinsically beautiful, rather than beautiful because it lasts so long?

Why, furthermore, should love depend on the mortality of the loved one? Is this realism or cynicism? It is rarely the case that love lasts forever. Perhaps a long-lived society would have to learn to deal with this rather than hold out for an unrealistic ideal? Or perhaps it could find a way of living up to the ideal?

> ## Box 12.8 Activity: Group discussion
>
> Look at Figure 12.2. Ask participants to consider whether a group of 'immortals' would have reason to produce such a statue.
>
>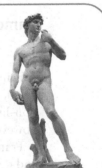
>
> Figure 12.2
> Michelangelo's David.
> ©iStockphoto.com/irakite.

(iv) Virtue and moral excellence

Immortals, says Kass, cannot be noble. To be noble is to 'rise above our mere creatureliness', it is to be prepared to give not just our lives, but also to 'spend the precious coinage of our time for the sake of the noble, the good and the holy'. If we give up mortality, we also give up the possibility of being noble.

But why can't someone who lives for a very long time give up their life to a cause? Might there not be something even *more* noble about giving up your life to a cause if that life would otherwise be immortal? Once we are immortal age will not weary us (even if the years could still condemn) so we'd be giving up something arguably even more precious than was given up by the young soldiers who died in the trenches. Would it be less noble?

But it is true perhaps that giving up *time* to worthy causes wouldn't be quite so noble when there is so much more time to give? Would it be less noble to spend, say 10 weekends working in a hospice when, instead of having roughly 60 years' worth of weekends (3,120 weekends) in a working lifetime, we'd have roughly 930 years' worth of weekends (48,360 weekends)? There seems to be some reason here to say 'yes' it would be less noble.

But it would still count as 'noble' wouldn't it? And what about someone who spend 4000 weekends working in the hospice? Why wouldn't that count as noble? Do we think Bill and Melinda Gates are less noble for giving away millions of dollars worth of their money because they have so much more money than the rest of us? To the extent that our nobility is measured in the percentage of our time/money that we give to others, adding to that time or money will not, in principle, detract from our nobility so long as we also add to the time/money we give away.

> ## Box 12.9 Activity: Essay writing
>
> Write a short essay (500 words) on:
>
> *Would immortality be the end of nobility?*

Immortality and humanity

Kass, when he talks of the threat of 'losing our humanity', is speaking metaphorically. A being who has lost interest in, and become disengaged from life, who is unmotivated, and lacking in aesthetic appreciation and moral virtue is not (necessarily) a non-human in any *literal* sense. A feral child[28] would be like this, perhaps, but however *dehumanised* it would still be *human*.

Francis Fukuyama, however, argues that to interfere with the processes of aging and dying will literally precipitate a change of *species,* instead of being human we will become *post-human* or *transhuman*. Just as *Homo sapiens* emerged from *Homo erectus* because (archaeologists think) of their large brain size so, because of immortality, the *post-human* will emerge from *Homo sapiens,* not because of the blind processes of evolution, but because of the intentional decisions of human beings.

Box 12.10 Philosophical background

The question of whether things have *natures* or *essences* is an old philosophical question.[29] If it is in the very nature of a triangle to have three sides, then nothing that doesn't have three sides could be a triangle. Or it is essential to being water, perhaps, that a liquid have the chemical structure H_2O, so nothing that isn't H_2O could be water.

We can apply this question to individual things (to you for example) and to types of things (to human beings). So we can ask whether there is any property such that if you lacked it you wouldn't be *you* but someone else (we know this wouldn't be your DNA because you might have an identical twin) and we can ask whether there is any property such that if a thing lacked it that thing couldn't be human.

Some properties, on this story, are contingent – such that having that property is not essential to being that (type of) thing. Other properties are essential – such that having that property *is* essential to being that (type of) thing.

Against the idea that things have essences, therefore, is the idea that *every* property is contingent, so there could be triangles that don't have three sides, or liquids that are water without having the chemical structure H_2O.

The position taken by Fukuyama is clearly an essentialist position (he believes that things have essences), in particular he believes it is not possible to be human without being susceptible to a process of aging that culminates in death.

But even if Fukuyama is right should this prompt us to conclude that it is morally unacceptable to intervene in the aging process? None of us, presumably, regrets the demise of *Homo erectus*? Why worry about the demise of *Homo sapiens*, then, especially if the post-humans are as much of an improvement on *Homo sapiens* as *Homo sapiens* was on *Homo erectus*?

This is the view of Nick Bostrom of Oxford University.[30] He welcomes the idea that we might become post-human, arguing that being post-human will be much better than being human. Bostrom believes, in effect, that Fukuyama's arguments are a version of the 'it isn't natural' argument. Why should we worry about improving ourselves in such a way as to transcend our nature as human beings, once we have accepted that, generally speaking, there is nothing morally questionable about our improving on nature?[31] But before we accept Bostrom's claim, let's look more closely at Fukuyama's argument.

The underpinnings of morality

Fukuyama argues that there is something extremely important about our common humanity, and that this something constitutes excellent reason not to interfere with it. It is our common humanity, Fukuyama points out, that grounds modern morality, underpinning our whole conception of rights and responsibilities.

The Universal Declaration of Human Rights, he argues, applies to each and every one of us in virtue of the fact we are human. We abhor acts of genocide, for example, because we recognise that differences of race or ethnicity are less important than sameness of species. We deem it unfair to withhold the vote from women or black people because, again, we recognise that differences of sex and colour are less important than sameness of species. Hugely important moral advances have been made over the last century, Fukuyama emphasises, precisely because we have come to see the importance of our common humanity.

Implicit in the idea that it is our common humanity that underpins our moral rights and responsibilities is the idea that we are not under the same sort of obligations to those from other species. Of course, this can be questioned (see Chapter 20) but as things stand nothing but a human being is accorded rights, and only human beings are deemed to have responsibilities. Even if we do see ourselves as having some sort of responsibility to members of species other than our own, it is only human beings – *things like us* – that we recognise as moral beings.

On this understanding of our rights and responsibilities, says Fukuyama, the idea that some of us will *stop* being human cannot be viewed with equanimity.[32] It calls into question our very notion of how far our rights and responsibilities extend. Can we just assume that once some of us have transcended our humanity and become post-human, those of us who have retained our humanity will accord to the post-humans the same rights?

More to the point, perhaps, can we simply assume the post-humans will see their obligations as extending to those who are not like themselves? Will our so-called *human* rights become *post-human* rights? Might this mean that humans will take on the status currently accorded to non-human animals?

Imagine what a human will look like to a post-human. He or she will have had at most 20 years' worth of education as compared to, say 200 years'. He or she will flourish as a mature creature for, say, 50 years before deteriorating, then dying. Such a lifespan will seem pitiable to one who flourishes for 900 years or more, not least because almost all of these pitifully short lives will be spent raising children. Would it be possible for the post-humans to view the humans as anything more than pets? Could they conceivably treat humans as their *equals*, as their *moral* equals?

To the extent it is our common humanity that underpins our conception of our rights and responsibilities, our conception of what it is to be *like us*, then allowing some people intentionally to transcend this common humanity might seem to undermine the very ground of our moral sense.

Bostrom believes Fukuyama's worries are unfounded because 'a well organised society can hold together even if it contains many possible coalitions of people sharing some attribute such that, if they ganged up, they would be capable of exterminating the rest'.[33] Bostrom believes that the steps society currently takes to prevent discrimination of various kinds could and would be extended to protect humans from any tendency on the part of post-humans to enslave or kill them.

But isn't the ability of a society to do this predicated precisely on the idea that despite our differences we are all *human*? The law does protect animals but not in the way it protects humans. Would we be happy about being protected in some future society in the way animals are protected in our society?

The differences between those who will live for 1,000 years and those who will live for 80 years seem so profound that it is not obvious that the two groups could interact and communicate in such a way that they could think of themselves as subject to the same rights and responsibilities. Their expectations, and the patterns of their lives, their experiences and hopes for the future would be quite different.

Would they – *could they* – live with each other? Work with each other? Marry or have children with each other? Would it be reasonable, for example, for the same laws to be applicable to both? Five years in prison would not have nearly the same impact on an 'immortal' as it would on a mortal. Nor would 6 months' community service.

Of course different races and ethnic groups already have a tendency to live largely separately, limiting their meaningful communications and interactions. But it is not obvious there is any practical reason for this over and above cultural convention. There is also reason to think that as they get used to interacting they start to interact socially, and even to marry each other.

But how practical would it be for humans and post-humans to have any meaningful interaction given the characteristic that separates them? If there is no meaningful interaction, furthermore, wouldn't that destroy the sense of commonality that underpins our conception of *human* rights?

It is true, furthermore, that our laws succeed to some extent to stop different ethnic groups slaughtering or enslaving each other. But there are significant and distressing exceptions. The UN was helpless to stop the slaughter in Rwanda.[34] In Bosnia, the common humanity of all participants was insufficient bar to the atrocities.[35] How much worse could this get if the participants weren't even bound by a common humanity?

> **Box 12.11 Activity: Personal reflection**
>
> Do you think that humans and post-humans could live together under the same laws? Would they extend to each other the same rights and responsibilities, and the same moral consideration?

The arguments against the moral acceptability of significantly increasing longevity that we have been considering seem to have more to them than we might have thought on first consideration. But they are not conclusive. Perhaps we would successfully manage the change to post-humanity with grace and charity, merely expanding our moral domain to include post-humans as well as humans? Perhaps we would extend our interests and activities in such a way as to live worthwhile lives, however long they are. Nothing in the arguments of those we have considered actually rules out these possibilities, or therefore, the moral acceptability of extending our lifespan.

Aubrey de Grey, however, believes he has some excellent arguments for the claim that it *is* morally acceptable, indeed morally *obligatory*, to intervene in the aging process. Let's turn to these arguments.

Two arguments for extending lifespan

We saw above that de Grey believes that we will, with a little ingenuity be able to solve all the practical problems with which we opened this chapter. He also believes he can undermine the claims of Kass and Fukuyama by showing that intervening in the aging process is a moral imperative. de Grey has two arguments for the claim that we are morally required to 'cure' death in the elderly. Here is the first:

'Put yourself in the position of someone powerful – the Prime Minister of France, for example – in, say, 1870 or so, when Pasteur was going around saying that hygiene could almost entirely prevent infant deaths from infections and death in childbirth. In your position, you have some influence over how quickly this knowledge gets out – and, thus, how quickly lives start being saved. But you realise that the sooner people start adhering to these principles and washing their hands and so on, the sooner the population will start exploding on account of all those children not dying. What would you have done: got the information out as soon as possible, or held it back as best you could in order to delay the population crisis? I have yet to meet anyone who says they would have done the latter. With curing aging, there is no difference. None. So, specifically: sure, there may well be some sort of population explosion, just as there was following the elimination of all those deaths – and we may respond by reducing birth rate as quickly as we did then, or we may take longer – but the first priority is to end the slaughter. Everything else is detail.' de Grey, http://www.sens.org, accessed 5 May 2010.

Is de Grey right to think that no one would have dreamed of halting programmes to prevent infant deaths even if they thought it likely that the population would explode as a result? If so, they must have thought that this population growth and its attendant problems would just have to be dealt with. Why should we think it is any different when it comes to preventing deaths in the elderly?

Box 12.12 Activity: analysing arguments

de Grey's first argument is another argument from analogy. Working in pairs set out the argument logic-book style and evaluate it as weak or strong. You can read about arguments from analogy in Box 11.5.

de Grey's second argument can be set out logic-book style as follows:

Premise one: It is morally obligatory to cure diseases.
Premise two: If we cure the diseases of aging we will become immortal.
Conclusion: It is morally obligatory to act in such a way that we will become immortal.

It seems clear that if all these premises are true de Grey's conclusion will also be true.

Premise two is clearly an empirical question. de Grey believes that if we learn how to repair the damage that accumulates as we age, and replace worn parts, the human body, like a well-maintained classic car, would go on forever. Others, however, believe that somatic cells have an upper limit to the divisions they can make (the so-called 'Hayflick effect'[36]) because the telomeres that protect the ends of chromosomes[37] get too short to do their job.

Some people believe, in fact, that we have already found our natural lifespans at 80ish,[38] others that the average lifespan will be pushed up to 120.[39] Either way, our deaths are, as Kass and Fukuyama would have it, inevitable and part of our physical nature. People who believe this argue that in the search for the fountain of youth the best we can do is *compress morbidity*, to keep ourselves as youthful as possible until the inevitable end.

If, however, de Grey is right and immortality is the inevitable result of curing the diseases of aging then far from transcending our humanity in becoming immortal, we would be fulfilling it, showing what human beings are actually capable of, what we have always been capable of were it not for the diseases that beset us before we knew how to cure them.

Clearly, however, only time, and science, will tell us whether or not dying is inevitable, or whether 'immortality' is not only achievable, but an integral part of the true human condition.

Premise one, however, is straightforwardly a philosophical question. Are we morally obliged to cure diseases? Could we imagine a situation in which a disease is such that we have morally good reasons not to cure it? What if a disease were only to strike murderers, taking effect during the act of murder? Would we want to cure this disease? What if curing a disease were so costly as to make it impossible for us to do other things? What if population growth was threatening our very existence? More importantly, for our purposes, what if curing the diseases of aging were to lead to immortality? Considering all the problems discussed in this chapter would this be enough in itself to make it morally acceptable *not* to cure the diseases of aging?

> **Box 12.13 Activity: Small group discussion**
>
> *If curing the diseases of aging were to make us immortal this would be a good reason to deny that we have a moral obligation to cure disease.*
>
> Divide participants into groups of four to discuss this question. Each group should then feed back their conclusion to the group as a whole. The whole group might then debate the question.

This concludes our discussion of aging, and the possibility of curing death. Next we shall consider biotechnology in the context of death itself.

Summary

In this chapter we have:

- considered the possibility that we will one day 'cure aging' and reflected on the social and personal consequences of a significantly increased lifespan;

- considered whether the tragedy of the commons gives us reason to reject utilitarian arguments for increasing lifespan;

- identified some deontological arguments against increasing lifespan, both claiming it would dehumanise us, one metaphorically, the other literally;

- examined de Grey's claim that no-one would have wanted not to cure infant death because of the social problems that would result from over-population, and that curing death in the elderly is no different.

Questions to stimulate reflection

Would society be able to cope with increasing human lifespan to 1,000?

Would we be able to maintain our engagement with life if we lived for 1000 years?

To what extent does our motivation come from the fact we live a finite time?

Could an immortal being also be a human being?

Are our moral rights and responsibilities inextricably linked to our being human?

Could mortal beings and immortal beings successfully share a society?

Is aging a natural condition or a disease?

Are there any diseases it is not morally obligatory to cure?

Additional activities

Read Swift's account of the Struldbrugs in Swift's *Gulliver's Travels* (http://www.searchengine.org.uk/Fiction/GulliversTravels/p3c10.htm) then discuss it with friends.

Ask family and friends whether they'd like to live forever, and if not why not. You might also ask them if they'd be prepared to give up having children or live on a very low calorie diet for the chance of living forever.

Write a short story about a world in which people live to 150 (or 1,000).

Conduct some research into the economics of immortality. Give a presentation of the results.

Write a list of pros and cons of living to 1,000, and/or to 150.

Discuss with friends the idea of posthumanism or transhumanism: what do most people think of the idea?

Conduct some web-research on Juan Ponce de León y Figueroa. Find out his connection with the fountain of youth.

Notes

1 http://en.wikipedia.org/wiki/Fountain_of_Youth. A Wikipedia account of the fountain of youth.
2 http://www.scientificamerican.com/article.cfm?id=the-truth-about-human-agi. A 'position statement' on aging from *Scientific American*.
3 http://www.mfoundation.org/index.php?pagename=video_faq_4. A video on 'the seven deadly causes of aging' by Aubrey de Grey.
4 http://www.ted.com/speakers/aubrey_de_grey.html. TED on Aubrey de Grey.
5 http://www.sens.org/media. Videos of Aubrey de Grey explaining his work.
6 http://news.bbc.co.uk/1/hi/uk/4003063.stm. A BBC news report on this claim.
7 http://news.bbc.co.uk/1/hi/uk/4059549.stm. One critic of de Grey.
8 http://www.thecentenarian.co.uk/. The website of the *Centenarian*, which offers advice on living to 100 and over.
9 http://www.telegraph.co.uk/finance/personalfinance/2883789/The-Struldbrugs-of-Luggnagg-and-an-age-old-problem-foretold.html. A *Telegraph* article on the downside of increasing longevity.
10 http://www.guardian.co.uk/books/2002/may/13/health.highereducation. Extracts from Francis Fukuyama's book *Our Posthuman Future: Consequences of the Biotechnology Revolution* (2003, Picador). Extract three is on extending longevity.
11 http://www.garretthardinsociety.org/articles/art_tragedy_of_the_commons.html. Garrett Hardin on the Tragedy of the Commons, from the Garrett Hardin Society.
12 http://www.cabinetoffice.gov.uk/about-cabinet-office.aspx. The website of the UK Cabinet Office.
13 http://www.ncbi.nlm.nih.gov/pmc/articles/PMC1228271/. Gray, C. (1997) 'Are we in store for some intergenerational warfare?' *Canadian Medical Association Journal*, **157**(8): 1123–1124.
14 http://www.timesonline.co.uk/tol/comment/columnists/anatole_kaletsky/article7142095.ece. A *Times* article on intergenerational conflict.
15 http://news.bbc.co.uk/1/hi/magazine/3550079.stm. The BBC on 'grey power'.
16 http://www.dailymail.co.uk/news/article-1258406/Rise-grey-power-ministers-90-year-olds-sit-juries.html. A 2010 initiative to get 90 year olds on jury service.
17 Fukuyama, F. (2003) *Our Posthuman Future: Consequences of the Biotechnology Revolution*. London: Picador.
18 http://www.methuselahfoundation.org/. de Grey's account of how he would solve the practical problems of significantly increasing lifespan.
19 http://www.maxlife.org/faqs.asp#q3. Another organisation that believes we can overcome the problems of 'maximum life'.
20 Kass, L. (2002) *Life, Liberty, and the Defense of Dignity: The Challenge for Bioethics*. San Francisco: Encounter Books.
21 http://www.guardian.co.uk/commentisfree/2010/apr/15/transhumanism-biological-immortality. A *Guardian* article about immortality. http://www.timesonline.co.uk/tol/comment/columnists/guest_contributors/article703117.ece.

22 http://www.independent.co.uk/news/science/never-say-die-who-wants-to-live-forever-2018292.html. An article by one who agrees with Kass.

23 http://www.dailymail.co.uk/news/article-431827/Would-die-boredom-lived-ever.html. The *Daily Mail* on boredom and immortality.

24 http://citywire.co.uk/money/the-economics-of-immortality/a399808. An interview with de Grey in which he claims that immortality would solve the pension crisis.

25 http://www.guardian.co.uk/money/2010/jun/24/state-pension-age-rise-plan. A report on union claims by charities and unions that it is 'unfair' to raise the retirement age to 66.

26 http://www.guardian.co.uk/uk/2005/nov/18/genetics.science. A report on a breakthrough in extending lifespan. http://www.telegraph.co.uk/health/7898775/The-Calorie-Restriction-dieters.html. A *Telegraph* report on two people living on a very low calorie diet.

27 http://www.uknetguide.co.uk/Lifestyle_and_Leisure/Article/Id_rather_be_dead_than_celibate-101884.html. UKnetguide report that two out of five Britons would give up sex to live to 100.

28 http://www.bbc.co.uk/dna/h2g2/alabaster/A269840/. A BBC report on feral children.

29 http://plato.stanford.edu/entries/essential-accidental/. The *Stanford Encyclopedia of Philosophy* on essence (essential versus accidental properties).

30 http://www.nickbostrom.com/. Nick Bostrom's website.

31 http://www.nickbostrom.com/papers/dangerous.html. A paper on transhumanism by Bostrom (non-philosophers won't find it difficult).

32 http://www.bluelight.ru/vb/showthread.php?t=181632. Fukuyama's essay on Transhumanism.

33 http://www.nickbostrom.com/ethics/dignity.html. Nick Bostrom's essay on 'Posthuman Dignity' (not difficult for non-philosophers).

34 http://news.bbc.co.uk/1/hi/1288230.stm. A BBC report on genocide in Rwanda.

35 http://news.bbc.co.uk/1/hi/world/europe/675945.stm. BBC report on the massacre in Srebrenica.

36 http://www.molecularstation.com/wiki/Hayflick_limit. Information on the Hayflick Effect from Molecular Station.

37 http://learn.genetics.utah.edu/content/begin/traits/telomeres/. An account of the supposed link between telomeres and aging from Learn Genetic at the University of Utah.

38 See Carne, B. and Olshansky, S.J. (2002) *The Quest for Immortality: Science at the Frontiers of Aging.* London: W.W. Norton and Company.

39 http://web.mac.com/sjayo/SJayOlshansky/Live_to_150.html. A radio interview with S. Jay Olshansky who denies the possibility of significantly increasing lifespan.

Further reading and useful websites

Appleyard, B. (2007) *How to Live Forever or Die Trying: On the New Immortality.* New York: Simon and Schuster.

De Grey, A. and Rae, M. (2008) *Ending Aging.* New York: St. Martin's Press.

Post, S. and Binstock, R. (2004) *The Fountain of Youth: Cultural, Scientific and Ethical Perspectives on a Biomedical Goal.* Oxford: Oxford University Press.

Kass, L. (2002) *Life, Liberty, and the Defense of Dignity: The Challenge for Bioethics.* San Francisco: Encounter Books.

http://www.debatingmatters.com/topicguides/topicguide/aging/. A topic guide
    and resources on debating whether increasing lifespan is a good thing or not from
    Debating Matters.
http://www.imminst.org/. The Immortality Institute, an organisation dedicated to
    advocating and supporting research into unlimited lifespans.
http://video.google.com/videoplay?docid=6581761732541483047&safe=active#. A video
    from the Immortality Institute on life extension.

13

Death and killing: the quality and value of life

Objectives

In reading this chapter you will:

- reflect on the nature of death;
- consider the pros and cons of changing our standard of death;
- consider whether 'quality of life decisions' should replace 'standard of death' decisions;
- learn about the different types of euthanasia;
- reflect again on our three moral theories and their views on the intentional killing of human beings;
- consider whether any type of euthanasia should be legalised.

You might think that death wouldn't change much whatever biotechnology does. But over the last 50 years advances in biotechnology have triggered a great deal of philosophical thought about death, and not just amongst philosophers.

The 'standard' of death

Sixty years ago death was easily determined. Once a person had stopped breathing, had no pulse and was turning stiff and greyish-white, he was dead. If he was still breathing and had a pulse, he was alive. Implicit in this was a certain way of determining death and a certain understanding of the nature of death. The irreversible cessation of the cardiopulmonary system was the 'standard' for death.

During the 1950s and '60s two technological advances, artificial respiration (AR)[1] and heart transplantation,[2] brought this standard of death into question.

During the 1950s AR made it possible for us to support the functioning of someone's cardiopulmonary system in the hope the heart would start beating spontaneously again. Often it did. But sometimes it quickly became clear that the patient would never again live a productive life however long – and expensively – we kept his heart pumping.

In the 1960s it became possible to transplant donor hearts into those whose own hearts were failing. This needed donors who were dead: taking the heart from a patient whose cardiopulmonary system was still functioning, even artificially, would be killing that patient.

On one hand, therefore, we had people with viable hearts and lungs and no hope of living a productive life. On the other we had people who would die unless they were given viable hearts and lungs. What was to be done?

In 1968 doctors at Harvard Medical School[3] suggested that death should be determined not by the irreversible cessation of the cardiopulmonary system but by the irreversible cessation of *brain* function.

On this standard if a patient's brain has stopped functioning the patient is dead. It is not, therefore, *killing* the patient if we allow his heart to stop, or even if we actively stop it. This change in the standard of death made it morally and legally permissible to remove functioning cardiopulmonary systems from patients whose brains are dead and transplant them into those who would otherwise die.

The brain, however, is a complex organ. It can die in parts. Must the whole brain be dead before we can say that a person is dead? Or is death a function of the death of part of the brain?

Box 13.1 Factual information: The brain

The lower brain: consists in the brain stem which controls the things we do unconsciously, like breathing, heartbeat and our reflexes. So long as the lower brain functions a person will breathe spontaneously, cough, react to light and swallow.

The higher brain: consists in the cerebral hemispheres, including the cerebral cortex. The higher brain underpins consciousness, enabling us to experience the world around us, to feel pleasure and pain and to form desires, goals and intentions.[4]

If death is determined by the death of part of the brain there are two broad possibilities: that death is attendant upon death of the lower brain or of the higher brain.

If we were to say that death consists in death of the lower brain this would have the advantage of being continuous with the cardiopulmonary standard of death: death of the lower brain leads inexorably to the irreversible cessation of the functioning of the cardiopulmonary system. The disadvantage of defining death thus is that a person's lower brain might be dead yet the person still be conscious. Do we really want to count as *dead* someone with whom we could, in principle, hold a conversation?

Box 13.2 Case studies: 'Locked-in syndrome'

In 1995 at the age of 43 Jean-Dominique Bauby, editor of the French magazine *Elle*, had a massive stroke. Shortly afterwards he was diagnosed with 'locked-in syndrome' (*coma vigilante*).[5]

Bauby's mind was functioning normally, yet the only part of his body over which he had intentional control was his eyes.

By means of an alphabet board and blinking Bauby managed to write the book on which the film *The Diving Bell and the Butterfly*[6] was based.

Bauby died of pneumonia 2 days after the publication of his book.[7]

If, on the other hand, we are to say that death consists in death of the higher brain this would have the intuitively acceptable advantage of ensuring that anyone whose consciousness was irretrievably lost would count as dead. But this would also mean we would count as dead people whose lower brain was alive. We would, therefore, be free to bury or cut the heart out of people who are warm and breathing, who cough when lifted, react to light and go through waking/sleeping cycles. Would *you* want to cut the (beating) heart out of such a person?

A person whose whole brain is dead, on the other hand is not, and never again will be, conscious and he or she will look and feel dead in the traditional sense. There is no counterintuitive consequence of setting the standard of death for normal human beings as death of the whole brain. Even if, thanks to artificial respiration, such a person's heart is beating, they are a healthy colour, and feel warm to the touch, the appearance of life is illusory, an artefact of technology.

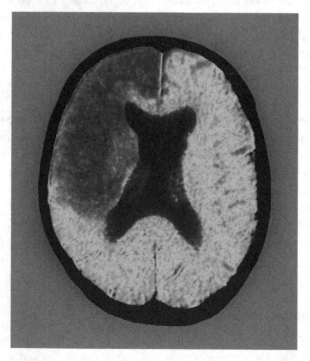

Figure 13.1 Computed tomography (CT) scan in axial section of the brain showing death of cerebral tissue (at upper left). © Zephyr/Science Photo Library.

The new standard of death, the whole brain standard, seems tailor-made for modern technology.[8]

> ### Box 13.3 **Activity: Review writing**
>
> Show participants a DVD of *The Diving Bell and the Butterfly* and ask them to write 500 words in the character of Jean-Dominique Bauby about the situation in which he finds himself.

Death versus 'quality of life' judgements

In his book *Rethinking Life and Death*[9] Peter Singer argues that, faced with the new technologies of the 1950s and '60s, we should have decided that the lives of those whose higher brains have died are not worth living, and that it is morally acceptable to kill them. Killing such people, he notes, would free organs for transplant and hospital beds for others as effectively as redefining death.

Such a move would not involve our having to accept that a warm person whose heart was beating was already dead (as a higher brain standard of death would require). It would instead involve the recognition that actively killing such a person is morally acceptable because their lives, without the possibility of consciousness, are worthless.

According to Singer we only refuse to countenance intentionally killing such people because we are trapped in old-fashioned absolutist[10] thinking about life's being intrinsically valuable *whatever* its quality. But this, he insists, is wrong: it is morally, and should legally be, permissible, to kill anyone who has irreversibly lost consciousness.

Singer is arguing for the moral – and legal – permissibility of euthanasia, the killing of someone for the benefit of that person. In particular Singer is arguing for the moral, and so the legal, permissibility of *non-voluntary euthanasia*. Here are the different types of euthanasia:[11]

Assisted suicide: killing yourself with the assistance of people who know they are helping you die.
Voluntary euthanasia: being killed by others at your own request.
Non-voluntary euthanasia: being killed by others, despite your inability to express a view on whether or not you want to die, because your quality of life is unacceptably low.

Some would add to this list *involuntary euthanasia,* where someone is killed despite having expressed the wish to live. Involuntary euthanasia seems indistinguishable from murder: even if a person is in great and un-relievable pain, if he wants to live, his right to life over-rides any belief on our part that death would be beneficial to him.

It is difficult not to sympathise with Singer's claim that those who have irreversibly lost consciousness have lives that are not worth living. In such a life there won't be any pleasure, pain, joy, laughter, tears or sorrow. There will be no plans, goals, intentions or actions; this person will never again *do* anything at all. What, we might ask, is the point of such a life? In the box you will find a case study of a person who, after an accident, lived such a life.

Box 13.4 Case study: Anthony Bland

On 15 April 1989 Tony Bland, aged 17, went to watch his team play in the FA Cup semi-final. The match was played in Sheffield at the Hillsborough Football Stadium. When the match started thousands of fans had not managed to get to their seats. The pushing started.

Hundreds of fans were crushed against the barrier erected to stop them getting into the ground. Ninety-five people died.[12]

Tony Bland didn't die. But his lungs were crushed, preventing oxygen from reaching his brain. As he was carried from the ground his lower brain was still alive and well. But his higher brain was dead.

Until 1993, Tony Bland lay in hospital being fed through a tube that went down his throat into his stomach. He dribbled and vomited during this process, and he reacted also to the changing of the catheter which removed his urine. His limbs became contorted and his arms rigidly flexed across his chest.

To this, and to the agonies of his family, Tony Bland was oblivious. His consciousness had been irreversibly lost on that April day 4 years earlier.[13]

So long as Tony Bland's lower brain was alive he did not meet the whole brain standard of death. Killing him, of course, was against the law.

In 1993, however, the Law Lords ruled that although it was not legally permissible to kill Bland, it wasn't legally necessary to keep him alive. This ruling permitted medics to stop artificial feeding. Tony Bland was allowed to starve to death.[14]

The Law Lords' ruling was a seminal one. It was the first time the law had explicitly recognised the legal permissibility of allowing someone to die. Had they not done so Tony Bland might be alive today.

Box 13.5 Philosophical background: The act–omission doctrine

According to this doctrine we are morally responsible for our acts but not for our omissions.[15]

This means that the doctor who strolls, rather than runs, to the room in which the elderly demented person is dying of a heart attack, is not guilty of killing that person. The doctor did not kill that person. He did nothing. It was the heart attack that killed him.

For activities involving this doctrine see Boxes 4.6 and 9.14.

Singer applauds the Law Lords' decision to allow Bland to die. But believes they didn't go far enough. If we recognise that a life is not worth living, he asks, why shouldn't we recognise it is morally acceptable actively to end it?

That Singer is arguing for *non-voluntary* euthanasia is clear. Had Bland ever signed an 'advance directive' expressing the wish not to be given life support should he irreversibly lose consciousness, his life support could have been withdrawn without a court order: he would *himself* have decided that life wasn't worth living. But not many 17 year olds sign advance directives.

Box 13.6 Factual information: Advance directives

An advance directive is a legal document in which a person sets out his wishes on how his appointed 'attorneys' (representatives) should organise his life, health, property and affairs, should he become mentally incompetent.[16]

In the UK this document is known as a Lasting Power of Attorney (LPA).[17] It becomes valid only when the writer becomes mentally incompetent (as judged by two doctors).

In the LPA a person can ask that he not be given life support should he irreversibly lose the capacity for consciousness.

Singer's argument is persuasive. The Law Lords themselves expressed disquiet at their judgement. As Lord Browne-Wilkinson put it:

'How can it be lawful to allow a patient to die slowly, though painlessly, over a matter of weeks from lack of food, but unlawful to produce his immediate death by a lethal injection, thereby saving his family from yet another ordeal to add to the tragedy that has already struck them? I find it difficult to find a moral answer to that question. But it is undoubtedly the law and nothing I have said casts doubt on the proposition that the doing of a positive act with the intention of ending a life is, and remains, murder.'[18]

In these words Lord Browne-Wilkinson underlined the fact that in the UK there is no distinction in law between euthanasia and murder. In the UK intentional killing *of any kind* is illegal – even if the alternative is allowing someone slowly to starve to death.

But is this law justifiable? Doesn't the Bland case demonstrate that non-voluntary euthanasia ought to be legalised? Is Singer right, furthermore, to think the law is based on the 'old-fashioned' absolutist belief that life is intrinsically valuable whatever its quality?

Box 13.7 Activity: Informal poll

Ask participants to answer 'yes' or 'no' to the following question before they read the rest of this chapter:

Should the law be changed to allow the intentional killing of those who have irreversibly lost the capacity for consciousness?

> After the poll has been conducted participants might list their reasons for their decision so they can be re-visited at the end of the chapter.

Assisted suicide and voluntary euthanasia

The UK law that forbids all intentional killing has also come under fire from people who object to the fact that assisted suicide and voluntary euthanasia are illegal.[19]

In both these types of euthanasia, unlike non-voluntary euthanasia, it is the person who dies who decides his life is not worth living. Even if we are not prepared to decide, on behalf of another, that their lives are not worth living, we might think it reasonable to allow mature competent adults to decide on their own behalf that their lives are not worth living. If so, the argument goes, we must equally obviously allow them to act on that decision even if they need help to do so.

The question of legalising assisted suicide and voluntary euthanasia may soon become pressing. If, as we saw in Chapter 12, technology could soon make us 'immortal' any trepidation we might feel about this will be mitigated by the possibility of seeking help to end our lives should we find ourselves unable to die by our own hands.

Until 1961 attempted suicide was punishable in the UK by death. Recognising the absurdity of this suicide was decriminalised. UK law now recognises the legal right of subjects to act on the decision that their own life is not worth living. But the Suicide Act of 1961 extends this right only to those able to end their lives by their own hand. Should they need help to die they must continue to live whatever their quality of life and however much they wish to die. Or they must be prepared to allow others to risk their own freedom by assisting them.

The risk is not negligible: the penalty in the UK for assisting a suicide is 14 years' imprisonment.

In 2000 this law came under pressure from a woman who tested the law in the hope of being allowed to die with her husband's help at a time of her own choosing. You can read about this in Box 13.8.

Box 13.8 **Case study: Diane Pretty**

In 1999 42-year-old Diane Pretty was diagnosed with motor neurone disease (MND). This incurable neuro-degenerative disease causes weakness and wasting of muscles, resulting in loss of mobility in limbs, and difficulties in speech, swallowing and breathing.

Fearful of death by choking, common in MND, Pretty went to the House of Lords to argue that the law violated her right to commit suicide at the time of her own choosing with the help of Brian, her husband of 23 years.[20]

The House of Lords rejected her argument, claiming that human rights legislation is designed to protect life, not to end it. This ruling was later upheld by the European Court of Rights.

Two days after her case was rejected in Europe, Pretty died.[21]

In recent years the situation in the UK has been complicated by the existence of Dignitas,[22] an organisation that helps people to die if they are able and willing to travel to Switzerland where assisting suicide is legal. Over 100 Britons have died under the auspices of Dignitas.[23]

It has not, however, escaped notice that if someone helps a person travel to Switzerland to make use of the services of Dignitas they are, in effect, helping that person to commit suicide. No one who has done this has ever been prosecuted. This failure to prosecute was recently underlined by the controversial case described in Box 13.9.

Box 13.9 Case study: Daniel James

At 23, Daniel James became the youngest Briton to die with the help of Dignitas. Daniel chose to die because he could not come to terms with needing 24-hour care after becoming a tetraplegic when his spine was dislocated in a rugby accident.

Before the accident Daniel had been a fit young man who played rugby for his university and for England Under 16s.

Daniel's parents, Mark and Julie, had accompanied him to Switzerland and stayed with him as he died. On their return to the UK they discovered someone had reported them to the police for assisting a suicide.[24]

The James' case was highly controversial. It was argued that Daniel had not had enough time to come to terms with his condition before he died, and that he needed help, not to die, but to live with his disability.

A spokesman for the Director of Public Prosecutions eventually said it had been decided it was not in the public interest to prosecute Daniel's parents despite evidence they had contravened the law.[25]

It wasn't long before another test case was brought. This time the case requested that the law against assisting a suicide be clarified. Debbie Purdy, a 46 year old from Bradford diagnosed with multiple sclerosis, wanted to know under what conditions her Cuban husband, Omer Puente, would be prosecuted should he help her to travel to Switzerland.[26]

Purdy won her case. In 2009 the Director of Public Prosecutions issued guidance on how decisions would be made on whether or not to prosecute a person who helped someone else commit suicide, either with the services of Dignitas or without.[27]

This victory, however, represents nothing more than a clarification of the law. It is not a *change* in the law. In the UK assisted suicide and voluntary euthanasia are still illegal.[28] This does not mean, however, that prosecution is inevitable. The new guidelines enable people to make a principled judgement about whether or not it is likely they'll be prosecuted if they help a loved one to commit suicide.

Once again we might ask whether the law forbidding euthanasia is justified, especially if we regularly fail to *apply* it when it is broken.[29]

The intrinsic value of life

If you read the section on deontology in Chapter 4 you will know that some deontologists would insist that, because human life is intrinsically valuable, it is absolutely wrong to kill another person even for that person's benefit. It is this 'old-fashioned absolutist belief' that Singer – a utilitarian – believes to be behind the fact euthanasia is illegal in the UK. Clearly anyone who believes killing is absolutely wrong will think this is as it should be.

It is not clear, however, that it is *only* this deontological argument that is behind the law. We could also offer a utilitarian argument to the effect that the decriminalisation of euthanasia would open the floodgates to the possibility of murder's being committed with impunity.[30]

The slippery slope to involuntary euthanasia

Imagine that a daughter has killed her elderly demented mother by smothering her with a pillow. Imagine also that she offers one of these motives for her act:

(i)   she was helping her mother achieve her own wish to die;
(ii) she was ending her mother's life because it had become worthless.

In the first case the daughter claims to have assisted a suicide, or engaged in an act of voluntary euthanasia. In the second case the daughter claims to have engaged in an act of non-voluntary euthanasia.

Whichever the claimed motive for the daughter's action we are left with several questions.

(i)   Was the claimed motive for the daughter's action the *real* motive?
(ii)   Was the daughter's belief her mum wanted to die true or at least such that it was reasonable to act on it?
(iii) Was the daughter's belief her mother's life wasn't worth living true?

Let's consider these questions in turn.

Identifying intentions

The daughter is claiming she acted for her mum's benefit. This might be true. But here are some other motives from which she might have acted. She might have:

(i)   lost her temper;
(ii)   wanted to relieve herself of the burden of her mum's care;
(iii) been impatient to inherit her mum's money.

How do we know the daughter is not trying to conceal the fact she straightforwardly murdered her mum?

To underline the difficulty of determining the intentions with which someone acts we need only consider the fact that it is sometimes difficult to determine the intentions with which we *ourselves* act. Have you ever wondered whether you deserve the praise you are getting for an action you have performed? Perhaps you have modestly accepted the praise whilst entertaining a sneaking suspicion that the motives for which you acted were not actually deserving of praise?

It is very rarely the case that we have only one reason for performing a particular action. The important question is which of these many reasons was causally implicated in producing the action. In the case we are imagining the daughter may have had *all* the motives offered for killing her mum: so was her act an act of euthanasia? Or was it an act of murder? Which motive actually caused her to act?

Of course the real problem arises when the act was a straightforward act of murder that the murderer is trying to conceal. Wouldn't we, by decriminalising euthanasia, be making it easy to conceal murder under the umbrella of euthanasia?

One problem with decriminalising euthanasia, therefore, is that euthanasia, by its very nature, is a matter of the intentions with which a person acts and the extreme difficulty of determining the intentions with which another acts.

> ### Box 13.10 Activity: Revision
>
> Read Box 4.6 on page 41 (deontology activity). Ask yourself whether it would be possible to tell which of the people had which intention. Reflect again on whether the nature of the intention with which these people acts is important in evaluating the moral acceptability of the action.

Identifying desires

Other problems arise when we ask whether the daughter was right to think her mother wanted to die, or if she did want to die, *why* she wanted to die, and whether it was reasonable to act on that desire. Once a person is dead, in the absence of an advance directive, we cannot determine what their desires were except through the reports of others. Nor can we determine the nature of, or reason for, any desire to die they might have had.

Perhaps the daughter's belief her mum wanted to die was nothing more than a projection of *her own* belief that life with dementia is not worth living? Perhaps it was nothing more than a reflection of the daughter's exhaustion, and desire that her mother *should* die? Perhaps her mum had been trying to make her daughter feel guilty by saying – falsely – that she wanted to die? Perhaps the mother really did want to die just before the daughter killed her, but the desire would have gone by daybreak?[31] Perhaps the mother did want to die, but only because her daughter was making her feel like a burden?

In these situations the daughter's belief that her mum wanted to die is either false, caused by the pressure the daughter herself was putting on her mother, or such that it was no more reasonable to act on it that it would be to act on a child's claim *he* wants to die. In these situations did the daughter commit euthanasia? Or murder?

Another problem with decriminalising euthanasia, therefore, is that it can be very difficult to decide whether a person really wants to die, why they want to die, and whether it is reasonable to act on their desire.

> ## Box 13.11 **Activity: Group discussion**
>
> Imagine a classmate, Sam, has been claiming that she wants to die since the break-up of an important relationship 2 years ago.
>
> Many of you, believing Sam is clinically depressed, have tried to persuade her to go to the doctor for anti-depressants. But Sam doesn't believe in taking drugs and won't go.
>
> Does Sam really want to die? Would it be morally permissible to help Sam to die? Should it be legally permissible to help Sam to die?

Judgements about the quality of another's life

A different problem arises, in the case of non-voluntary euthanasia, when we ask whether the daughter was right to think her mother's quality of life so poor that she was better off dead. We might argue that, given the dementia, the quality of her life must at least have been severely compromised.

But immediately we are teetering at the top of the slippery slope. Are we to condone the killing of anyone who has dementia or any other condition that 'severely compromises' the quality of life? But who is to judge when the quality of another's life is severely compromised? It is salutary, in this context, to consider the findings revealed by recent technological breakthroughs in brain scanning.[32] Consider the case study in Box 13.12.

Box 13.12 **Case study: Rom Houben**

After a car crash aged 20 Rom Houben spent 23 years in what doctors believed to be a permanent vegetative state (PVS).[33] In 2008 a brain tomography scan demonstrated that his cerebrum was functioning normally. Shortly afterwards it was discovered that he was able intentionally make miniscule movements of his toe and right forefinger.

Three years later, after intensive therapy, Houben uses a computer to communicate: 'At last', writes Houben 'my views can be heard and my feelings expressed'.[34]

In 1996 research involving 40 patients suggested that 43% of those diagnosed with PVS in fact had locked-in syndrome.[35] A decade later it is still thought that 40% of PVS patients are being misdiagnosed.[36]

In Rom Houben's case we needed technology to tell us that his quality of life was better than we thought: that *to him* his life was worth living.

In other cases it is not technology we need so much as empathy. Healthy people nearly always overestimate the difficulties of living with disease and disability. If we were to condone the killing of anyone (supposedly) believed by a healthy person to be living a severely compromised life, many people whose lives are *to them* worth living might find their lives in danger. Maybe a diagnosis of dementia, when euthanasia is decriminalised, will become effectively a sentence of death?

Another problem with decriminalising euthanasia, therefore, is that it is extremely difficult – especially when we are healthy – to make sound judgements about the quality of life experienced by another.

> **Box 13.13 Activity: Discussion**
>
> In pairs, participants should discuss what it would be like to have locked-in syndrome.
>
> After 5 minutes ask participants to rate, on a scale from −5 (very low) to +5 (very high), the quality of life they believe they would have with locked-in syndrome.
>
> Once ratings are in compare them with ratings taken from people who actually have locked-in syndrome. (As reported by Dr Ashraff Ali, a consultant in neurorehabilitation at the Royal Hospital for Neurodisability in South London, most such patients rate their quality of life to be around 3 or 4.)
>
> Open to the whole group a discussion of any discrepancy between the ratings.

Eliminating the possibility of abuse

In the light of all these difficulties it might seem obvious that what we should do is *legalise* euthanasia, rather than *decriminalise* it (see Box 13.14).

Box 13.14 Factual information: Legalisation versus decriminalisation

To **decriminalise** an action is to take it out of the scope of the law. To decriminalise euthanasia would be to compare it to the selling of sweets. Anyone in Britain can sell sweets to anyone else, in any amount, at any time, for whatever they can get for them.

To **legalise** an action is to regulate it by law. The sale of alcohol in the UK is regulated: it can only be sold to those over 18, many need a licence to sell it, and it cannot be sold outside certain hours.[37]

If we legalise euthanasia we would be able at the same time to regulate it in such a way as to eliminate the possibility of the abuses described above. Wherever euthanasia is legally permitted, it is also highly regulated for precisely this reason.[38]

In the Netherlands, for example, euthanasia continues to be illegal, but no one is prosecuted for it so long as he is a qualified doctor and he satisfies the conditions the state lays down. By such means the state forbids the non-medically qualified from committing euthanasia, and reserves the right to prosecute doctors who fail to satisfy the conditions outlined in Box 13.15.[39]

Box 13.15 Factual information: The Netherlands Criminal Code Article 293

Doctors are exempted from criminal liability for helping someone to die when (and only when) they:

(i)   are convinced the patient has made a voluntary and well-considered request to die (possibly in writing before they became incompetent);
(ii) are convinced that the patient is facing interminable and unendurable suffering (mental or physical);
(iii) have informed the patient about his situation and his prospects;
(iv) are certain the patient is convinced that there is no solution acceptable to him except death;
(v)   have consulted at least one other independent doctor who has seen the patient;
(vi) have given his written assessment of the care requirements as referred to in the points above;
(vii) have helped the patient to die with due medical care.

This holds only for those of 18 years and over. Under this age parents must either be involved in the decision (if 16 or 17), or are required to approve of the decision (if under 16).

But at least euthanasia *is* permitted in the Netherlands: mentally competent adults *are* free to choose to die at a time of their own choosing so long as the conditions laid down by the law are satisfied. The question we might want to ask ourselves, therefore, if we are utilitarians like Singer, is whether permitting euthanasia under regulation designed to prevent the abuses possibly attendant on decriminalising it, would be more utility-producing that legally banning it.

Box 13.16 Activity: informal poll

Ask participants to answer 'yes' or 'no' to the following question before they read the rest of this chapter:

Should euthanasia be legalised under regulations designed to eliminate abuse?

After the poll has been conducted participants might be asked to list their reasons for voting as they voted and these reasons noted so they can be re-visited at the end of the chapter.

Regulation and euthanasia

In order properly to weigh the utility of permitting euthanasia under regulation as in the Netherlands against the utility of its being illegal as in the UK, it is necessary to reflect on how the law against euthanasia works in practice.

The first notable effect of the law is that everybody in the UK who is suspected by the authorities of having intentionally killed another person will appear before a court of law. As every death must be certified by a doctor, this means that any death a doctor is not happy about will be reported to the authorities. This is a major incentive against killing someone else unless you:

(i)   are confident you can fool a doctor;
(ii) have the collusion of a doctor;
(iii) are willing to face a court of law;
(iv) are willing secretly to dispose of a body.

Assuming that people likely to engage in euthanasia are unlikely to be confident of fooling doctors or practised in the secret disposal of bodies, if euthanasia is committed in Britain it is likely to be with the collusion of a doctor, or by someone willing to have their actions scrutinised by a court. Let's have a look at these possibilities.

Medical collusion

It would be a hard-hearted doctor who did not sympathise with a person who, faced with the pointless agony of a beloved parent, ended the life of that parent. It would be naïve to think that doctors never use their discretion in such cases to certify death without notifying the authorities.

In Britain this has recently become more difficult because of the unmasking of Dr Harold Shipman who murdered 177 of his patients before being caught.[40] Now in cases of unexpected death the agreement of two doctors is needed before a death certificate will be accepted by the authorities. If this is not forthcoming the coroner will order a post-mortem. If an unexpected death is a case of euthanasia, therefore, the collusion of two doctors is needed to escape facing legal scrutiny. Again it would be naïve to think this never happens: doctors, more than anyone else, are aware of the realities of the deathbed.

Next we should remember that it is not necessarily illegal to allow someone to die even if it is always illegal to kill them. In recognition of this many people, as the result of an agreement between family and doctor, have died of a lung infection that could easily have been treated by a course of antibiotics. Doctors, furthermore, are not above finishing their coffee then strolling to the room in which a person is dying of a heart attack, nor do they always expect to be called before, rather than after, a death.[41]

There is another distinction that, like the act–omission distinction, facilitates the ending of a life that is no longer worth living but without intentionally killing anyone. The 'doctrine of double effect' (see Box 13.17) enables us to distinguish between intended consequences and foreseen but unintended outcomes.[42]

Imagine that the act of giving an injection of morphine has two results. The first is that a person's pain is relieved. The second is that the person dies of an overdose of morphine. So long as the doctor intended only to relieve pain does the fact that the doctor foresaw that the injection would also kill his patient make him or her guilty of murder?

According to the letter of the law it does not. You commit murder only when you perform an act that (i) directly results in someone's death, and (ii) you performed that act intending that the person should die. In this case the first condition was satisfied but the second condition wasn't: the death of the patient may have been a foreseen outcome of the act but it wasn't the intention with which the act was performed. The doctor gave the injection with the intention of relieving pain.

Box 13.17 Philosophical background: The doctrine of double effect

Imagine you are standing on a bridge. You see a train hurtling down the railway track below and realise with horror it will hit the five men working on the track. Beside you is a lever that will divert the train onto another track. But if you divert the train it will kill a rambler who is strolling along listening to his iPod.

What should you do?

Most people argue you should divert the train, thereby suggesting it is better to kill one person than to allow five to die.

On the other hand faced with the possibility of a doctor's killing one tramp in order to use his organs to save five others, most people argue that the five should be allowed to die, rather than the one be killed to save them.[43]

What is the difference?

The doctrine of double effect purportedly explains the difference in our intuitions by claiming that:

- In the train case we act with the intention of saving the five, we merely foresee *and do not intend* the death of the one. This makes our action morally acceptable.
- In the doctor case we actively intend the death of the one because it is only by means of causing his death that we can save the five. This makes our action morally unacceptable.

Such examples of medical collusion demonstrate that euthanasia's being illegal in the UK neither means that euthanasia does not happen in the UK, nor that there aren't all sorts of ways, short of euthanasia, in which lives can be brought to an end.

It is interesting in this context to note that medical practitioners in the UK, as represented by bodies such as the Royal College of Medicine, consistently oppose the legalisation of euthanasia.[44] They are afraid it would undermine the commitment of medics to the saving of life, that euthanasia would soon become the cost-effective way to treat the elderly and the infirm, and/or that it would discourage the search for more effective palliative care[45] or pain-relieving drugs.[46]

> ## Box 13.18 Activity: Personal research
>
> In the US state of Oregon,[47] where physician-assisted suicide is legal, 45% of patients given good palliative care changed their minds about euthanasia.[48]
>
> Can you find any other empirical evidence to help weigh the utility of regulating euthanasia against the utility of banning it?

In weighing the utility of regulating versus banning euthanasia, therefore, we might ask whether medical collusion is more or less likely to be forthcoming where euthanasia is illegal, than where it is legally regulated, and how our answer affects our calculation of utility.

> ## Box 13.19 Activity: Informal poll
>
> Participants should answer 'yes' or 'no' to the following question before they read the rest of this chapter:
>
> *Is medical collusion as likely to happen where euthanasia is legally regulated as it is where euthanasia is illegal?*
>
> Participants might list their reasons for their vote so they can be re-visited at the end of the chapter.

Willingness to face scrutiny in a court of law

As we have seen it is undoubtedly the case that people – both medical practitioners and ordinary people – sometimes act on their belief that euthanasia is morally acceptable even when it is clearly illegal. Much of this goes on under the radar of the authorities.

Occasionally, however, people make no attempt to hide the fact they have broken the law. In Box 13.20 you will find a case study of one who openly admitted to having committed euthanasia.

Box 13.20 **Case study**

In 2005 Donald Mawditt, aged 72, called 999. When help arrived it was too late. Mawditt told paramedics that he had given Maureen his 'soul mate' and wife of 50 years, diazepam to tranquilise her, then strangled her with a carrier bag and 'held it there for 5 minutes' after she had stopped breathing.

Maureen, a grandmother of four, was 70. She was terminally ill with a failing heart and liver. She was doubly incontinent, incoherent, had spasms and lapsed in and out of consciousness. She had begged her husband to strangle her, a plea that had been heard by their doctor.

As Mawditt was taken from his house by police, he kissed his wife's body and said 'goodbye, my darling'. Mawditt was charged with murder, but pleaded guilty to manslaughter.

Judge Crowther sentenced Mawditt to a 3 year conditional discharge, saying:

'You have caused the death of your wife at a time when her life had become intolerable. It is sometimes described as mercy killing. Our law does not recognise that as such and our social ethos is such that the taking of a life can never be condoned. Even in such cases punishment is required to mark the gravity of the matter and to enable the perpetrator to pay a proper penalty for the act. You are plainly no risk to society, so I come to the conclusion that the proper disposal is one that at first sight is utterly exceptional but to which I am driven by logic: you will never be punished for this act save insofar as your suffering has been punishment in itself.'

Mr Mawditt's daughter Karen said, 'If dad had chosen to lie to the police he would never had been charged with the killing. I admire my dad for what he did.'[49]

In such cases there is usually a public outcry. People make it clear in no uncertain terms that a person in this situation is not to be treated as a murderer. Usually they get their way. In such situations, as with Mr Mawditt, the court often hands down a suspended sentence, lets someone off on the grounds of temporary insanity or otherwise absolves them of guilt.

It would seem that even where the law clearly and unambiguously states that all intentional killing is prohibited, there is room for the law to recognise a distinction between murder and euthanasia in the sentences handed down.

Another question we might ask therefore in weighing the utility of regulating versus banning euthanasia, is whether the courts will be able to have the same discretion in passing sentence where euthanasia is regulated by law as they do where euthanasia is illegal.

> ### Box 13.21 Activity: informal poll
>
> Participants should answer 'yes' or 'no' to the following question before they read the rest of this chapter:
>
> *Would the courts have the same discretion in sentencing were euthanasia to be legally regulated as they do where euthanasia is legally banned?*
>
> Participants might list their reasons for their vote so they can be re-visited at the end of the chapter.

The time has come to make up our minds. It is clear that if, like some deontologists, we believe that euthanasia is *never* morally acceptable, we will believe it should remain illegal.

If, on the other hand we believe that euthanasia is at least sometimes morally acceptable, we might, on utilitarian grounds, believe that euthanasia should be:

(i) decriminalised: such that anyone is free to kill anyone else so long as that person wants to die or his quality of life has fallen below a certain point;

(ii) legalised: with regulations tight enough to ensure that no one is killed unless they want to die or their quality of life has fallen below a certain point;

(iii) illegal: because there are ways of making sure that anyone who really wants to die, or whose quality of life has fallen below a certain point, can die without making euthanasia legal.

> ### Box 13.22 Activity: Virtue ethics and euthanasia
>
> A group of participants should imagine that they are a committee of the 'great and the good' appointed by the government to advise it on whether or not euthanasia should be decriminalised or legalised (and if so how regulated). We can imagine that each of the committee members has the reputation of being a virtuous person.
>
> Committee members might be given roles to play as follows:
>
> **Chairperson:** This person's job is to chair committee meetings, keep members to the agenda, make sure the committee stick to their remit and to present the final report.
>
> **Note-taker:** This person's job is to keep the minutes of the meeting(s), and to produce a report of the meeting.

Other participants should be asked to act as witnesses called up before the committee to make arguments for or against imposing legalising euthanasia. These members should represent the following organisations:

Faith groups

Disability rights organisations

Organisations concerned with the rights of the aged

Civil liberties organisations

Medical practitioners' organisations

Lawyers and judges

Participants should be given time to conduct some research and prepare their arguments, then a meeting of the committee should be held. Witnesses should be called one by one until all have been heard. The debate should then be opened to the committee.

This concludes not only our discussion of euthanasia but also our consideration of the social and ethical issues that are generated by biotechnology at the beginning and end of life.

Summary

In this chapter we have:

- considered how technological advances made desirable a change to the standard of death;

- learned about the different types of euthanasia and revisited the deontological belief that it is always and everywhere wrong to kill however benevolent the motive;

- been introduced to arguments for the moral permissibility of non-voluntary euthanasia, assisted suicide and voluntary euthanasia;

- become acquainted with the distinction between decriminalisation and legalisation;

- noted that decriminalising euthanasia might result in many acts of murder being committed under its umbrella;

- seen that legalising euthanasia would permit it to be regulated in the hope of eliminating the possibility of abuse;

- learned about the act–omission doctrine and the doctrine of double-effect and seen how doctors and families collude in ensuring that loved ones don't suffer more than necessary even where euthanasia is illegal;

- weighed the utility of legalising euthanasia versus those of leaving the law as it is;

- considered how a virtue ethicist would view the legalisation of euthanasia.

Questions to stimulate reflection

Does believing that euthanasia is *morally* permissible entails believing that euthanasia should be *legally* permissible;

Are there deontologists who do not accept that 'do not kill' is a moral absolute?

Are utilitarians committed to believing euthanasia should be legalised?

What is the difference between decriminalising something and legalising it?

Are the doctrines of act versus omission and double-effect merely devices for allowing a deontologist to escape the consequences of his absolutist beliefs?

Is it hypocritical of a society effectively to turn a blind eye to euthanasia whilst maintaining its illegality?

Is there any way of eliminating the possibility of abusing laws permitting euthanasia without introducing stringent regulation?

Would a virtue ethicist legalise euthanasia?

Additional activities

Find out more about the standard of death by researching and writing a short (1,000) word essay on how to determine death.

Talk to your family and friends about assisted suicide. Would most legalise or decriminalise it? What are their reasons?

Write a 1,500-word essay on assisting suicide and the law.

Read about the case of Daniel James (Box 13.9). Do a web-search on the case. Do you think Daniel made the right decision?

Whichever side you are on, produce a presentation arguing for the *other* side.

Organise a debate on the following motion: 'This house believes that the law should accept that when life has no quality it is morally permissible to kill a person.'

Watch this debate on euthanasia from Australian television: http://fora.tv/2009/02/03/IQ2_Debate_Should_Euthanasia_Be_Legalized. Which side would you vote for?

Notes

1 http://my.clevelandclinic.org/healthy_living/healthcare/advance_directives/hic_ understanding_life_support_measures.aspx. An account of artificial life support measures from the Cleveland Clinic in the United States.

2 http://news.bbc.co.uk/1/hi/england/cambridgeshire/7117750.stm. A BBC retrospective on the first ever heart transplant.

3 A definition of irreversible coma. *Journal of the American Medical Association* (1968), **205**:337–340.

4 http://www.bbc.co.uk/science/humanbody/body/interactives/organs/brainmap/. A BBC Science and Nature website on the human brain.

5 http://www.ninds.nih.gov/disorders/lockedinsyndrome/lockedinsyndrome.htm. Information on locked-in syndrome from the US National Institute of Health.

6 Bauby, J.D. (1997) *The Diving Bell and the Butterfly.* New York: Alfred A. Knopf.

7 http://www.independent.co.uk/news/people/obituary-jeandominique-bauby-1272406. html. Obituary of Jean-Dominique Bauby from the *Independent* newspaper.

8 http://news.bbc.co.uk/1/hi/6987079.stm. A BBC report of a call to change the definition of death.

9 Singer, P. (1996) *Rethinking Life and Death: The Collapse of Our Traditional Ethics.* New York: St. Martin's Griffin.

10 See the section on deontology in Chapter 4.

11 http://www.bbc.co.uk/ethics/euthanasia/. The BBC Ethics guide on euthanasia.

12 http://www.thefirstpost.co.uk/46969,sport,football,hillsborough-disaster-pictures. The Hillsborough Disaster in pictures from *The Week* magazine in the UK.

13 http://www.spuc.org.uk/about/no-less-human/Bland.pdf. An article with full details of the Tony Bland case from the Society for the Protection of the Unborn Child.

14 http://news.bbc.co.uk/onthisday/hi/dates/stories/november/19/newsid_2520000/2520581. stm. A BBC retrospective on the judgment in the case of Tony Bland.

15 http://www.bbc.co.uk/ethics/euthanasia/overview/activepassive_1.shtml. The BBC gives a good account of the act–omission doctrine on this page.

16 http://www.direct.gov.uk/en/Governmentcitizensandrights/Death/Preparation/ DG_10029429. Information on advance directives from the government in the UK.

17 http://www.bbc.co.uk/blogs/theoneshow/2010/01/power-of-attorney-top-tips.shtml. A video on lasting powers of attorney from the BBC's *The One Show.*

18 Airedale NHS Trust v. Bland [1993] AC 789.

19 http://www.dignityindying.org.uk/. The Dignity in Dying Organisation of the UK.

20 http://www.guardian.co.uk/society/2002/mar/20/health.uknews. A *Guardian* report on the Pretty case.

21 http://news.bbc.co.uk/1/hi/health/1983457.stm. A BBC report of Pretty's death.

22 http://news.bbc.co.uk/1/hi/world/europe/2676837.stm. A BBC report on the operations of Dignitas.

23 http://www.dignitas.ch/index.php?lang=en. The Dignitas Organisation website.

24 http://www.dailymail.co.uk/news/article-1078531/We-help-paralysed-son-die-Anguish-parents-quizzed-police-taking-crippled-rugby-player-suicide-clinic.html. *Daily Mail* report on the Daniel James case.

25 http://www.telegraph.co.uk/news/majornews/3689907/Parents-of-rugby-player-in-Dignitas-assisted-suicide-will-not-face-charges.html.

26 http://www.independent.co.uk/news/people/profiles/debbie-purdy–omar-puente-a-matter-of-love-and-death-1522544.html. Details of the Debbie Purdy case from the *Independent*.

27 http://www.telegraph.co.uk/news/newstopics/politics/7317372/Assisted-suicide-questions-and-answers.html. A *Daily Telegraph* Q&A on the guidelines.

28 http://www.cps.gov.uk/publications/prosecution/assisted_suicide_policy.html. The DPP guidelines.

29 http://newsforums.bbc.co.uk/nol/thread.jspa?forumID=7459&edition=1&ttl=20100820154228. The BBC 'Have Your Say' on assisted suicide.

30 http://www.telegraph.co.uk/news/uknews/law-and-order/7865305/Legal-assisted-suicide-creates-slippery-slope-to-doctors-killing-without-consent-expert-claims.html. An argument to the effect that legalising assisted suicide will produce a slippery slope.

31 http://www.telegraph.co.uk/health/3343327/Depression-is-not-a-good-reason-to-die.html. An account of depression causing someone temporarily to wish to die.

32 http://www.wellcome.ac.uk/News/2009/News/WTX056177.htm. A warning about the use of brain scanning to determine consciousness.

33 http://www.guardian.co.uk/world/2009/nov/23/man-trapped-coma-23-years. A *Guardian* report on Rom Houben.

34 http://news.bbc.co.uk/1/hi/world/europe/8526017.stm. A BBC correction of original reports on Rom Houben.

35 http://www.bmj.com/cgi/content/full/313/7048/13. The misdiagnosis of PVS.

36 http://www.timesonline.co.uk/tol/life_and_style/health/article3004892.ece. An update on misdiagnoses.

37 http://www.bayswan.org/defining.html. The first two paragraphs of this paper nicely capture the difference between legalisation and decriminalisation.

38 http://euthanasia.procon.org/view.resource.php?resourceID=000136#11. International regulations on euthanasia.

39 http://www.telegraph.co.uk/news/worldnews/europe/netherlands/7841696/Euthanasia-cases-in-Holland-rise-by-13-per-cent-in-a-year.html. A report to the effect that euthanasia cases have been increasing in the Netherlands.

40 http://news.bbc.co.uk/1/hi/in_depth/uk/2000/the_shipman_murders/news_and_reaction/default.stm. A BBC report on the Shipman murders.

41 See the discussion of the act–omission doctrine in Chapter 4 and Box 13.5.

42 http://www.bbc.co.uk/ethics/euthanasia/overview/doubleeffect.shtml. The BBC on the doctrine of double effect.

43 http://www.open2.net/ethicsbites/trolleys-killing-double-effect.html. Read about the Trolley Problem on Ethics Bites.

44 http://www.timesonline.co.uk/tol/news/uk/health/article715074.ece. A *Times* report of doctors insisting the RCM abandon its neutral stance on euthanasia.

45 http://euthanasia.procon.org/view.subissues.php?issueID=000422. The ProCon site on palliative care.
http://www.guardian.co.uk/society/2007/feb/28/socialcare.guardiansocietysupplement3. A *Guardian* article on palliative care.

46 http://www.carenotkilling.org.uk/about/. The 'Care not Killing' website.

47 http://www.oregon.gov/DHS/ph/pas/faqs.shtml. An Oregon government information site about the Death with Dignity Act.

48 http://www.euthanasia.com/charts.html. Some information on assisted suicide in Oregon.

49 http://www.telegraph.co.uk/news/uknews/1497507/Husband-who-killed-his-soul-mate-goes-free.html. A *Daily Telegraph* report on the Donald Mawditt case.

Further reading and useful websites

Gorsuch, N. (2009) *The Future of Assisted Suicide and Euthanasia*. Princeton, NJ: Princeton University Press.

Paterson, C. (2008) *Assisted Suicide and Euthanasia: A Natural Law Ethics Approach (Live Questions in Ethics and Moral Philosophy)*. Farnham, UK: Ashgate.

Penney, L. (2007) *Assisted Dying and Legal Change*. Oxford, UK: Oxford University Press.

http://euthanasia.procon.org/. The ProCon website on euthanasia

http://www.debatingmatters.com/topicguides/topicguide/assisted_dying/. The Debating Matters topic guide on euthanasia.

http://news.bbc.co.uk/hi/english/static/health/euthanasia/basics.stm. BBC fact files on euthanasia.

Part III | In the Midst of Life

Questions

Do you think that human beings should use biotechnology to enhance themselves?

Do you think everyone's genome should be freely accessible to all? Should it be available to the person whose genome it is? To the authorities?

Can we prevent the techniques of synthetic biology being used for the purposes of terrorism?

Should we try to solve the crises in global food and energy security by genetically modifying crops?

Do individuals own their own genes and tissues? Should companies be able to patent genes? Should provision be made under patent law for making patenting drugs available more cheaply for the world's poor?

How, in relation to biotechnology, should we manage relations between the developed and the developing world? Is it morally acceptable to apply one set of standards to the developing world and another set to the developed world?

Is it morally acceptable to experiment on non-human animals, to genetically modify them, use them for sport or keep them in zoos?

Does the environment have intrinsic value, or is it valuable only instrumentally? Either way do we have moral duties towards the environment? If so what are these duties?

Introduction

In Part III we shall consider those advances that fall outside the areas of the beginning and end of human life. These are the issues that, as full adults in the midst of life, we have a duty collectively and individually to consider as citizens and subjects who participate in making the decisions about how biotechnology should be used.

In the role of decision-makers we are responsible for our own futures, for the future of other human beings, for the future of the non-human animals that share our environment, and for that very environment. In Part III we shall be discussing this responsibility.

This responsibility is far-ranging. It requires us, as far as we are able, to inform ourselves of new developments and of how they might be used, and to reflect on the social and ethical issues they generate. We shall be considering these issues under four headings: (i) our duties to ourselves, (ii) our duties to each other, (iii) our duties to non-human animals and (iv) our duties to the environment.

In Section 4, our duties to ourselves, we shall look, in Chapter 14 at biological enhancement, in Chapter 15 at the collection, storage and use of bioinformation, and in Chapter 16 at the uses of biotechnology for hostile purposes, both legal (in warfare) and illegal (in terrorism). In Section 5, our duties to each other, we shall discuss, in Chapter 17, genetic modification and food and energy security, in Chapter 18, bio-ownership and patenting and, in Chapter 19, human justice, how bio-technological advance affects relationships between the developed and developing worlds. In Section 6, our duties to nature, we'll discuss, in Chapter 20, whether or not non-human animals have rights and the implications of our answer for their use in agriculture, entertainment, zoos and experimentation. Finally in Chapter 21, we'll consider whether the non-living environment is intrinsically or instrumentally valuable, and the ramifications of our answer for how we ought, or ought not, to act. We shall look in particular at the threats of species-extinction and climate change.

Section 4
Our duties to ourselves

14

Human enhancement: the more the better?

Objectives

In reading this chapter you will:

- consider whether it is morally permissible to use biotechnology for the purposes of human enhancement;
- reflect on the precautionary principle in respect of genetic enhancement;
- consider whether the enhancement/therapy boundary is a moral boundary;
- reflect on whether enhancement is consistent with being 'true to oneself';
- consider whether the use of enhancement in sport is cheating;
- reflect on whether enhancing our children is consistent with our unconditional love for them;
- examine the social ramifications of permitting enhancement;
- reflect on the fact that 'evolution' is now partly in our own hands.

How would you like to be taller, blonder, more intelligent or have a better memory? Sound good? Well just around the corner (if you believe the hype) there's a positive cornucopia of enhancers on their way: smart drugs that will enhance your cognitive abilities or your moods,[1] genetic engineering that will increase your immunity or make it easier for you to lose weight and bio-nanotechnology that will give you artificial muscles,[2] enable you to monitor your health by means of an implant or the fabric of your clothes[3] or make it unnecessary for you ever to clean your house.[4]

In some cases it'll be too late for you. But you'll still be able to enhance your children. No longer will you be able to choose their characteristics only by your choice of partner, you will also be able to choose the genes, drugs or nano-implants that will make it more likely your children are tall, intelligent, sporty, musical or whatever you'd like them to be.

Not everyone views these developments with equanimity. Will they herald the loss of the unconditional love we currently have for our children? Will those of us who don't want, or can't afford, to enhance ourselves, lose out? Will *everyone* end up tall, blond and beautiful? Some have more pressing worries: are the developments safe?

Can we really intervene genetically to change just one characteristic, or develop enhancing drugs without undesirable side effects?[5]

As things currently stand we have little idea of the genetic bases of such characteristics as intelligence, sporting prowess or musical talent. It is also clear that all such characteristics depend on whole clusters of genes. Such 'genetic holism' means that it will always be difficult to be certain of the effects of any genetic intervention, whether engineered or pharmaceutical.

Box 14.1 Factual information: Genetic holism, malaria and sickle cell anaemia

Anyone carrying just one copy of the gene mutation implicated in sickle cell anaemia has a 'heterozygote advantage' in being protected against malaria: the malaria parasite cannot attack the red blood cells that are, as a result of this mutation, slightly malformed (though not fully sickle-shaped).[6]

Understanding of this warns us to take care in engineering the genes implicated in sickle cell anaemia. Removing the defence against malaria would not necessarily be beneficial even if it cured or alleviated the effects of sickle-cell anaemia.

How many other conditions are 'paired' in this way?

The problem of genetic holism would, of course, be exacerbated if we are engineering germ cells rather than somatic cells (see Box 14.2). Could we ever feel safe enough to make changes that will affect future generations, when we have no idea what environmental changes our children's children will experience, nor of how their genes might mutate? Can we be certain the virus vectors used to 'deliver' new genes are harmless? Might our grandchildren regret our willingness to engage in germ-line engineering?[7]

Box 14.2 Factual information: Genetic engineering

There are two types of cell which might be engineered genetically:

Germ cells (sperm and eggs) carry 23 chromosomes each. They combine in reproduction to produce a new organism. To engineer these cells is to produce a change that will be passed down the generations.

Somatic cells (ordinary body cells) carry the full complement of 46 chromosomes. To engineer these cells is to produce a change that will die with the person whose cells are being altered.[8]

Given these facts our discussion will necessarily be speculative. In our usual spirit of pragmatic optimism, though, we will assume that science will prevail in making the technology safe. So the question is: should we take advantage of the enhancement opportunities offered by biotechnology or are there moral pitfalls in such activities?

Box 14.3 Activity: Personal reflection

Reconsider the precautionary principle (Chapter 6, pp. 79–85). Do you think that the problem of genetic holism should prompt us to lean on that principle in banning the engineering of (i) germ cells, (ii) somatic cells?

Many people use 'therapy' to characterise acts intended to eliminate disease and disability (such as PGD – although PGD is hardly therapeutic for the embryos discarded), and 'enhancement' for acts intended to enhance desirable characteristics. We shall adopt this convention and define 'enhancement' according to the definition in Box 14.4:[9]

Box 14.4 Definition: Enhancement

An intervention is an enhancement if and only if it is motivated by the desire to improve some characteristic or condition *beyond* that which is required for good health or normal functioning.

Some have argued that the distinction between therapy and enhancement acts as a moral boundary: therapeutic interventions being morally acceptable, enhancements morally unacceptable. Others have offered two reasons against this claim:

1. the idea, considered in Chapter 11, that disease and disability are partly determined by culture;
2. the fact that treating the distinction between therapy and enhancement as a moral boundary will lead to injustices.

Imagine that we discover a way to ensure heterosexuality.[10] If we think of this as a therapy it would, on this story, be morally permissible. If we think of it as an enhancement it would be morally impermissible. Is homosexuality a disability or is it normal? It is easy to imagine the disagreements such an issue would stimulate.

Box 14.5 Activity: Group activity

Francis Fukuyama suggests the following thought experiment:

'Assume that in 20 years we come to understand the genetics of homosexuality well and devise a way for parents to sharply reduce the likelihood that they will give birth to a gay child. This does not have to presuppose the existence of genetic engineering, it could simply be a pill that provided sufficient levels of testosterone in utero to masculinise the brain of the developing foetus. Suppose the treatment is cheap, effective, produces no significant side effects and can be prescribed in the privacy of the obstetrician's office. Assume

> further that social norms have become totally accepting of homosexuality. How many expecting mothers would opt to take this pill?'[11]
>
> How many participants agree with Fukuyama that most would take the 'pill'? What are the ramifications for the therapy–enhancement distinction, especially in those countries where discrimination on the grounds of sexuality is illegal?
>
> Note: biotechnology is fast finding ways of enabling gay and lesbian people to have their own biologically related children (see Part II, especially Chapters 9 and 10).

So long as there is disagreement over what can be counted as a disease or disability treating the therapy/enhancement distinction as a moral boundary will not be straightforward.

This is further illustrated by a situation that demonstrates the possible injustices that could arise.

Buchanan *et al.* ask us to imagine two boys, Billy and Johnnie.[12] Billy is only 5'2" tall because he has a genetic problem resulting in a deficiency of growth hormone. His condition can easily be treated by means of human growth hormone, and as a therapeutic intervention this is morally unremarkable.

Johnnie is also only 5'2" tall. But Johnnie's height is a simple function of the fact his parents are both very short. Johnnie's lack of inches could as easily be remedied by human growth hormone (HGH) as Billy's. But the intervention in his case would be an enhancement because 5'2" is just within the normal height range. On the view we are considering it would be morally unacceptable to treat Johnnie.

But is this right? Both boys are going to be equally disadvantaged in our heightist society. They would benefit equally from treatment with HGH. Neither is in the least bit responsible for their condition, and both conditions are genetically based (if we assume Johnnie's parents' shortness has a genetic basis). Are we really morally justified in refusing treatment to Johnnie just because the treatment would be an enhancement rather than a therapy?

If you think that Johnnie should be treated, or at least that it wouldn't be wrong to treat him, then you believe at least some enhancements are morally acceptable (or even morally required) and you cannot treat the therapy/enhancement boundary as a moral boundary.

The acceptability of enhancement

We might say it is blindingly obvious that enhancement is morally acceptable.[13] After all we have been enhancing ourselves and our children since the beginning of time. Nowadays we do not merely adorn our bodies, remove our bodily hair and paint our faces, we inject botox to rid ourselves of wrinkles, take steroids to pump up our muscles, syphon fat from our thighs to make ourselves thinner and pop blue pills to make sure of our sexual pleasures.

We also aim to enhance our children's characteristics every time we refuse a drink, or take extra calcium or fish oil capsules in pregnancy. We do the same when we have them vaccinated or move to the suburbs to give them more room. Almost everything parents do, qua parents, is aimed at improving their child's chances in life.

Given this, it would seem that if there was ever a time to discuss the moral acceptability of enhancement that time is long gone.[14]

Biotechnology and enhancement

To this claim, however, it might be objected that the enhancements we have gone in for to date are quite different from those offered by biotechnology.[15] Here are two types of argument for this claim:

(i) biotechnological enhancements threaten our very identities;
(ii) biotechnological enhancements will lead to unacceptable social injustices.

We'll consider both these objections in the order given.

(i) Enhancement and identity

We shall consider this claim in relation to three contexts:

1. the use of mood- or cognition-enhancing drugs by individuals;
2. the use of performance-enhancing techniques by athletes;
3. the use of biotechnological techniques to enhance children.

In each case the objection will be that use of such techniques threatens the very identity of the person being enhanced.

Context one: mood-enhancing drugs

Claim: If we take enhancing drugs to improve our mood or our cognition we are making ourselves into different and inauthentic people, we are not being true to ourselves.

The thought is that if, when we are depressed, we engage in enjoyable activities and succeed in lifting our moods we are engaging in self-improvement.[16] This is laudable. Similarly, if in pursuit of improving our cognitive skills we do su doku or crosswords, our actions are praise-worthy because they are a way of improving ourselves and self-improvement is a good thing.[17]

But if we improve our moods by taking Prozac, or we enhance our cognitive skills by taking Modafinil, we are not engaged in self-improvement, we are being *inauthentic,* untrue to ourselves. Far from being laudable, this is morally unacceptable.

Box 14.6 **Factual information: Cognitive enhancers**

Ampakines: developed for the treatment of Alzheimer's disease but known to have cognitive enhancing effects.

Donepezil: a cholinesterase inhibitor that increases the concentration of acetylcholine, thereby enhancing the power of electrical transmission between brain cells. Used to treat dementia, but known to enhance the brain function of the healthy.

Modafinil: developed to treat narcolepsy, clinical trials have shown it to boost cognitive performance in healthy young people and the sleep-deprived.

Ritalin: a treatment for attention deficit hyperactivity disorder (ADHD) in children. Used frequently by students to improve concentration and alertness.

Propranolol: a beta-blocker that neutralises distressing memories and reduces the symptoms of post-traumatic stress disorder.

Mem compounds: three separate compounds under development as possible treatments for Alzheimer's disease. Animal studies suggest that they can help to restore memory.

It should be emphasised that the long-term effects of such drugs in the healthy are not known, but that there have been indications that they should not be used by those vulnerable to mental disorder.[18]

The first response we might make to this claim is to ask *why* taking Prozac or Modafinil makes us *different*, whilst engaging in pleasurable or cognitively challenging activities merely makes us *better*?

·One answer might be that in taking drugs we are changing properties *essential* to ourselves whilst in engaging in challenging or pleasurable activities we are changing only our *contingent* properties.

The question of whether we have essential properties is a big one in philosophy.[19] An essential property is one that persists through change. When you were born you were about 45.72 cm tall. You are now probably over 1.524 metres. But it is *you* who was once 45.72 cm and is now over 1.524 metres, you have persisted through this change, so your height cannot be one of your essential properties. Height is therefore a contingent property, one you can acquire and lose whilst remaining you.

We might respond to this claim, however, by suggesting that it cannot be that taking such drugs changes one of our essential properties: after all *you* took the Prozac and it was *your* mood that lifted.

But this misunderstands the claim the true import of which depends on distinguishing between ourselves as persons and as human beings. It is indubitable that the same human being persists through the taking of Prozac or Modafinil, the question is whether the same *person* persists.

Box 14.7 **Philosophical background: Personal identity**

The question of *personal identity*, of what it is that makes you *you* is an important philosophical question.[20] Here are some of the answers philosophers have given:

Memory: you are who you are because you have the memories you have (so if another person had *all* your memories, that other person would *be* you).

Brain: you are who you are because you have the brain that you have (so if your brain were transplanted into another person's body that person would become you).

Most philosophers now deem these theories too simplistic.[21] Can you imagine why?

But even having made this distinction we are left with the question of why we should believe that engaging in pleasurable or challenging activities merely changes our contingent properties and makes us *better* people, whilst taking drugs changes our essential properties and makes us *different* people.

Might we say that the former changes our view of the world and/or of ourselves (contingent properties), whereas taking drugs changes our *biochemistry* (an essential property)?

There are two (related) reasons for rejecting this thought: the first is our rejection of the biological determinism underlying it. The second is that engaging in these activities changes our biochemistry as effectively as taking drugs does.

We have seen throughout this book that our biology does not determine who we are. Our identities are as much a function of nurture as of nature. Epigenetics tells us quite clearly that our biology can be a function of our experiences in just the way that our experiences can be a function of our biology.[22] The experiences we have, and the actions we perform, contribute to determining which of our genes is expressed, and to the way in which they are expressed. We persist through changes in our biology just as we persist through changes in our environments.

This is illustrated in the case we are considering. When we engage in pleasurable or challenging activities in the hope of lifting our moods or improving our cognitive skills we thereby alter the biochemistry in our brains. In enjoying pleasurable experiences, for example, we are increasing the uptake of serotonin in our brains, something that is known to lift our mood.[23] Exercise can have the same effect, as can achieving a desired end or being with a loved one.

If changing the biochemistry in our brains changes an essential property and makes us different people, therefore, engaging in pleasurable pursuits does this just as effectively as taking drugs and by the same means.

It would seem that if we rest the claim that taking biotechnological enhancers changes our identities on the idea that our biological properties are essential to us so we do not, as persons, persist through changes to them, this claim is simply false.

> **Box 14.8 Activity: Group discussion: pharmaceutical enhancement and character**
>
> *Taking Prozac has the same effect on our brains as having fun. Therefore there cannot be a moral difference between the two.*
>
> The group might be divided according to their own views on this subject or they might be assigned sides to take.

We might, however, find another argument for this claim in Aristotelian virtue ethics (see Chapter 4, pp. 33–37). According to Aristotle, human beings can fulfil their potential and achieve *eudaimonia*, the proper end for human beings, only if they exercise the virtues. This involves:

- identifying the right things to do;
- doing the right things;
- doing the right things for the right reason.

No one, according to the Aristotelian, starts off knowing which actions are right, this is knowledge that we acquire by observing and emulating virtuous people (if we are lucky, our parents and teachers). No one is able immediately always to do the right thing either. We acquire this ability by acquiring the right habits. Just as a naturally strong person will become unfit if he succumbs to the temptation to be lazy, so a person will become dishonest if he succumbs to the temptation to lie for personal gain.

According to Aristotle, becoming virtuous and fulfilling our human potential necessarily involves putting in a sincere and sustained effort to identify the right goals, and the exercise of tenacity and self-discipline in pursuit of those goals. On this view our characters are in our own hands, we make ourselves into the people we eventually become by making the choices we make. By giving into temptation we allow ourselves to become one sort of person. By resisting temptation we enable ourselves to become different sorts of people.

Virtue theory fits rather nicely with the epigenetic facts. In arguing that our characters – who we *are* – are as much of a function of what we do and the experiences we have as they are of our biological starting point, Aristotle is claiming that our characters are a function of nature and nurture (and the exercise of our own free will).

With this in mind might we say that taking a mood-enhancer like Prozac, or a cognitive-enhancer like Modafinil, counts as giving into temptation?

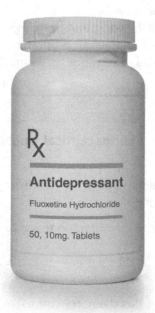

Figure 14.1 ©iStockphoto.com/James Steidl.

Are we, over time, likely to become different people because we take Prozac to lift our moods rather than go out with friends? Will taking Modafinil to enhance our cognitive skills lead to our becoming one sort of person whilst doing crosswords and su doku leads to our becoming a different sort of person? Might we claim that if we rely on engaging in pleasurable or challenging experiences to lift our moods or enhance our cognitive skills we will become *better people* than we will if we simply take drugs? Might drug-taking effectively *prevent* us from becoming virtuous people and achieving eudaimonia?

The Aristotelian account offers us a way of giving substance to the charge that taking pharmaceutical enhancers threatens our identities in a way that engaging in traditional pursuits doesn't.

> ### Box 14.9 Activity: Paired discussion
>
> Does virtue ethics suggest that we should *never* take cognitive enhancing drugs because doing so might weaken our character?
>
> Might the Aristotelian 'golden mean' provide an answer (see page 34)?

Context two: performance-enhancers in sport

Claim: If an athlete takes the hormone EPO (erythropoietin) to increase his endurance he demonstrates the fact he can't win by *himself*.

This suggests that when an athlete takes a performance-enhancing drug like EPO he is cheating. Cheating is unacceptable because it amounts to the admission that an athlete cannot win without pharmaceutical help. In effect the athlete steals the prize from the 'clean' athlete who would otherwise have won.[24]

But why should we think that an athlete is cheating if he takes EPO? Taking EPO has exactly the same effect on the body that training at altitude does. Both raise HCT levels (the percentage of red blood cells) and so the efficiency in which oxygen is transported around the body, thereby increasing endurance. Why should achieving this by one means be cheating, achieving it by another means not cheating?[25] The winner, after all, is the one who gets to the finishing point first, not the one who gets there first as a result of one activity rather than another.

We might say that the athlete cheats because he acts illegally. Taking EPO to increase endurance is not, after all, permitted by the rules. Training at altitude is. This is clearly a reason to believe that taking EPO is morally unacceptable whilst training at altitude is morally acceptable.

But this merely begs the question: why is EPO banned? We can see that if drug taking is cheating it should be banned. But our interest is in *why* it is cheating.

We might appeal to the health-threatening aspects of drugs and say we want success in sport to be determined by ability not by a willingness to risk health (or character). But, as Julian Savulescu of Oxford University argues, this is an argument only for banning drugs that are unsafe or the taking of drugs in amounts that are unsafe.[26]

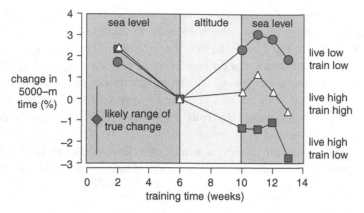

Figure 14.2 Training at altitude. Graph shows percentage change in 5000-m time from baseline performance (at 6 weeks) in three training groups. Baker, A. and Hopkins, W.G. (1998) Altitude training for sea-level competition In: *Sportscience Training & Technology.* Internet Society for Sport Science (http://sportsci.org/traintech/altitude/wgh.html).

It is not, for example, an argument for banning EPO. The risks associated with raising HCT too high are the same whether as a result of training at altitude or taking EPO, or indeed training in a hypoxic chamber, which is permitted after a ruling of the World Doping Agency in 2006. If athletes increase their HCT over 55% they risk a heart attack however their HCT was raised. If they keep their HCT levels below 50% they are safe whether they take EPO or train at altitude. A concern for the health of athletes suggests we should ban both training at altitude *and* taking EPO where these activities raise HCT levels too high, but that there is no need to ban either training at altitude *or* taking EPO where these activities do not raise HCT levels too high.

Banning only those drugs that are unsafe, as recommended by Savulescu, would have several benefits:

- the authorities would only have to test for HCT which is easier and cheaper than testing for EPO;
- the current tests for EPO can be easily avoided by means of plasma expanders and diuretics, so testing for HCT would be fairer;
- it would save a lot of money in attempts to find better tests for EPO;
- it would remove the counterintuitive impact of its being legal to boost HCT to 56% by training at altitude but illegal to raise it to 41% using EPO;
- it would enable athletes from those developing countries that are not at high altitude to avoid the expense of training at altitude;
- it would mean that honesty is not penalised by rules that cannot be properly enforced.

If all (and only) safe drugs were permitted this would avoid all the contortions the authorities currently go through to ensure a level playing field. It would also provide incentives to drug companies to produce safe drugs, rather than drugs that cannot be detected.[27]

So far, then, we have not found a reason for thinking that an athlete's winning with the help of pharmaceuticals should be counted as cheating any more than his winning as a result of training in the traditional way.[28]

It is not every drug, however, that has a non-pharmaceutical alternative. An athlete who doesn't want to take EPO would not be at a disadvantage under the 'safe drugs allowed' regime so long as he or she was able and willing to train at altitude. But the regime would also permit any steroid use moderate enough to avoid liver damage. What if an athlete wasn't willing to take steroids even knowing he wasn't risking his health by doing so? What if he or she wasn't convinced that taking steroids in small quantities was safe? Surely such an athlete would either be forced to take such drugs, or be at a disadvantage?

We might argue that if the drugs in question are not health-threatening why should we worry about everyone's being effectively forced to take them? Drug-taking for athletes would simply be comparable to alcohol-avoidance for drivers: if you want to engage in this activity you are 'forced' to fulfil certain conditions.

If, however, we were right to suggest above that taking pharmaceutical enhancers could be character-threatening, could this give athletes reason to desist even if this would put them at a disadvantage? What about those who dislike taking drugs even if they are said to be safe? Are we really to force such people out of competitive sport? If so permitting safe enhancers could leave us with a playing field that would be level only for those who felt able to use drugs.

How many athletes would find the temptation to succeed in their sport overwhelming, despite concerns about the impact of drug-taking on their characters or a dislike of drug-taking in general? Perhaps those who cared about their characters and those who are sceptical about 'safe' drugs would soon be forced out of professional sport? Perhaps success in professional sport would soon be determined by a willingness to take risks with one's character, or a willingness to believe the claims of drug companies, rather than by ability? Would we get the same enjoyment from watching sport if we knew that this was the case?

Our knowledge that this is the case might affect more than our enjoyment in watching sport. At the moment we treat successful sportspeople as role models for the young. Would we still want to do this if we knew that every athlete was taking drugs, even if the drugs he was taking were safe?[29] Perhaps we would also have to insist that the only drug-taking permitted is that consistent with the formation of a good character? Imagine the difficulties we would have in deciding what this amounts to!

But would an athlete's character be threatened by having to take safe performance-enhancing drugs for the purposes of competing in his sport? Can't we just recognise that if athletes want a chance of winning they have to take safe performance-enhancing drugs just as they have to train and adhere to a good diet. Is there any reason we should think of this as threatening to the athlete's character?

It might help us to think about this to recognise that non-pharmaceutical enhancers have also been believed to amount to cheating.[30]

In 2008 an unprecedented 108 world records were smashed by swimmers. This was possible because modern swimsuits use nano-particles to mimic the modified scales found on sharks. These 'dermal denticles' reduce drag and turbulence, whilst the polyurethane layers have ultrasonically bonded seams to ensure that the suits fit like a second skin and compress the muscles. Wearing one of these suits enables a swimmer greatly to improve his or her hydrodynamics and so their chances of winning. The swimsuits confer such an advantage that any swimmer unwilling to wear one is seriously disadvantaged.[31]

The Olympic Gold Medal winner Rebecca Adlington, however, refused to wear the new swimsuit saying:

'I would never in a million years take drugs to help me, so why would I wear a suit just to improve my performance? It's just not who I am.'[32]

Why exactly does Adlington think it is wrong to wear one of the new swimsuits? Does Adlington think she would not *herself* be winning? Might wearing a performance-enhancing swimsuit weaken character? Can our characters be weakened as effectively by wearing a performance-enhancing swimsuit as by taking a performance-enhancing drug? Or could it be that taking performance enhancing drugs solely for the purposes of sport are not character-weakening? Is Adlington being over-scrupulous?[33]

> ## Box 14.10 Activity: Essay writing: drugs in sport
>
> Participants should research and write a 1500-word essay on one of the following:
>
> 1. Athletes who refuse to enhance themselves by legal means deserve to lose.
> 2. Taking cognitive enhancers before an exam is cheating.
> 3. There is no difference between using a performance-enhancing drug and using a performance-enhancing swimsuit, and both are acceptable.
>
> The claims could instead be used to stimulate group discussion.

Context three: enhancing children

Claim: If we engineer the genes of children to raise the probability of their having desirable characteristics we thereby demonstrate that we don't love them for *themselves*.

This example suggests that biotechnologically enhancing our children is tantamount to acknowledging that we do not love them unconditionally. In the words of the Nuffield Council for Bioethics,[34] enhancing our children might be seen as demonstrating a lack of the 'natural humility' a parent should have in loving his child irrespective of that child's characteristics.

Clearly we do not want to suggest that use of the modern techniques of enhancement alter the properties essential to a child's being the child it is, whilst using traditional techniques changes only its contingent properties. Such a claim would immediately fall foul of the arguments given above for the claim that our biological properties are no more essential to us than our non-biological properties.

Nor does this suggestion seem to rest on the idea that such enhancement weakens a child's character. The character-weakening effects of biotechnological enhancement, if they exist, stem from a person's *choosing* to use them when he would be better putting in an effort by engaging in some traditional technique. When we enhance our children the choice is ours not theirs.

This very fact might be cited as reason for thinking it is wrong to enhance children: perhaps we should not enhance children until they can consent to being enhanced?

But how can a parent avoid enhancing their children without consent? Socialising a child essentially involves enhancement, if only by traditional means, and this must necessarily start before a child can consent. It would be a brave parent who declined to enhance their child until that child could consent.

There is a case to be made, however, for the idea that we should enhance our children only when there is reason to believe that the child would consent to such enhancement were he in a position to do so. For example, we vaccinate a child, despite his objections, because we believe – with reason – that were the child in a position to judge the child *would* consent. Could it be that whilst we can reasonably presume that our children would consent to traditional techniques of enhancement, we cannot reasonably presume this in the case of modern enhancers?

Buchanan *et al.*[35] warn us that relying on the presumption of consent is risky. This is because people have a tendency to endorse the way they were brought up even if these ways were not optimal; their love (or fear) of their parents precludes criticism. Clearly a child's later endorsement of his parents' techniques is not, therefore, sufficient to justify the claim these techniques were morally acceptable. Nor is it necessary: a child may greatly object to the fact his streak of cruelty was modified by his upbringing. We do not think we thereby have evidence for believing his upbringing was wanting.

Julian Savulescu thinks it is actually morally *required* of us to enhance our children by whatever means possible. Savulescu thinks that to refuse to enhance a child when it would have been possible to do so is actively to choose for your child a future worse than that you could have chosen. To do this, he argues, is morally reprehensible.

But is the fact parents consider something to be an enhancement a *sufficient* reason for believing an intervention is morally acceptable? Should everything a parent considers to be an enhancement be considered an enhancement by others? What if the state disagrees? What if other people disagree? Whose views should be counted in deciding whether or not an intervention is an enhancement?

We can imagine situations, for example, when parents might want to use enhancers for their own sake rather than for the sake of the child. Here are two scenarios that suggest this could be the case:

1. Imagine a child who is extremely boisterousness, not because he has anything wrong with him, but because that's his nature. Should his parents use Ritalin to curb his boisterousness?

Mightn't this enhancement suggest that these parents love their child only when he is calm and well-behaved?

2. Imagine we discover a set of genes that correlates with musical talent. Imagine further a couple, neither of whom is musical, who want a musically gifted child. They try IVF and PGD but none of their embryos has the required genes. Eventually they decide to genetically engineer the genes for musical talent into two of their embryos.

Mightn't this enhancement suggest that these parents will love only a musically talented child?

> ### Box 14.11 **Activity: Personal reflection**
>
> Do you agree parents should be given free rein to enhance their children? If not how would you regulate parental uses of enhancement?

(ii) Enhancement and social injustice

Our second general reason for being wary of biotechnological enhancements is that they will be relatively expensive. It seems reasonable to think that only the rich will be able to afford them. This means that we could end up with a two-tier society.

You might respond with the reasonable claim that we already have a two-tier society: wealthier parents can pay for independent education, orthodontists, extra-curricular tuition and designer clothes, whilst the poor must put up with state education, NHS dentists (if they can find them), after-school clubs and Matalan. Given that we already seem to think that two-tier societies are morally permissible, why should the fact that biotechnological enhancement might exacerbate this be a problem?[36]

This reply has some force. Especially when we consider that the state funds traditional enhancements (for example music lessons) up to a certain standard for the less wealthy. It would presumably do the same for the new enhancements, especially those conducive to social cohesion and advance. Were we, for example, to discover ways safely to enhance such general capacities as intelligence, health, fitness or memory, it would clearly be in the interests of the state to pay for everyone to be enhanced by such means.

Enhancing everyone's health would save huge amounts of money lost to the economy in sickness. It would also, in those countries that pay for healthcare, make paying for healthcare less expensive. Enhancing everyone's intelligence and memory would also seem beneficial for the state (although there could be drawbacks to such enhancements – high intelligence correlates with high suicide rates – and what if we were to remember every nasty thing that had ever happened to us?).

The state guaranteeing a decent basic minimum of goods such as education, health-care and income, by taxing the rich and using that money to support the poor, ensures that inequalities of social goods do not get serious enough to generate social unrest.

Why shouldn't the same system support a distribution of biotechnological enhancement equal enough to preclude social division and unrest? Perhaps therefore issues of social justice should not prevent us from embracing biotechnological enhancement?

It is possible, though, that in responding thus we could be grossly underestimating the inequalities that could result from permitting the non-traditional types of enhancement.

Consider a distinction between the 'social lottery' (determined by financial inequalities), and the 'natural lottery' (determined by genetic inequalities). There is undoubtedly a social lottery and it is undoubtedly the case that we accept winners and losers in this lottery. We may believe it unfair, but in the western world, where governments ensure a decent minimum to all, this unfairness does not become so unacceptable we feel we must do something about it.

But to what extent is our acceptance of the inequalities of the social lottery dependent on the fact that we believe that *natural* lottery, the distribution of talents and abilities, *is* fair? Might it be that our acceptance of the social lottery is dependent on our belief that, thanks to state subsidy, a poor but clever person has as much chance of getting to university as a rich but stupid person? If so social stability is ensured by our belief that the combination of a fair natural lottery and state funding generates a playing field level enough for the poor to compete fairly with the rich.

If this is the case then if, by virtue of biotechnological enhancements, it starts to look as if the *natural lottery* is becoming as unfair, as it is becoming indeed a function of the social lottery, social unrest might follow.[37]

At the moment rich and poor alike can work only with the material they have. If a child has a low IQ this might be mitigated by an excellent education and a sinecure in daddy's company, but the IQ itself can't be changed. If, however, we come to understand the genetic bases of such general characteristics as intelligence, and we acquire techniques by which to enhance such characteristics, the rich will be able to ensure not just that a child with low IQ will be comfortable, but that no child of theirs will *have* a low IQ.

The rich will no longer have to accept whatever hand they're dealt, they'll be able to take steps to guarantee that all their children have – in spades – whichever characteristics society deems most desirable.

To permit biological enhancement would be to accept that it is no longer a matter of luck that one has whatever talents and desirable characteristics one has. Such things would be a matter of the economic power of one's parents or perhaps their good management and willingness to forgo other good things in life for the sake of their children. The (relatively) rich would be able to buy not just social goods such as education and healthcare, they'd also be able to buy goods we currently think of as natural, such as good health and intelligence. Permitting people to enhance their children threatens to eliminate the natural lottery, at least for those able and willing to act on this option.

This could have a serious impact on society. At the moment, for example, it is not unreasonable to claim that the relatively wealthy predominate in our universities because their excellent education makes them *seem* more intelligent. In future such a claim might be unreasonable because being rich will mean that you *are* more intelligent. And why would employers take a risk on hiring the poor when employing the relatively wealthy would guarantee they'd be employing those with the talents they need? The rich and the poor would no longer be in the same boat when it came to luck: very little would *be* a matter of luck, at least for the rich.

> ### Box 14.12 **Activity: Group debate**
>
> *This House believes that the state must regulate enhancement to avoid the natural lottery becoming as unfair as the social lottery.*
>
> Participants might be put into groups and directed to take a certain side, or left to choose their own sides.

The bifurcation of society

To permit biological enhancement, therefore, could be to end up with a society in which rich people are tall, beautiful, intelligent, sporty and musical, not to mention well-educated and employed, and poor people, unless they're lucky, are short, ugly, stupid, uncoordinated, tone-deaf and unemployable. We could end up with a society in which the rich and the poor are so different that they are virtually two different *species*.[38]

We have already discussed the difficulties that could arise if society started to bifurcate in this way when we discussed the possibility of significantly increasing longevity. But the technology of enhancement exacerbates this issue.

Imagine, for example, that groups spring up, membership of which depends on the value placed by parents on given enhancements. The sports-minded, for example, might enhance their children's sporting ability to the extent that there'd be no point in anyone else competing. The musically minded might enhance musical ability to the extent that no one else would bother auditioning for the choir or orchestra. Society might start to look as if it depended not so much on a division of *labour* as a division of *nature*.

It wouldn't necessarily be the talents that were enhanced either. Some groups might choose to ensure that their daughters are modest and unassuming and that their sons are warrior-like and competitive. Other groups might choose to engineer out the competitive spirit, or engineer in a tendency to religious belief. After a few decades of this society could start to fragment in such a way that various different parts of society would have very little in common. At the same time, those within each group could have a *huge* amount in common. Perhaps even enough to threaten biodiversity within the group.

But are these concerns serious enough to suggest that the state should ban, or regulate, enhancement?

> **Box 14.13 Activity: Creative writing**
>
> Could permitting parents a free rein with enhancement lead to the bifurcation of society?
>
> Write a 500-word essay imagining the effects this could have on society.

There are certainly some enhancements the state might reasonably ban. It might, for example, reasonably ban enhancements that could lead to a ratcheting up of the social norm that would be socially self-defeating. Imagine, for example, if everyone were to enhance the height of their children by three inches. This would be ergonomically expensive – all public seating would have to be altered to ensure comfort – and of no benefit to anyone.

The fear of racheting up the norm could also prompt the regulation of the use of pharmaceutical enhancers such as Ritalin and Prozac. If everyone used Ritalin to socialise their boisterous boys the normal boisterousness of boys will start to seem *abnormal*. If everyone used Prozac as soon as they were anything but cheerful this could lead to the idea that it is abnormal to be a bit down.[39] Is this acceptable or should we just accept that boisterousness and being a bit down occasionally are part of the human condition?[40]

The elimination of suffering

This last consideration prompts a deeper question, one that is relevant to both enhancement and the questions about PGD in Chapter 10: how far is it reasonable to go in enhancing the characteristics we like, and eliminating those we don't like? Is it our hope, for example, that we might eliminate suffering altogether?

You may have read *Brave New World* (if not, I do recommend it[41])? If so, you will remember the 'soma' that everyone took to ensure they were permanently happy?[42] There was a governmental edict to the effect that all desires had to be satisfied within a certain time, so that no-one ever yearned for anything. Did you, or do you, think this is a desirable state of affairs?

Most people think that the ordinary citizens in the year of Our Ford 632 were less than human in their total acceptance of and satisfaction with their condition. Perhaps suffering of some kind is an essential part of becoming truly human? Many people have believed that it is by experiencing adversity that we grow in psychological strength. Would we forget how to strive for anything if everything is always as we want it to be? If it is true, as people have long believed, that character-development depends on the exercise of tenacity and self-discipline in the overcoming of hardship, what will happen if we eliminate hardship? Will we also eliminate character?

Or are all such thoughts just an indication of lack of imagination? Perhaps this traditional view of suffering was just a function of people putting a brave face on things: as suffering *couldn't* be eliminated, let's make a virtue out of a necessity. Now we *can*, in principle, eliminate suffering, do we *really* think it is a good thing?

> ### Box 14.14 Activity: Group discussion
>
> Imagine that we can remove all suffering from the world. Should we do so?
>
> The discussion should be open to the whole group, each of whom can argue as they choose. This website might help: http://www.bltc.com/.

The issues attending the possibility of biological enhancement are big ones. Many of these enhancements are very much still on the drawing board. But others are with us already. Consideration of the problems outlined above suggests that discussion of the moral ramifications of our use of such techniques can't start too soon.

Summary

In this chapter we have considered the moral acceptability of enhancement. In particular we have:

- learned of the distinction between somatic and germ-cell engineering;
- reflected on genetic holism;
- considered whether the therapy/enhancement boundary is a moral boundary;
- wondered about the threat to identity posed by
  - cognitive and mood enhancers as used by individuals;
  - performance enhancers in sport;
  - parents' enhancement of children.
- considered the notion of social injustice in
  - the distinction between the social and the natural lottery;
  - the possibility of a bifurcation in society;
  - the desirability of eliminating suffering altogether.

Questions to stimulate reflection

'It is morally acceptable to use biotechnology for therapeutic purposes, but not for the purposes of enhancement'. Do you agree?

Is it morally acceptable to genetically engineer non-heritable changes, but not heritable ones?

Is it morally irresponsible to engineer our genes before we know how our genes interact with each other?

Coffee is a cognitive enhancer, why should Modafinil be different?

Should we allow athletes to use performance-enhancing drugs so long as they are safe?

Would enhancing our children demonstrate that we do not love them unconditionally?

Would permitting enhancement lead to the natural lottery becoming as unfair as the social lottery?

Might different groups, by enhancing themselves in accordance with their own values, become different species?

Might widespread pharmaceutical intervention result in our losing sight of what it is to be human?

Additional activities

Participants might write 100 words on how each of our three moral theories would view (i) enhancers in sport, (ii) designer babies.

Conduct an informal poll amongst friends and family on people's views on designer babies.

Hold a debate on the use of enhancers in sport.

Find out more about the ban on technological swimsuits. Do you agree with it?

Conduct some research on attitudes to human suffering. Is it an essential part of the human condition?

Imagine you are taking an exam in the morning and you haven't managed to sleep. Should you take Modafinil to help you? Write a list of the pros and cons of doing so.

Use your imagination to write 1,000 words on what life would be like if everyone genetically enhanced their children.

Notes

1 http://www.thesite.org/workandstudy/studying/studentlife/smartdrugs. An account of smart drugs by the Site.Org.

2 http://nanotechweb.org/cws/article/tech/24508. A report on artificial muscles by nanotechweb.

3 http://www.physorg.com/news147928092.html. A report on 'smart clothing' from Phyorg. com.

4 http://nanogloss.com/nanotechnology/nanotechnology-cleaning/. From the Introduction to Nanotechnology website.

5 http://newsforums.bbc.co.uk/nol/thread.jspa?forumID=6630&edition=1&ttl=20100823105602. A BBC Reith lecture on the ethics of genetic enhancement.

6 http://malaria.wellcome.ac.uk/doc_WTD023878.html. Information on malaria and the sickle-cell trait from the Wellcome Trust.

7 http://today.ninemsn.com.au/article.aspx?id=284244. A radio interview on human genetic enhancement.

8 http://www.geneticsandsociety.org/article.php?id=286. Information about the difference between germline engineering and somatic cell engineering from the Genetics and Society website in the United States.

9 http://www.hum.utah.edu/~bbenham/2510%20Spring%2009/Gene%20Therapy/Resnik-therapyenhancement%20morality.pdf. A philosophical paper about the therapy enhancement distinction (not difficult for non-philosophers).

10 http://www.newscientist.com/article/mg20227094.000-harnessing-science-to-create-the-ultimate-warrior.html. A BBC report on the genetics of homosexuality.

11 Fukuyama, F. (2002) *Our Post-Human Future: Consequences of the Biotechnology Revolution.* London: Picador, pp. 39–40.

12 Buchanan, A., Brock, D. W., Daniels, N. and Wikler, D. (2001) *From Chance to Choice: Genetics and Justice.* Cambridge: Cambridge University Press, pp. 115–118.

13 http://www.time.com/time/health/article/0,8599,1921027,00.html. An article on human enhancement from *Time* magazine.

14 'Stronger, smarter, nicer humans' Julian Savulescu's 'Sydney Ideas Lecture' on Human Enhancement, originally broadcast on ABC Radio National in Australia, 19 August 2007. http://www.debatingmatters.com/topicguides/topicguide/designer_babies/. Lots of news articles both for and against 'designer babies' from Debating Matters.

15 http://www.biology-online.org/2/13_genetic_engineering.htm. Biology-Online on the advantages and disadvantages of genetically engineering humans.

16 http://www.guardian.co.uk/society/2008/jul/27/mentalhealth.drugs. A report of a government exhortation to smile rather than take Prozac.

17 http://www.telegraph.co.uk/news/uknews/1548910/Intelligence-drugs-could-be-common-as-coffee.html. A *Telegraph* article on cognitive enhancers.

18 http://www.thedoctorschannel.com/video/1640.html?order=title&page=25&specialty=4. A Doctors' Channel video on the contraindications of Modafinil.

19 http://plato.stanford.edu/entries/essential-accidental/. The *Stanford Encyclopedia of Philosophy* on the distinction between essential and accidental properties.

20 http://www.iep.utm.edu/person-i/. The *Internet Encyclopedia of Philosophy* on personal identity.

21 http://philosophybites.com/2008/11/christopher-shi.html. A podcast of philosopher Christopher Shields talking about personal identity for Philosophy Bites.

22 http://www.bbc.co.uk/sn/tvradio/programmes/horizon/ghostgenes.shtml. A BBC Science and Nature report on epigenetics.

23 http://www.chm.bris.ac.uk/motm/serotonin/depression.htm. Serotonin and mood from the University of Bristol.

24 http://www.open2.net/ethicsbites/sport-genetic-enhancement.html. Philosopher Michael Sandel on performance-enhancing drugs in sport for Philosophy Bites.

25 http://blip.tv/bion/human-enhancement-biotechnology-in-sports-15-03-11-part-5-professor-julian-savulescu-4976680. Podcast of philosopher Julian Savulescu talking about enhancement in sport.

26 We should accept performance-enhancing drugs in competitive sports: debate. A debate between Julian Savulescu of Oxford University's Uehiro Centre and opponents including Dick Pound, Head of the World Anti-Doping Agency. http://www.youtube.com/watch?v=0hPFMDFacRA.

27 http://www.thehastingscenter.org/Publications/BriefingBook/Detail.aspx?id=2206. The Hastings Centre from the United States on sport and enhancing drugs.

28 http://www.timesonline.co.uk/tol/comment/columnists/guest_contributors/article4359068.ece. An article from the *Times* on the use of enhancers in sport.

29 http://www.debatingmatters.com/topicguides/topicguide/drugs_in_sport/. A Debating Matters reading list for performance enhancement in sport.

30 http://www.telegraph.co.uk/sport/othersports/swimming/5894600/FINA-under-fire-as-hi-tech-swimsuits-row-overshadows-World-Championships-in-Rome.html. A *Telegraph* article on enhancing swimsuits.

31 Lea, Randall, D. (2009) Ethical considerations of biotechnologies used for performance enhancement. *The Journal of Bone and Joint Surgery (American)*, **91**: 2048–2054, doi:10.2106/JBJS.I.00023. An article on the ethical issues of biotechnological enhancement.

32 http://www.guardian.co.uk/sport/2009/jul/19/rebecca-adlington-swimsuit-fina. A report on Adlington's attitudes to 'technological doping'.

33 http://online.wsj.com/article/NA_WSJ_PUB:SB10001424052970204313604574328372762265260.html. A Wall Street Journal Report on FINA's banning of the high-tech swimsuits.

34 http://www.nuffieldbioethics.org/go/ourwork/behaviouralgenetics/introduction. The report from the Nuffield Council for Bioethics.

35 Buchanan, A. *et al.* (2001) *From Chance to Choice: Genetics and Justice.* Chapter 5, p. 165.

36 http://www.newscientist.com/article/dn13879-comment-here-come-the-designer-babies.html. An article from the *New Scientist* on designer babies.

37 http://www.bbc.co.uk/dna/h2g2/A3136042. The BBC on John Rawls' 'natural lottery' (and other ideas).

38 http://news.bbc.co.uk/1/hi/uk/6057734.stm.

39 http://ieet.org/index.php/IEET/more/3277/. An article from the Institute of Ethics and Emerging technologies.

40 http://www.dailymail.co.uk/femail/article-1074175/How-I-weaned-son-Ritalin-proved-discipline-IS-better-drugs.html. A *Daily Mail* article on a mother's taking her son off Ritalin.

41 Huxley, A. (1932 [1998]) *Brave New World.* New York: Harper Perennial Modern Classics.

42 http://www.huxley.net/soma/somaquote.html. Quotes about soma from *Brave New World*, from Huxley.net.

Further reading and useful websites

Green, R.M. (2009) *Babies by Design: The Ethics of Genetic Choice.* New Haven, CT: Yale University Press.

Harris, J. (2007) *Enhancing Evolution: The Ethical Case for Making Better People.* Princeton, NJ: Princeton University Press.

Murray, T. and Miah, A. (2004) *Genetically Modified Athletes: Biomedical Ethics, Gene Doping and Sport: The Ethical Implications of Genetic Technologies in Sport.* London: Routledge

Sandel, M.J. (2007) *The Case Against Perfection: Ethics in the Age of Genetic Engineering.* Cambridge, MA: Harvard University Press.

http://www.debatingmatters.com/topicguides/topicguide/designer_babies/. A 'Debating Matters' topic guide to designer babies.

Allen Buchanan, Beyond Humanity? The Ethics of Biomedical Enhancement-Lecture 1 (avi)

Allen Buchanan, Beyond Humanity? The Ethics of Biomedical Enhancement-Lecture 2 (avi)

Allen Buchanan, Beyond Humanity? The Ethics of Biomedical Enhancement-Lecture 3 (avi)
    Three lectures on biomedical enhancement from the Uehiro Centre for Practical Ethics at the University of Oxford.

http://www.humanenhance.com/NSF_report.pdf. Twenty-five questions and answers on the ethics of human enhancement from the US National Science Foundation.

15

Bio-information: databases, privacy and the fight against crime

If you are not an identical twin, you will be distinguished from everyone else by 1% your DNA.[1] If there is a match between your DNA and a sample of DNA the source of which is unknown, you can be conclusively identified as the source of that sample despite sharing 99% of your DNA with every human being on the planet (and 98% of it with chimpanzees, and 60% with bananas). Your genome contains 3,000,000,000 base pairs. It differs from that of any other person, therefore, in about 6,000,000 locations.[2]

Your looks, your behavioural traits, your personality, your responses to drugs, foods and allergens are all a function of your unique set of genes, and the unique environment in which you grew up.

We are the product of both nature and nurture.[3] The debate has long raged about which is most influential. Fashions change. In Victorian times nature was deemed all. In the mid–late twentieth century it was 'conditioning' that was deemed important. Nowadays we recognise neither is primary: epigenetics tells us that our genes influence the way we respond to our environments and our environments influence the way our genes are expressed.[4] If we want to understand ourselves we must learn about nature *and* nurture.

Over the last few decades our understanding of the nature side of the spectrum has been greatly facilitated by:

- the mapping of the whole genome;
- the mapping of the location of many common genetic variations each potentially a 'bio-marker';
- the development of 'genechips' that allow us to test simultaneously for 500,000 different bio-markers;[5]
- advances in bioinformatics, which allow us to capture, process, analyse and store information on the sequences, structure and function of genes;[6]
- the development of databases that enable us to analyse the interactions between genes, the environment and the phenotypical traits that interest us.

We are now able to test individuals and groups of people for many specific bio-markers, we can use individuals' genetic profiles as a means of conclusively identifying them, and individuals prepared to pay can have their genomes sequenced to learn about disorders to which they are susceptible, the better to make choices of lifestyle.

Box 15.1 Factual information: Genetic information

Sequencing: determines the exact sequence of a length of DNA.

Genetic profiling: sequencing the whole genome of an individual, usually for the purposes of identification or health management.

Genotyping: determines which genetic variants an individual possesses.

Genetic testing: testing an individual for specific bio-markers, usually because a problem is indicated. For example someone with Huntington's disease in the family might be tested for the HD gene.

Genetic screening: this involves testing whole populations or sub-populations for specific bio-markers, usually as part of a public health service, to identify those with conditions for which an affordable cure or therapy is available. In the UK, for example, new parents can have babies screened for phenylketonuria (PKU).

In this chapter we shall consider the social and ethical issues generated by bioinformatics, the capture, storage and use of information about our biological characteristics, in particular our DNA.

Bio-information and identity

If the police successfully harvest DNA from a crime scene they can in principle identify someone as having perpetrated the crime.[7] The use of such evidence to implicate someone in the crime depends on the existence of a match between that person's DNA and the DNA found at the scene.

Matches can be found by testing DNA samples from the scene of the crime against samples obtained from those suspected of the crime, those living or working near a crime who volunteer DNA for the purposes of elimination, and from samples held on police databases. In each case a failure to match a sample with the sample from the crime scene demonstrates innocence, a match the opposite. In every country that can afford such technology, DNA matching has supplemented fingerprinting as a means of helping the police identify the guilty.

But such methods are not uncontroversial. Let's consider a recent argument about the National DNA Database (NDNAD) in the UK.[8]

Box 15.2 Factual information: National DNA Database (NDNAD)

In a typical month matches between crime scene samples and the NDNAD link suspects to 15 murders, 31 rapes and 770 motor vehicle offences. For example:

- In 2006 the DNA of Mark Dixie, arrested after a minor scuffle at a pub, was matched to the DNA of the man who had murdered Sally Ann Bowman and raped her as she lay dying. Dixie is now serving 34 years in jail.[9]
- In 2004 Craig Harman threw a brick off a motorway bridge, causing Michael Little, a 53-year-old lorry driver, to have a heart attack. Harman left blood on the brick. Although it didn't match any DNA on the database, familial searching led to a relative whose DNA matched by 16 out of 20 points. This led to Harman, whose DNA matched perfectly. Harman was jailed for 6 years.
- In 2008 a mentally ill man called Sean Hodgson was released after 26 years in prison when his DNA proved that he could not have been the murderer of 22-year-old Teresa de Simone.[10]

In the US too DNA has been used to convict the guilty, but also to free 245 people innocent of the crimes for which they were convicted. For example:

- In 2010 Raymond Towler was freed after 30 years in prison for raping an 11-year-old girl. He had been convicted after being picked out at an identity parade by the victim.[11]
- In 2009 James Bain was freed after 35 years in jail in Florida for kidnapping, burglary and strong-arm rape.[12]

The NDNAD was established in 1995. It was the first, and remains the largest, criminal database in the world. In the UK anyone associated with a crime – suspects, victims, witnesses – will have a sample of their DNA taken. Until recently, all these DNA samples have been added to NDNAD. Many of the individuals with samples or profiles on the database have never even been cautioned by the police never mind convicted of a crime; 39,000 of them are children.[13]

Because DNA is extremely stable it can be stored indefinitely. DNA profiles can be stored even after the sample from which they were derived has been destroyed. At the end of 2008 the NDNAD held over 4 million samples.

In 2008 however the European Court ruled the NDNAD illegal.[14] Test cases had been brought by two individuals who had been suspected, but not convicted, of a crime. Both objected to their DNA being added to the database. The European Court judged that the retention of their DNA was a violation of their right to privacy, that it was 'blanket and indiscriminate', a 'disproportionate interference' and 'unnecessary in a democratic country'.

> ### Box 15.3 Activity: Devil's advocate
>
> Do you think the European Court was right to argue that the DNA of those who haven't been convicted of a crime should not be kept on the NDNAD?
>
> Having decided on the view to which you tend, consider the arguments that someone holding the opposite view might use against you. Do any sway you?

The case against the NDNAD was being considered by the European Court having previously been dismissed by the UK's highest court of appeal: the Law Lords. We have looked at the European Court's reason for its ruling. Let's now consider the Law Lords' reason for *their* ruling.

The Law Lords rejected the appeal because the ground of the appellants' claim was that they had never been convicted of a crime. To accept this, their lordships argued, would be to accept that those who *had* been convicted of a crime are less 'innocent', of a *new* crime, than those who have not been convicted of a crime in the past. This, they pointed out, violates an assumption fundamental to British law: the assumption that *everyone* is innocent until proven guilty.[15]

That this is an important plank of British law is undeniable. In Britain the previous convictions of anyone being tried for a crime are revealed only under very specific conditions. It is thought that if members of the jury know the defendant has previously been guilty of a similar crime, they would convict defendants, not on the basis of the evidence presented, but on the basis of their previous guilt.

The purpose of the NDNAD is to solve crimes for which no one has been convicted. For such crimes *everyone* must be assumed to be innocent. There can be no grounds, therefore, for distinguishing some on the database as 'innocent' and others as 'guilty'. On the basis of this the Law Lords dismissed the case insisting that the claimants' privacy was not unacceptably invaded by the fact their DNA was held by the NDNAD.

> ### Box 15.4 Activity: Small group discussion
>
> The European Court argued that those never convicted of a crime have the right to privacy and that this is violated by keeping their DNA on the NDNAD.

The Law Lords argued that the NDNAD exists to help solve crimes for which no one has been convicted. As everyone must be deemed innocent of such crimes, no distinction can be made between the DNA of those who have, and those who haven't, been convicted of a crime.

Divide participants into small groups and ask the groups to discuss which side they are on. Groups should appoint a spokesperson to report back to the group.

A universal database?

The Law Lords decided that the DNA of those never convicted of a crime could stay on the NDNAD. They could just have easily have decided that it was a violation of *everyone's* privacy to have their DNA recorded. The Law Lords did not ask that the NDNAD be dismantled as a threat to privacy because they recognise the value of the NDNAD for preventing and solving crime.

In 2008 alone, for example, 17,614 crimes including 83 killings and 184 rapes were solved as a direct result of the NDNAD. If a database with 4 million samples on it is so useful, why shouldn't we have a database with 61.5 million samples? Why shouldn't we, in other words, have a universal database, on which *everyone's* DNA is recorded? Every crime committed by a British subject who leaves DNA at the scene could be solved within hours.

Constructing such a database would be easy. In recent years DNA has been collected from millions of people. Every new baby has its heel pricked so its blood can be tested for PKU. The results are recorded on 'Guthrie cards' and kept in the hospitals in which the infant was born. Soon newborns showing signs of liver disorders will be tested for 92 different genetic conditions.[16] Few adults will not have had blood, urine or tissue taken at some point, and these samples, or the profiles generated by them, will also be recorded.

The collection of such samples and the profiles they generate has been standardised to facilitate data-sharing, and computerisation has made such data-sharing easy. If all such databases were effectively to become extensions of the NDNAD, the police would soon be able to check crime scene samples against pretty well the whole population.

In fact, why stick at a *national* database? Criminals do not respect national boundaries. The threat of international terrorism is a huge incentive for nations to share their records, at least with friendly countries. Why not aim for an *international* database?[17]

What a tool bioinformatics could be in the global fight against crime and terrorism!

An Orwellian nightmare

The idea of a universal database, however, prompts anguish from civil rights organisations. To such organisations the idea of their own government's having access to everyone's DNA, never mind other governments sharing that access, is a nightmare of Orwellian proportions. A universal DNA database is something to fear, they say, because:

(i)   the information held on it will be so rich;
(ii) this information could be used to limit options;
(iii) the information could be politically incendiary;
(iv) such databases could result in a genetic underclass;
(v)   such databases would threaten our privacy;
(vi) such databases are inherently insecure;
(vii) a benign government could become malign.

Let's look at each of these reasons for fearing a national or international DNA database.[18]

(i) DNA is information-rich

Possession of your DNA profile would allow the authorities to do far more than check your DNA against crime-scene samples. Even in our current state of understanding they would be able to determine your family relationships. They would know, for example, who had fathered your baby, whether it has half-siblings, and whether the man you think of as 'dad' really is your father.

The authorities would also have access to information about your present and future health. They will know whether you will develop Huntington's disease, or are susceptible to heart disease, breast cancer or Alzheimer's. As we discover (if we ever do) the genetic bases of tendencies to violence, to intelligence, to sporting prowess, etc., all our personalities, capabilities, proclivities and behavioural traits will become an open book.

This is the sort of information we might not even want to share with our best friend or family. We might not even want to know this information *ourselves*. In principle, though, a universal database would make *all* of it accessible to the authorities.

(ii) Limiting options

Imagine that we could identify musical ability at birth. Might the government then argue that it wastes money to provide music lessons for everyone? Maybe those without the genes for sporting prowess would soon be restricted to classes in keep fit; the sports hall, swimming pool and games pitches would be reserved for those with these genes.

> ### Box 15.5 **Activity: Paired discussion**
>
> If you found that you didn't have the genes for musical ability would this dissuade you from learning to play an instrument or from joining a choir?
>
> Do you think it would dissuade others?
>
> Do you think the government should fund the musical education of those whose genes suggest they have no musical talent?

If we had the genes for intelligence, furthermore, might the government decide that some individuals aren't worth educating beyond a basic minimum? In *Brave New World* nutrients were withheld from the 'epsilons' so there would be someone to do the 'grunt work'. In *our* brave new world the government wouldn't even need to *do* anything to produce epsilons, it would just identify them from their DNA.

What if the authorities could identify children with the genes coding for mono-amine oxidase and tryptophan hydroxylase, both enzymes linked to specific cases of violent behaviour?[19] Would they be required to attend classes in anger management and relaxation? If their violent tendencies seemed to be being expressed might they be imprisoned despite the fact they haven't done anything wrong?

Many have thought a universal database could be the first step to a society in which decisions about what will happen to us are made by government rather than by our parents or ourselves.

> ### Box 15.6 Activity: Creative writing
>
> If a 'murder' gene were found, one that correlated almost exactly with a pathological inability to empathise with others and an enjoyment of torture and killing, would this justify treating a child as a criminal and imprisoning it, despite its being, at the time of incarceration, entirely innocent?
>
> Write a 500-word story from the point of view of such a child or one of its parents.

(iii) The 'politically incendiary'

What if, once everyone's DNA was on the database, it became clear that certain groups shared a genetic inheritance? What if, for example, it became clear that women do not, on the whole, have the genes that correlate with scientific ability? What if blacks, on the whole, have the genes for criminality?

This possibility was noted by the cognitive scientist, Stephen Pinker, in response to this question:

'What is your dangerous idea? An idea you think about that is dangerous not because it is assumed to be false but because it might be true.'[20]

In the past women and black people have been discriminated against *because* they were members of these groups. Most of us believe such discrimination was based on blind prejudice. But if there are demonstrable genetic differences between these groups and other groups, and these differences correlate with behaviour and abilities that were cited as reason for such discrimination, could science prove blind prejudice right?[21] Pinker believes this could prove politically incendiary.[22]

Francis Fukuyama expresses a different worry. He believes such issues can't even be discussed in current intellectual communities because everyone is afraid of being accused of prejudice. He thinks this might lead to claims that there are scientific facts that shouldn't be made public.

Might Plato's idea of the 'noble lie', a lie told for the good of society, be revived?[23] Perhaps there *are* occasions when lies *should* be told, or at least truth suppressed, for the greatest good of the greatest number?

Box 15.7 Activity: Group discussion

On 14 January 2005 Larry Summers, then President of Harvard, made a speech that included the following two sentences:

> 'It does appear that on many human attributes – height, weight, propensity for criminality, IQ, mathematical ability, scientific ability – there is relatively clear evidence that ... there is a difference [between] a male and female population.'[24]

> 'There is reasonably strong evidence of taste differences between little girls and little boys that are not easy to attribute to socialisation.'

In February 2006, partly as a result of such remarks, Summers was forced to resign.

Consider what would happen if science were to provide genetic evidence for Summers' claim about the differences between the male and female mind.

The discussion might be facilitated by means of the following questions:

- Could genetic evidence show that *all* men have scientific ability or that *no* woman does?
- If women were demonstrated to be statistically less likely to have scientific ability does this suggest that less money should be spent on science education for women or that *more* money should be spent on women to bring them up to scratch?
- Should such findings dissuade women from considering a career in science?
- Would such findings be so 'politically incendiary' they should be suppressed?
- Is there any scientific finding so politically incendiary it should be suppressed?

(iv) A genetic underclass?

The worries considered so far have been predicated on the government's ready access to your DNA. More worries emerge if we consider the possibility that access to your DNA might go further than the government.

Insurance companies claim – correctly – that much of the information available on a DNA database is already available from medical records and family histories. They also suggest that access to DNA databases could bring down the cost of insurance.[25] Why should you insure yourself for anything, after all, but accident and the few conditions to which your genes make you susceptible? If you could convince the insurance company that your lifestyle minimises the few risks you do face the price might go even lower.

Some insurance companies already pay larger annuities to people who smoke or engage in other life-threatening behaviour. Such people, they reason, will not need their pensions for as long as others. Perhaps your poor genes will ensure you a wealthy, albeit short, retirement?

But not everyone embraces such a rosy view of what would happen if insurance companies had access to bio-information. In the United States the use of bio-information by insurance companies has been banned for fear some people would become uninsurable.

Employers might also find bio-information valuable.[26] Might you become unemployable because your genes suggest you have a health risk? Might you be unable to pursue a particular career because your genes suggest you would be a health and safety hazard for the company?

What if it became possible for potential partners to check out your genes? Might the person you love decide you are too much of a risk?

> **Box 15.8 Activity: DVD-watching**
>
> Get hold of a DVD of the film GATTACA and arrange a showing of it followed by a group discussion of how likely it is that such a scenario could become a reality.

(v) The luxury of complete privacy

Would you like to be one of those celebrities who cannot so much as look out of their window or chat to a neighbour without its being recorded? Or do you prefer your obscurity? How much do you value your privacy? After the fall of Ceausescu in Romania, many Romanian citizens said that the worse thing about his reign had been the constant surveillance: 'the government knew everything about you at every moment' complained one.

Perhaps the idea we are ever free of surveillance is an illusion anyway, with CCTV, mobile phones, credit cards and laptops with internet connections.[27] But imagine if the government could trace you from the DNA you leave on everything you touch. Would you ever again feel you had escaped from prying eyes?

> **Box 15.9 Activity: Creative writing**
>
> Write a short story – perhaps a funny one – in which you imagine you are trying to escape from your life, but are constantly surprised by people who know your name and all sorts of personal information about you.

(vi) The security of bio-information

Naturally those who are in favour of universal databases to fight crime will argue that the information on these databases is completely secure. That, indeed, it is secure *even from the government*. Only those fighting crime will have access to such databases.

But we are all aware that data can be lost, sold or misused. In 2009, for example, the UK's Joseph Rowntree Reform Foundation published a report 'Database State' which examined 46 UK government databases and found all but 6 to be insecure.[28] The evidence on which this report was based (and the impartiality of those compiling the report) has been questioned, but who are we to believe? In Box 15.10 you will find some examples of situations in which the security of data was far from ideal.

On the other hand it seems that many young people are unconcerned about their privacy. Judging from entries on Facebook many are quite happy to see their personal details and even their indiscretions plastered over the web. Perhaps privacy isn't an issue?[29]

Box 15.10 Factual information: Sensitive data in the UK

The Driver and Vehicle Licensing Authority (DVLA) in the UK has made £9 million from selling vehicle owners' contact details to private parking companies.[30]

In 2008 contact and other details of 25 million people receiving UK child benefit were burnt, unencrypted, onto a CD and sent off in the post without registration. They disappeared.[31]

In just one year 1500 UK passports were lost in the post.[32]

The details of 3 million UK learner drivers were lost when a computer hard drive went missing from a US contract company working for the UK DVLA.[33]

In 2007 the Medical Training Application Service published on an insecure website the personal details, including details of the sexuality, of 1000 junior doctors.[34]

(vii) Benign versus malign government?

Even if everyone's DNA were available on one universal database *our* government, most of us like to think, would not misuse it in any of the ways described above.

But governments change. Few people in Germany in the early 1930s realised how their government was changing. Can we be certain that we will *always* be governed by people who would never misuse the information available on a universal database?

Box 15.11 Activity: Group discussion

This house believes that a universal database would be a serious threat to civil liberties.

Sides might be allocated to participants, or they might choose their own sides.

Governmental efficiency

. . . .

You might be unconvinced by those who put these objections to the idea of a universal database. Such people, you might think, must be very cynical. In fact, you would add, there is everything to gain from the government's having ready access to a universal database.

Think how often, for example, the authorities have to check your identity: when you pay your taxes, draw benefits, travel abroad, enter a government building or other secure area, undergo a criminal record check or take a government job. A universal database of bio-information would make this incredibly easy. One day we might not even have to carry identity cards, our irises would do the trick.

Such a database would greatly facilitate governmental planning. The authorities would no longer have to base future public services on educated guesswork, it will *know* how many people are likely to develop heart disease or Alzheimer's. It will be possible also to target those who are at most risk. Five year olds known to be susceptible to heart disease, for example, could be given early encouragement to adopt appropriate lifestyle choices.

Perhaps too if we ever find the genes associated with, for example, swimming or mathematical prowess, the authorities, knowing how many children have such genes, could plan public swimming pools more effectively and train the right number of maths teachers?

A DNA based identity card linked to all the records the government holds on us would be so much more efficient (and be so much less open to abuse) than expecting us to remember unique identifying numbers.

With all these benefits potentially available many who argue for universal databases cannot see why anyone should object to them. Why, they ask, should you be frightened of the authorities being able to identify you by your DNA unless you have something to hide?[35]

> **Box 15.12 Activity: Paired reflection**
>
> Imagine it is the year 2035 and that we have successfully identified many of the genetic variations correlated with personality, behavioural traits, susceptibilities to disease, responses to drugs and allergens, etc.
>
> Further imagine that a sample of everyone's DNA is held on a database to which all government departments have access.
>
> Working with a partner:
>
> (i) list the benefits that could be derived from governmental access to such a database;
> (ii) list the problems, if any, that might arise from governmental access to such a database.

Personalised medicine

Even if the idea of a universal database is rejected, many individuals would be interested in having their own genomes sequenced. What a luxury, you might think, to know in advance to which illnesses you are susceptible. How much more enjoyable would that pizza or those nights out be if you knew you had no susceptibility to alcoholism[36] or heart or liver disease?[37]

In 2010 the going rate in the US for genome sequencing is $9,500–32,000. But the cost is expected to drop below $1000 within the next few years.[38] It is possible, anyway, to find out a lot about your genome by means of 'genotyping' (see Box 15.1) which is already fairly cheap. Many companies offer this service to the public, and many individuals buy it, either to discover whether they have or carry a particular condition, or to manage their health more effectively.

It is also possible, by such means, to determine your likely response to various drugs. For example the psychiatric DNA test GeneSightRx will already help medics know whether 26 psychiatric drugs, including Seroxat and Prozac, are likely to work for you.[39] This is a boon when it is estimated that a third of psychiatric drugs are of no benefit to the person for whom they are prescribed.

It also introduces the possibility of 'bespoke' drugs. Many cancer drugs, for example, work only for those with particular DNA. Patients whose tumours test positive for BRAF might get PLX 4032, for example, whilst those whose tumours test positive for EGFR will get erlotinib instead.[40] When we consider the number of deaths from adverse reactions to prescription drugs[41] we can see that such advances are likely to be hugely advantageous.

Box 15.13 Definition: Pharmacogenetics/pharmacogenomics

The merger of pharmacology and genetics into a field that pertains to the hereditary responses to drugs. For example, after the administration of a muscle relaxant drug, a patient may have difficulty breathing due to a genetically determined defect in metabolising (processing) the muscle relaxant.

The term 'pharmacogenetics' dates to 1962 when Dr Werner Kalow published *Pharmacogenetics: Heredity and the Response to Drugs* (Philadelphia, PA: W.B. Saunders and Co.)

Pharmacogenetics is used interchangeably with the newer term 'pharmaco-genomics.'[42]

In the future it seems likely that you will be able to carry a card that your doctor will slot into a reader, the better to determine which drug would suit you best and in what dosage. Prescription will no longer be a hit and miss affair.

Not everyone, however, thinks personalised medicine is a good idea. Many people prefer blissful ignorance. Who wants to spend their life worrying about a possibility that may never become actual? Wouldn't a life spent under the Damocles sword of the possibility of early onset Alzheimer's be blighted?[43]

> ## Box 15.14 Activity: Personal reflection and presentation
>
> Would you want to know if you had the combination of ApoE4 and TOMM40 that greatly increases your chances of inherited Alzheimer's?[44]
>
> Over the next week keep a notebook in which to jot down thoughts about how you would respond to such a discovery. Be alert to mentions of Alzheimer's in the news or the papers, talk to people whose relatives have Alzheimer's, check out the websites of organisations devoted to Alzheimer's.
>
> At the end of the week give a short (5 minute) presentation of your decision and the reasons for it.
>
> Alternatively a poll might be conducted and used to stimulate a group discussion.

Another problem could arise from the discovery that you carry something inherited or with a familial tendency.[45] To discover you are a carrier of cystic fibrosis, for example, is to discover your siblings are also likely to be carriers.[46] Would you want the responsibility of having to inform them of this fact? Could you live with yourself if you didn't? Might the government compel you (or your doctor) to inform them?[47] Is this reasonable? Should you have your children sequenced, the better to manage their health in childhood? But what if, when grown, they would rather not have known about their health risks?

Box 15.15 Factual information

Sergey Brin, the co-founder of Google™, had his genome sequenced and learned he had the mutation of gene LRRK2 that confers a 20–80% increased risk of Parkinson's Disease.[48] He has donated $4 million to subsidise a study of 10,000 Parkinson's patients.

Brin is married to Anne Wojcicki, the co-founder of 23andMe,[49] a private company that markets, for £399 a time, genetic scans that assess the chances of developing 105 diseases from breast cancer to baldness.

The Parkinson's patients who volunteer for the study will pay only $25 for the scan. Their genomes and detailed lifestyle questionnaires, will then be compared to those provided by those customers of 23andMe who do not have Parkinson's.

Brin and Wojcicki have already volunteered their son's DNA for the study.[50]

There is also the possibility of lifestyle guilt. We all probably feel guilty enough already when we do things we know are not good for us, or don't do things that are good for us. Who wants to feel lifelong guilt for not doing everything they can to mitigate risks they *know* they run? Very few smokers are ignorant about how they could improve their future health. This makes many feel extremely guilty. Yet still they don't act. Won't many people end up feeling permanently guilty?

In the States doctors have argued that individuals should be prevented from learning about their own DNA because they will not be able to handle such knowledge. A Congressional inquiry was instituted in Congress in 2010 and the Food and Drug Administration has written to sequencing companies warning them they are selling a medical device without prescription.[51] Many, however, believe that this is a paternalistic attitude and that individuals have a right to pay to see their own DNA, even if they might not like what they learn.

One thing they might learn, of course, is that the son or daughter they have brought up as their own is not, in fact, their own. One father who made this discovery described it as 'crushing' and although he told his 17-year-old 'daughter' that it wouldn't change anything, he admits that 'it does, though, of course it does'.[52]

Imagine the anguish this father must feel. Is this a good reason to ban the possibility of individuals learning about their own DNA?

Box 15.16 Activity: Web-wandering

All participants should wander round the web looking for incidents where an individual's knowledge of their genome has not been an unmitigated blessing. Bring the results back to the group for a 'show and tell'.

In the UK there is a thriving debate about whether the National Health Service (NHS) should pay for treatment for illnesses caused by such things as smoking and obesity.[53] If someone could have done something to prevent themselves getting these illnesses, the claim goes, they have forfeited the right to have their treatment paid for out of the public purse. In countries without a welfare state health insurers might also impose a premium on those who choose not to give up their bad habits. Would it be fair for the state to refuse to refund treatment in such cases?

Box 15.17 Activity: Discussion topic

George Best, called by many the greatest ever English footballer, was an alcoholic. He had a liver transplant in 2002 but he couldn't stop drinking and died in 2005, aged 59, of cirrhosis of the liver.[54]

Best was able to afford private healthcare. But others aren't. Should drinkers who refuse to give up drinking be treated on the NHS for drinking-related conditions?

If they are alcoholics does this alter the situation?

Biobanks

Personalised medicine will be a distant dream until we properly map the common genetic variants against the phenotypical characteristics that express them. It is only if we can collect DNA samples from huge numbers of people, and map them against the lifestyles and characteristics of these people, that we will find the correlations that we need to make predictions about susceptibility to disease, responses to drugs, tendency to violence and so on. Armed with these correlations we will be able to develop better diagnostic tools, better therapies and target drugs to the individuals for whom they are most likely to work.

But given the fears associated with DNA databases, and even an individual's acquiring information about his own genome, how are we ever going to persuade enough people to give samples of their DNA?

There is an obvious way to secure the benefits of DNA databases without paying the feared costs: we need a DNA database, accessible to researchers, in which every sample is given *anonymously*. Such a database would be of no use to the police or the authorities for whom the identification of individuals is paramount.[55]

Box 15.18 Factual information: The 'HapMap Project'

The International HapMap is a resource freely available to those searching for the genetic variations that correlate with increased susceptibility to various conditions.[56] It could not have been constructed unless many people had donated their DNA to the project. It is unlikely so many people would have donated their DNA had they not been assured of anonymity.

Genetic variations that are near each other on a chromosome tend to be inherited together. A 'haplotype' is a region of such linked variants.

In a given population 55% may have one version of a haplotype, 30% another, 8% another, and the rest a variety of less common haplotypes.

Researchers wanting to find the genetic variants correlating with, say, high blood pressure, can use the HapMap to search for haplotypes common in those with hypertension, but uncommon in those without it.

Millions of individuals worldwide have now donated their DNA anonymously to national and international 'biobanks'. Amongst the largest such biobanks is Iceland's. Run by deCODE genetics (until it went bankrupt in 2009) all the citizens of Iceland since 1703 until the present time have given tissue, blood and urine samples, details of lifestyle and environment and medical records, to the Icelandic biobank. This makes it one of the most useful research resources of all times. Citizens can actively opt out, but 95% of the current population is included. There are also large biobanks to be found in Canada, Estonia and the UK.

Everyone donating DNA and medical details to these biobanks does so under conditions of 'informed consent', where the information includes the fact that no one

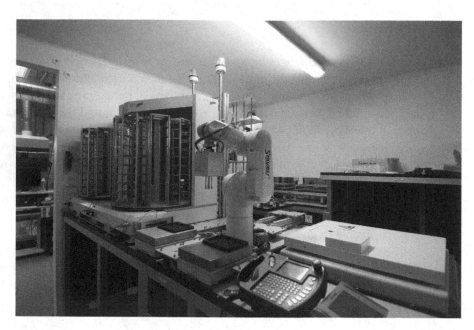

Figure 15.1 Equipment for handling multiple samples at UK Biobank, Cheshire, a project which stores and protects a vast bank of medical data and material from volunteers. © Wellcome Images, London.

connected with the study will be able to identify the individual who donated the DNA. Clearly records *are* kept of who donates the DNA, but they are kept in such a way that they are not accessible to those doing the study or anyone else unless there is specific reason to search them out.

Unfortunately, this anonymity is not foolproof. In 2003 Sweden's foreign minister, Anna Lindh, was assassinated. The Swedish Police found the assailant's DNA on the knife used to kill her. Using the Guthrie cards collected by Sweden's hospitals a match was found with a Serb national, who was subsequently arrested and convicted of Lindh's assassination. Guthrie cards have also been used successfully by police in New Zealand and Scotland. Who is to say that biobanks will not be used in the same way?

Box 15.19 **Factual information: deCODE genetics**

In 2009 deCODE, the company responsible for Iceland's biobank, and also a pioneer in personal DNA testing, filed for bankruptcy.[57]

This has caused consternation about the data held by deCODE. An American Investment company, Saga Investments, has agreed to buy deCODE's core science operations, so it is likely the data will end up in their possession.[58]

But those who gave DNA samples to deCODE did not sign up to allow this information to be passed on.[59]

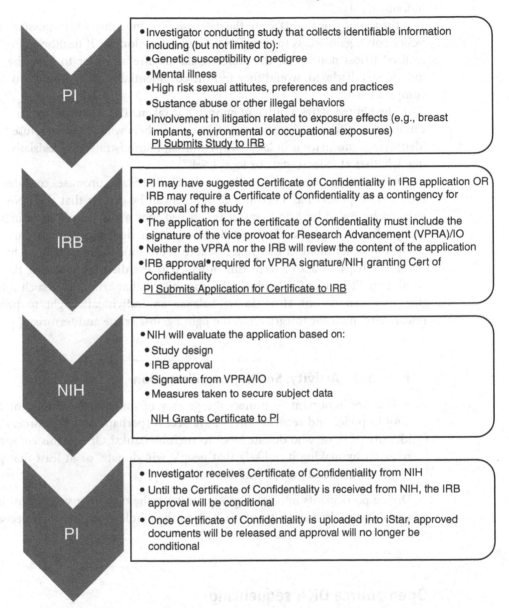

Figure 15.2 Steps to obtaining a Certificate of Confidentiality from the National Institute of Health (NIH) (http://www.usc.edu/admin/provost/oprs/research/confident.html).

In the UK the police can go to court to get access to DNA databases held by hospitals and other institutions. Healthcare professionals can go to court to bar such access. But there is no guarantee they will succeed. The individuals whose DNA is on the database for which access is requested, furthermore, have no say in the matter. The fact police can ask for such information is not on the consent forms that such individuals sign.[60]

If those who donated DNA to the database *were* informed of the possibility that the police could gain access to their DNA, would they donate? If healthcare professionals realised (most don't) that the police could acquire an order to have the details of individuals disclosed, would they feel the confidentiality they promise to subjects is compromised?

In the United States a different approach is taken. The National Institute of Health can issue 'certificates of confidentiality' to researchers who can then refuse to disclose identifying information in 'any civil, criminal, administrative or legislative proceeding, whether at federal, state or local level'.[61]

This means that when a researcher in the United States promises confidentiality, so long as that project has a certificate, subjects can be certain that the DNA they give will not be traced back to them. It is believed that many people from marginalised groups donate DNA that they would not otherwise donate because of this.

On the other hand, if the police believe they could solve a heinous high profile crime, perhaps an act of terrorism in which many died, by violating the terms of confidentiality for the individual who committed that crime, is it such a bad thing that they can do so? How do we balance an individual's right to privacy and researchers' need for integrity and the fight against crime and terrorism?

> **Box 15.20 Activity: Small group discussion**
>
> Is it more important to protect the privacy of individuals or to fight crime? Should police and security forces have access (perhaps on court order) to the identity of those who donate DNA to such biobanks? Or will this compromise research by making it unlikely that people will donate, or at least that people from marginalised groups will donate?
>
> Divide participants into small groups and ask them to discuss this issue and to appoint a spokesperson to report back to the whole group on their decisions.

Open-source DNA sequencing

Amongst the scientific community, however, there is a movement towards greater openness, a rejection, indeed, of the notion that DNA privacy is even important. Craig Venter the geneticist was the first individual to have his genome sequenced: he published the lot on the web.[62] He was followed shortly afterwards by James Watson, one of the co-discoverers of the double helix.[63]

George Church of Harvard University, also, has published his genome on the web, together with his medical details, and invited 100,000 volunteers to do likewise.[64]

Church launched his project with a pilot phase in which nine other high profile individuals – all of them with impeccable scientific credentials – openly published their own DNA profiles and medical records. No doubt encouraged by this 13,000 individuals are already on the waiting list for later phases.

In contributing to Church's 'Personal Genome Project'[65] volunteers (who must be from the United States) allow their DNA profiles to be added to 'open-source' software. This means that *anyone* can work on them (including employers and insurance companies). By permitting open access such people hope to solve the problems we want to solve sooner than we otherwise would.

If these influential and highly thought of scientists are prepared to eschew anonymity and publish their medical records and DNA profiles openly on the internet under their own names, perhaps the rest of us are worrying unnecessarily about privacy? Perhaps, in these days of Facebook and other networking websites, we'll all soon be clamouring to make our DNA public?

> ### Box 15.21 Activity: Discussion topic[66]
>
> Would the fact that so many respectable geneticists and other scientists have signed up to publish their DNA profiles and other details openly on the web encourage you to do likewise?
>
> Does their doing this suggest that none of these scientists is worried about the arguments of those concerned about civil liberties?
>
> Does this mean we shouldn't be concerned either?

Behind the relaxed attitude of such scientists is the idea that only ignorance grounds our perceived need for secrecy about our DNA. There are two sorts of ignorance they cite:

(i) the ignorance that generates a belief in genetic determinism;
(ii) ignorance of the fact that we leave our DNA everywhere.

The belief our genes *determine* our characteristics and behaviours, these scientists say, generates fear of allowing others access to our DNA. But as we know genetic determinism is false. If we could convince the public of this, they say, people might lose their fear of DNA databases.

This would almost certainly be the case, they add, if people realised their DNA is already accessible to everyone. Every time we drink, they point out, our DNA is left on the rim of the glass. It is hugely unlikely that anyone ever travels by bus without leaving their DNA on the bus when they alight. Why are we so worried about keeping our DNA private when anyone could gather it any time they liked?[67]

But is it really ignorance that is behind people's fear of DNA databases? Or might the factors noted above come into it too? Could it be suggested that it is all very well for high profile individuals with the clout of these famous scientists to make their details accessible to all, but the rest of us might not have it so easy. Any misuse of *their* data, after all, will be big news and is unlikely to harm them: they're unlikely, for example, to be short of a job and they could probably afford not to be insured. Can the rest of us afford to be as sanguine?

> **Box 15.22 Activity: Paired reflection**
>
> With a partner ask whether you think that those afraid of allowing others access to their DNA are being misled by a misplaced belief in genetic determinism or by a failure to recognise that they leave their DNA everywhere?

Our understanding of genetics, combined with bioinformatics, our increasing ability efficiently, quickly and cheaply, to analyse, store and use that information, is generating ethical and social issues that no generation before us has had to grapple with. It is only by thinking through these issues, for ourselves as individuals and for the societies (and the global community) to which we belong, that we will be able responsibly to deal with such issues.

Summary

In this chapter we have considered the moral implications of the collection, storage and use of bio-information. In particular we have:

- discussed whether the right to privacy of those not convicted of crime is violated by being stored on the UK NDNAD;

- seen that the idea of a national or international DNA database would generate the following fears for some people:
  - the richness of the information that could be accessed;
  - the possibility of options being closed off;
  - the possibility of discovering politically incendiary bio-markers;
  - worries about the emergence of a genetic underclass;
  - the fear of losing any chance of privacy;
  - the fear that bio-information would be lost, sold or misused;
  - the possibility of a new government's being malign.

- seen that other people believe it would have the following benefits:
  - easer and quicker solution to crimes;
  - prevention of crime;
  - increased national and international security;
  - increased efficiency of public services;
  - better planning of public services;
  - targeting of public services where they will do most good.

- considered the pros and cons of personalised medicine;
- reflected on the need for biobanks and the importance of anonymity;
- reflected on the tension between the desire for privacy and for security;
- asked whether our desire for privacy is based on ignorance.

Questions to stimulate reflection

'Nothing to hide, nothing to fear'. Should this allay fears about DNA databases?

Profiling every infant's DNA at birth and making their profiles available to every government department would greatly facilitate the efficient delivery of public services. Should we do it?

Would you want to know at 20 that you had a high chance of developing Alzheimer's Disease at 70?

Would it be reasonable for employers to employ only those whose genetic inheritance suggested they'd be good at the job?

Would it be justifiable for public health services to refuse to treat someone who, knowing they had a higher than usual risk of heart disease, had not made sensible lifestyle changes?

Were we to discover that women are not, of their very nature, as good at science as men, should this change our attitude to the teaching of science to women?

We leave our DNA everywhere all the time: is it reasonable to suppose we can keep it private? If not should this alleviate our fears about DNA databases?

Additional activities

Prepare a class project on the ethics of bioinformatics on the model of this: http://protist.biology.washington.edu/fingerprint/dnaintro.html.

Use these case studies to trigger debate: http://www.nuffieldbioethics.org/fileLibrary/doc/DNA_database_case_studies.doc.

A series of activities from real science: http://www.realscience.org.uk/science-discussion-girls-maths.html.

Pretend you are someone else trying to find out about *you*. How much of a profile of yourself can you build up from Facebook, Twitter, etc.?

Discover as much as you can about the health history of your family. What does it tell you about your own susceptibility to various conditions?

Find out about the UK Biobank on: http://www.ukbiobank.ac.uk/.

Notes

1 http://www.independent.co.uk/news/uk/crime/whodunnit-twins-deny-dna-theft-link-1934712.html.

2 http://www.nigms.nih.gov/publications/factsheet_geneticvariation.htm. A fact sheet on genetic variation from the US National Institute of General Medical Science.

3 http://www.timesonline.co.uk/tol/news/science/article5986239.ece. Nature and Nurture from the *Times* newspaper

4 http://www.nature.com/nature/supplements/insights/epigenetics/index.html. *Nature* on epigenetics.

5 http://www.dnalc.org/resources/animations/dnachip.html. An animation on gene chips from the Dolan DNA learning centre in the United States.

6 http://www.bioinformatics.org/wiki/Bioinformatics_FAQ. FAQ on bioinformatics from Bioinformatics.org.

7 http://www.exploredna.co.uk/dna-crime-scene-collection.html. Collecting DNA from a crime scene.

8 http://www.parliament.uk/documents/post/postpn258.pdf. A 'Postnote' on the NDNAD from the UK Parliament.

9 http://www.guardian.co.uk/politics/blog/2010/apr/09/reality-check-conservatives-dna-bowman. A *Guardian* report on the Bowman case.

10 http://www.telegraph.co.uk/news/uknews/law-and-order/5010003/Sean-Hodgson-Police-re-examine-cases-using-DNA-profiling.html. The *Telegraph* reporting on the Hodgson case.

11 http://www.timesonline.co.uk/tol/news/world/us_and_americas/article7120167.ece. A *Times* report on Raymond Towler.

12 http://www.msnbc.msn.com/id/34467096/. A report from Associated Press on James Bain.

13 http://www.statewatch.org/news/2009/sep/uk-home-office-ethics-group-dna.pdf. A report from the Ethics Group of the NDNAD.

14 http://www.bailii.org/eu/cases/ECHR/2008/1581.html. The European Court ruling.

15 http://www.genewatch.org/sub-563143. Everything you could want to know about the UK NDNAD from Genewatch.

16 http://www.bionews.org.uk/page_68686.asp?dinfo=Y7N4PAmZl5Sorwq27ejPeY3Y. An article about the new genetic tests.

17 http://news.bbc.co.uk/1/hi/uk_politics/3809575.stm. BBC report of a call for an international database.

18 http://www.liberty-human-rights.org.uk/issues/3-privacy/dna-database/index.shtml. The organisation Liberty on the NDNAD.

19 http://www.independent.co.uk/news/uk/do-your-genes-make-you-a-criminal-1572714.html. A report on a man who claims to have been born a killer.

20 http://www.edge.org/3rd_culture/dangerous07/dangerous07_index.html. The Edge Organisation's 'Dangerous Idea' site.

21 http://www.wired.co.uk/wired-magazine/archive/2009/11/features/hard-to-swallow-race-based-medicine?page=all. A report on 'race-based medicine' from *Wired*.

22 http://www.timesonline.co.uk/tol/comment/columnists/guest_contributors/article6952298.ece. An article arguing we shouldn't 'shoot the messenger' if we discover genes linked with criminality.

23 http://cco.cambridge.org/uid=3040/extract?id=ccol0521839637_CCOL0521839637A006. Cambridge Collection Online on the Noble Lie.

24 http://www.president.harvard.edu/speeches/summers_2005/nber.php. Transcript of Summers' speech.

25 http://www.timesonline.co.uk/tol/life_and_style/health/article5989433.ece. Bringing down the cost of insurance.

26 http://www.independent.co.uk/news/business/news/job-testing-may-create-a-genetic-underclass-635549.html. Employment and DNA.

27 http://www.telegraph.co.uk/technology/news/7054432/Terrorism-and-child-pornography-used-to-justify-surveillance-society-says-academic.html. The *Telegraph* on the surveillance society.

28 http://www.jrrt.org.uk/uploads/Database%20State%20-%20Executive%20Summary.pdf. Executive summary of Database State.

29 http://www.bbc.co.uk/blogs/haveyoursay/2010/08/are_you_ashamed_of_your_online.html. A suggestion that people will change their name as they come of age to rid themselves of their past.

30 http://www.thisismoney.co.uk/news/article.html?in_article_id=415902&in_page_id=2.

31 http://news.bbc.co.uk/1/hi/uk_politics/7103566.stm.

32 http://news.bbc.co.uk/1/hi/uk_politics/7103566.stm.

33 http://news.bbc.co.uk/1/hi/uk_politics/7147715.stm.

34 http://www.guardian.co.uk/technology/2007/apr/26/news.health. A report on the accidental release of details on junior doctors.

35 http://www.hgc.gov.uk/Client/document.asp?DocId=226&CAtegoryId=8. Report on databases from the Human Genetics Commission.

36 http://www.sciencedaily.com/releases/2004/10/041021084120.htm. Report on a genetic susceptibility to alcoholism.

37 http://www.medscape.com/viewarticle/723904. Report on the heritability of non-alcoholic fatty liver disease. http://www.parliament.uk/documents/post/postpn329.pdf. A Postnote on personalised medicine from the UK parliament.

38 http://www.newscientist.com/article/dn16552-genome-sequencing-falls-to-5000.html. Report on the cost of genome sequencing from the *New Scientist*.

39 http://www.timesonline.co.uk/tol/life_and_style/health/mental_health/article7078157.ece. *Times* report on GeneSightRx.

40 http://news.bbc.co.uk/1/hi/health/7034089.stm. A BBC report on bespoke drugs.

41 http://jama.ama-assn.org/cgi/content/full/279/15/1200. A report from the *Journal of the American Medical Association* on adverse reaction to drugs.

42 http://www.medterms.com/script/main/art.asp?articlekey=4858.

43 http://alzheimers.org.uk/site/scripts/documents_info.php?categoryID=200137&documentID=168&pageNumber=1. Information about early onset Alzheimer's disease.

44 http://www.facebook.com/note.php?note_id=109392478801.

45 http://www.bmj.com/cgi/content/full/321/7274/1464. A case study from the *British Medical Journal*.

46 http://www.aboutcysticfibrosis.com/cystic-fibrosis-in-children.htm.

47 http://www.ncbi.nlm.nih.gov/pubmed/11137485. A survey of attitudes about the duty to inform family members about relevant results.

48 http://www.guardian.co.uk/technology/2009/mar/15/sergey-brin-google-founder. A profile of Sergey Brin from the *Observer* newspaper.

49 https://www.23andme.com/. The website of 23andme.

50 http://www.nytimes.com/2009/03/12/business/12gene.html. A report of Brin's donation to Parkinson's research. http://www.mja.com.au/public/issues/175_07_011001/savulescu/ savulescu.html. A useful case study about getting children tested for Huntington's disease.

51 http://www.genomicslawreport.com/index.php/2010/07/21/14-more-fda-letters/.

52 http://women.timesonline.co.uk/tol/life_and_style/women/families/article7107079.ece. A *Times* report on this case.

53 http://www.bbc.co.uk/radio4/factual/costofhealth_20080708.shtml. A BBC radio programme about personal responsibility and the NHS.

54 http://www.bbc.co.uk/dna/h2g2/A33314997. A BBC profile of George Best.

55 http://www.genewatch.org/sub-507674. The Genewatch organisation on biobanks.

56 http://hapmap.ncbi.nlm.nih.gov/. Home page of the International HapMap Project.

57 http://www.nytimes.com/2009/11/18/business/18gene.html. A report on the bankruptcy of DeCODE Genetics.

58 http://www.news-medical.net/news/20100122/deCODE-genetics-completes-sale-of-its-Iceland-based-subsidiary-to-Saga-Investments.aspx. A report on the sale of decode genetics to Saga Investments.

59 http://www.actionbioscience.org/genomic/hlodan.html. An activity on this story from Actionbioscience.org.

60 http://www.telegraph.co.uk/health/7756320/DNA-database-created-from-babies-blood-samples.html. A report on the fact police can apply for access to hospital DNA records.

61 http://grants.nih.gov/grants/policy/coc/background.htm. Background information on 'certificates of confidentiality'.

62 http://www.technologyreview.com/biotech/19328/. A report from *Technology Review*.

63 http://www.technologyreview.com/Biotech/18809/. A report on the sequencing of James Watson's genome.

64 http://bigthink.com/georgechurch. George Church on the 'Big Think' website.

65 http://www.personalgenomes.org/. Project homepage.

66 http://www.economist.com/debate/days/view/284. Debate from *The Economist* on DNA and secrecy.

67 http://www.theaustralian.com.au/news/nation/push-for-jail-terms-for-theft-of-dna/story-e6frg6nf-1111117999454. *The Australian* newspaper considers whether DNA theft should become illegal (it is illegal in the UK under the Human Tissue Act 2004).

Further reading and useful websites

Collins, F. (2010) *The Language of Life: DNA and the Revolution in Personalised Medicine.* London: Profile Books.

Corrigan, O. and Tutton, R. (2004) *Genetic Databases: Socio-ethical Issues in the Collection and Use of DNA.* London: Routledge.

Widdows, H. and Mullen, C. (2009) *The Governance of Genetic Information: Who Decides?* Cambridge: Cambridge University Press.

http://www.hgc.gov.uk/Client/Content.asp?ContentId=122. Information about genetic testing from the UK's Human Genetics Commission.

http://www.wellcomecollection.org/whats-on/events/wellcome-debate.aspx. The Wellcome Trust: a debate on personalised medicine.

http://www.debatingmatters.com/topicguides/topicguide/genetic_screening/. Debating Matters Topic Guide on the genetic screening of infants.

16 Security and defence: security sensitivity, publication and warfare

Objectives

In reading this chapter you will:

- consider how biotechnological advances might be used for hostile purposes;
- reflect on the adequacy of current attempts to guard against this;
- learn about 'dual-use' technologies and the difficulties that attend them;
- consider the possible ramifications of 'open-source wetware';
- reflect on the possible impact of 'garage-biology' on our ability to keep ourselves safe;
- reflect on the extent to which we can sensibly assess risk in this area;
- identify and evaluate possible responses to the threat of bioweaponry.

In this chapter we shall be discussing the fact that biotechnology can be used for hostile purposes. In particular we shall be looking at the use of biotechnology to produce weapons with which to wreak havoc.[1] The intentional dispersal of the Ebola virus in a city, for example, would have appalling consequences.[2] So would the use of nano-vehicles to deliver toxic agents into the lungs of a platoon of soldiers[3] or the hostile release of harmful self-replicating organisms into the environment.[4]

Naturally nation-states and the international community have taken steps to guard against such possibilities. This started with the Geneva Convention in 1925 which banned 'germ warfare'. Since then, the 1972 Biological and Toxin Weapons Convention (BWC) and the 1993 Chemical Weapons Convention (CWC)[5] have prohibited the acquisition, retention or transfer of chemical and biological weapons and controlled materials relevant to their development. In the United States the possession, use and distribution of about 80 toxins known to be a potential threat to public health are controlled by the 'Select Agent Rules'[6] and a similar list of so-called 'Schedule 5' pathogens is kept in the UK. Since 1985 the 'Australia Group',[7] a voluntary and informal group of about 40 countries, have imposed export controls limiting the supply of chemical and biological agents, essential equipment, technology and know-how to countries suspected of pursuing biological and chemical weapons capability.

The effectiveness of biological weapons conventions

But such measures are of limited use. For one thing, 30 states have neither signed nor ratified the BWC. Amongst these are states, like Syria, that are believed to be actively pursuing a biological weapons capability.[8]

There is also the problem of compliance. Despite having ratified the BWC, North Korean armed forces are believed by South Korea to be capable of carrying out 13 different kinds of viral and bacterial attack using biological agents including cholera, yellow fever and typhus. It has been suggested that Iran, Cuba and Libya are all in breach of the BWC despite having ratified it.

Box 16.1 Factual Information: Non-Compliance with BWC

Perhaps the most flagrant breach of compliance was discovered in 1989 when Dr Vladimir Pasechnik,[9] the research director of a Soviet Biological Weapons facility, defected to the UK.

Pasechnik informed the west that the Soviet Union had, for years, been producing the smallpox virus in industrial quantities.

Despite the fact that Russia, after the fall of the Soviet Union, signed a Trilateral Agreement with the US and the UK to ensure that all such activities were verifiably ended, the agreement collapsed when Russia, believed to have continued the programme, refused access to their biological weapons installation.[10]

Until it is possible to verify non-compliance it would seem that these conventions are little more than window-dressing.[11]

But perhaps this is obvious? After all it is not only other states that pose a threat when it comes to biological weapons. In fact, since 9/11 many would say that the most serious threat to our security comes, not from other nation-states, but from terrorist organisations such as Al-Qaeda.[12] Such organisations are not, of course, even invited to sign the BWC, the CWC or any other treaty. Nor are they likely to do so. Their activities are outlawed under the 2006 Terrorism Act in the UK and the USA Patriot Act in the United States, but it seems unlikely that either act will be an effective deterrent.[13]

Box 16.2 Activity: Personal reflection

Is there any point to developing international treaties if they are not signed by every state, if they are not backed by effective procedures to verify compliance and if organisations below state level cannot be covered at all?

Biological weapons and terrorism

Some believe that no terrorist organisation has or will succeed in getting the wherewithal to develop effective biological weapons.[14] They point to the fact that even if such an organisation managed to get hold of a virus virulent enough to do significant damage, they would then have to 'weaponise' this virus, and deliver it under conditions that would facilitate its effective dispersal. Such things are not a simple matter. Turning a virus into a weapon, for example, involves stabilising the liquid or powdered pathogen, preserving its infectivity and virulence over time, storing and transporting it, finding an effective means of dispersal and then waiting for the meteorological and atmospheric conditions that will enable it to disperse effectively.

But might this underestimate the lengths to which terrorists would go, and the money and expertise available to them?[15] Throughout this book we have adopted a stance of pragmatic optimism, assuming that science will eventually find a way to do things it can't currently do. Perhaps the only sensible stance to take in connection with terrorists' ability to develop biological weapons is one of pragmatic pessimism?

It is already the case, in fact, that many of the barriers that might once have prevented a terrorist organisation from developing biological weapons are melting. For one thing it is no longer necessary for such a group to get hold of a natural virus in order to get started on its biological weapon. The relatively new discipline of synthetic biology would enable it to *make* a virus.

Box 16.3 **Factual Information: Synthetic biology**

Synthetic biology is the intersection of biology and engineering.[16] It is focused on the redesign and fabrication of existing biological organisms, and the design and fabrication of components and organisms that do not exist in the natural world.

Synthetic biology differs from genetic engineering in that the latter involves only the insertion and deletion of genes in existing organisms. Synbio (as it is called) is capable of producing entirely new organisms.

The potential benefits of this technology are many and varied. They include producing:

- single cell sensors to detect pollution, toxins or infectious tissue;
- organisms capable of breaking down environmental toxins;
- synthetic pharmaceuticals such as artemisinin, used in the treatment of malaria;
- biofuels, for example hydrogen;
- complex molecular devices for tissue repair/regeneration.

The combination of synbio and nanotechnology is a particular powerful one: the tiny 'machines' of nanotechnology could be used to 'deliver' the organisms created by synbio to precisely targeted regions of, for example, human or animal bodies.[17]

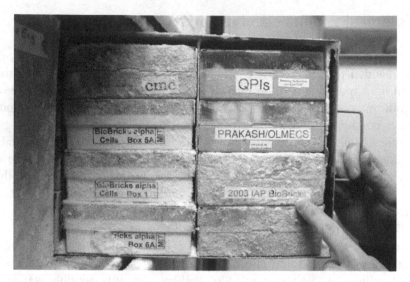

Figure 16.1 BioBricks. © Sam Ogden/Science Photo Library.

Synthetic biology uses engineering principles to design and construct biological systems. It can be used to construct synthetic versions of existing genomes, and also, in principle, to construct entirely new organisms, genomes that have never existed in nature. The hope is that by such means we can produce exactly the organisms we need: single-celled organisms perhaps that will 'eat' pollutants, organisms that will glow green when they come into contact with explosives or infection, or organisms that will attack cancer cells.

In pursuit of such aims scientists are working round the clock to produce cassettes of modular biological components, known as 'BioBricks',[18] that can be added to a 'chassis', a 'minimal organism'[19] consisting of only the genes necessary for life, to produce a new organism that will perform whatever function it is designed to perform. MIT keeps a registry of these BioBricks, as they are produced, and makes them available freely on the internet. Oligonucleotides (strands of DNA) are available to order commercially. So the scientist who wants to emulate God in His acts of creation has everything he needs.

But of course what we 'need' is a function of our aims, and it is not the case that everyone's aims are benign. In 2003 the Central Intelligence Agency released a report that concludes:

'Advances in biotechnology have the potential to create a much more dangerous biological warfare threat. The effects of some of these engineered biological agents could be worse than any disease known to man.'[20]

Of course creating a biological weapon from an entirely new virus is a major undertaking. It would be a matter of combining a number of genes that together would block the immunological defences of a host, infect him, cause illness or death and spread to others. This is a very tall order.

There isn't any need, furthermore, to create such a virus from scratch. All that's really necessary is to find an existing virus that suits your needs and synthesise that.

The idea of synthesising viruses, furthermore, is not just a futuristic dream. In 2001, at Stony Brook University in New York, a team of biologists synthesised the polio genome from scratch by stringing together commercially available oligonucleotides in accordance with a map of the RNA polio genome that they found on the internet.[21] The virus was confirmed to be both live and infectious when it paralysed mice.

Box 16.4 **Factual Information: Poliomyelitis**

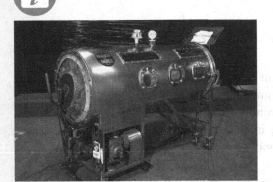

Figure 16.2 An Emerson respirator, known as an 'iron lung', used to treat polio patients. Courtesy of CDC/GHO/Mary Hilpertshauser.

Poliomyelitis was one of the most dreaded diseases of the twentieth century.[22] Highly infectious, thousands, mainly children, were crippled by it.

This terrible disease has been all but eradicated by the use of an effective vaccine that was discovered in the 1950s. So effective was this vaccine that few countries now carry significant stocks of it. The only countries in which polio is still endemic, in fact, are India, Afghanistan, Pakistan and Nigeria (and in India only 42 cases were recorded in 2010, a drop of 94 per cent from the year before).[23]

The scientists who synthesised the polio virus claimed to have done it as a warning to the effect that terrorists might be able to make a biological weapon without going to the trouble of getting hold of a natural virus.[24] Certainly they demonstrated very effectively the possibility that a deadly virus could be synthesised from scratch in such a way that it could, in principle, be 'weaponised'.

It might be suggested that no great harm would be done even if terrorists did synthesise a virus like polio. We do, after all, have a vaccine. It wouldn't take us long, in an emergency, to produce enough of the vaccine to at least mitigate the consequences of the hostile release of the virus.

But again such optimism might be misplaced. In Australia in 2001 a team of microbiologists, using genetic engineering techniques in an attempt to induce mouse infertility, accidentally produced a superstrain of mousepox.[25] This virus killed mice that were naturally resistant to mousepox, mice that had been vaccinated against it and even mice that had been given antiretroviral drugs.

The existence of a vaccine, therefore, merely requires a terrorist organisation to synthesise a vaccine-resistant strain of the virus, rather than just the ordinary one. The methods to do this have been improved since 2001 and the cowpox virus has also been synthesised in vaccine resistant form. Cowpox infects a range of animals, including human beings.[26] Like mousepox, cowpox is closely related to the smallpox virus, which, until it was eradicated in 1980, killed more people than any other disease in history. The smallpox genome, like the polio genome, is freely available on the web.

Although there is no treatment for smallpox there is a vaccine that could, should the situation demand it, be dusted down and used again.[27] But it wouldn't be much use against a genetically engineered superstrain of the virus. The fact that at 200,000 base pairs the smallpox virus is huge compared to the polio virus at 7,500 base pairs is no deterrent either given the speed with which the tools of synthesis are improving: it took several years to synthesise the polio virus, but it only took Craig Venter 2 weeks, in 2005, to synthesise the genome of a bacteriophage containing 6,000 base pairs.

Garage biology

These facts suggest that the risk from the new techniques of synthetic biology might not even come from organised terrorism. They might instead come from our own neighbourhood. Tucker and Zilinskas wonder if the real threat might not come from a clever graduate student who, working in his parents' garage, synthesises a deadly virus, either by accident or by design, and then allows it to escape, again by accident or design.[28]

In fact it might not even be a clever graduate student but just a clever young person fascinated by his ability to play with the building blocks of life as he once played with his Lego™ or Meccano™ set. We are all familiar with the idea of 'hackers', young people often without formal training who endlessly play with the building blocks of the digital world to design new software and programs. The tools that make this possible can be easily and cheaply secured on the web, and a grassroots community provides easy access to the required expertise.[29]

That the same is now true for the biological world is clear. There is already an active community of biohackers. They call themselves 'biopunks'[30] and they are constantly swapping expertise and information internationally by email and in their chat rooms. In 2007 a student from Boston University posted on the web a 'Primer for synthetic biology'[31] which describes in simple, non-technical language how to get started with biohacking. Such information, of course, is grist to the mill of terrorists.

But they – both terrorists and biohackers – need more than just the knowledge. They also need the materials and the equipment. Once again, however, this need be no hindrance. We have already seen that MIT's registry of BioBricks is available online freely to anyone who wishes to access it. Secondhand equipment – gene splicers, industrial grade fridges, etc. – can already be bought relatively cheaply on eBay and soon kits should be available commercially, which will also presumably work their way onto eBay.

The final piece of the jigsaw is the basic raw materials. But these are available commercially very cheaply (10 cents per base pair). That there are no barriers to non-scientists getting hold of them was demonstrated in the mid-2000s by an enterprising journalist from the UK's *Guardian* newspaper.

James Randerson succeeded in obtaining part of the smallpox virus with nothing more, as he put it, than 'an invented company name, a mobile phone number, a free email address and a house in North London.'[32] The strand of DNA arrived by post within days. Randerson did not have to prove a link to a legitimate organisation, nor was he questioned about why he wanted it. The sequencing company that supplied the DNA did not know why it was required, nor did it check. The sequence might, Randerson pointed out, have fallen foul of the Anti-Terrorism, Crime and Security Act 2001 had he not modified it to prevent it ever forming part of a functional gene. But the fact is that no check was made and none is required by the authorities.

In the light of Randerson's experience the *Guardian* asked three UK companies whether they ever screened their orders for sequences banned under Schedule 5. One did no screening at all, the others claimed to make checks and one had carried out a pilot study on screening. In Box 16.5 you can read a BBC news story about another journalist's journey into synthetic biology.

Box 16.5 Case study: How I obtained sarin ingredients

By Angus Stickler[33]

I started my search with a computer and the help of London University undergraduate Nigel Eady.

Nigel entered in the words 'sarin' and 'synthesis' to a basic search engine and immediately came up with a long list of links to information about sarin.

The first one took us to a website for Bristol University, where, on its first page there is a description of the various stages of making the compound (since removed).

With just three clicks, we've found a recipe for making sarin in five easy steps with four chemicals. Armed with this, we went in search of ingredients.

First, Derbyshire-based chemical company Fluorochem where all I had to do was give my credit card details and delivery address over the phone.

A box covered in orange toxic stickers arrived a couple of days later.

Swallow just 4 g of this chemical and you're dead. They sold me 250 g.

To be fair the managing director of Fluorochem did ask me what I wanted it for. I told him it was for research into the chemicals used in pesticide manufacture. He told me there was a problem – I wanted 500 ml – the smallest quantity they could provide was two and a half litres. It needed special delivery and that was expensive.

The company also wanted the order faxed through on headed note paper. He helpfully he told me what I should write.

A quick cut and paste to make up the fake BBC headed note paper, and I composed the letter.

'Dear Mr Birch,

Further to our conversation earlier, I would like to confirm the order. I recognise that this is hazardous material, and give an assurance that it will be handled and disposed of properly in accordance with COSHH procedures.'

The chemical was delivered within a week.

I pressed on and phoned through the orders for the last two chemicals. In total, a complete shopping list for sarin.

Fluorochem could only provide me with one of the chemicals, but I had found it elsewhere by then anyway. Again all I needed was my credit card and the fake letterhead to Molekula based in Dorset.

At no point did either of these companies check my credentials.

With a modicum of deception I was able to buy the precursors of a chemical weapon – a weapon of mass destruction.

Neither company has done anything improper. Both issued us with statements.

Fluorochem said: 'The Home Office has confirmed that none of the products supplied to you requires a licence.

'We fully comply with Home Office Guidelines on restricted chemicals. We conduct ourselves properly and professionally in these matters. We understand clearly the point your programme is making and in many ways welcome it.'

And Molekula said: 'Molekula makes every effort to screen all orders from individuals for all products which are considered to be of a sensitive nature. We only ship material to company addresses and do not supply to private residences.

'On the wider subject of chemicals with potential double use, we believe this thorny area is the responsibility of government agencies, whose role is specifically to protect the community from potential misuse and abuse.'

The name of the BBC gave me some credibility. But the corporation is not generally associated with chemical research. There are no laboratories here.

I used a credit card to buy the chemicals, not a company order form – even the headed note paper was doctored. If security checks were made, they failed.

The chemicals are now in my possession, locked away in a safety cabinet.

All a potential terrorist would need now, is the where-with-all to make the stuff. And you don't need to be a professor to work it out.

Our student Nigel Eady took me to his university's lab. He has an extractor fan, glass beakers and some condensing and cooling equipment.

'Standard chemical equipment which you could find in any school,' said Nigel. 'It's not really a high tech operation, or greatly technical knowledge that you need, or even complex apparatus to produce a compound like sarin.'

He said you could even make it in a well-ventilated garage.

We bought enough of these chemical precursors to make twice the amount of sarin used in the Tokyo subway attack.

The delivery method is tried, tested and easily improved upon.

The tube trains acting as pistons would force this home-made gas throughout the underground. Tens of thousands could be injured or die.

The only difference between the chemical used in Tokyo, or Iraq by Saddam Hussein, is that this time it could be bought, built and used in Britain.

In November 2005 *New Scientist* magazine surveyed 12 gene synthesis companies in the United States and in Europe asking whether they screened nucleotide orders for suspect sequences. Five said they screened all orders, four said they sometimes screened orders and three said they never did any screening.

The result surprised Eckard Wimmer, the scientist responsible for recreating the polio virus as a 'warning' to the authorities about how easily it could be done:

'It's surprising to me that after all these discussions for at least four years, that no more urgent recommendation has gone out to these companies saying that if you don't carry out more rigorous checks you may be in trouble.'[34]

One reason that so few companies screen might be because they are not impressed with the software available: if an ordered sequence is short, the likelihood it will match a piece of DNA banned under Schedule 5 is high. It is not clear how the company should respond to false positives other than by refusing the order. Such a move would not be competitively advantageous.

> ### Box 16.6 Activity: Web-wandering
>
> Put 'biopunk' into an online search engine and see what you can find out about the goings-on in the biohacking community.
>
> Bring your results back to the group and contribute to a group discussion on this issue.

So it is not just organised terrorists who might use biotechnology to produce bioweapons. How, we might reasonably ask, can we guard against misuse of a new technology when the people we have to be aware of include our neighbour's daughter, working on the creation of a new biological organism in her parents' garage? We might note uneasily that, according to a report in the UK's *Times* newspaper, in the United States two home grown labs have already been shut down.

Bioweapons and censorship of scientific publications

The ability of a determined terrorist organisation to synthesise a vaccine-resistant strain of smallpox, and the ability of an adolescent to produce a novel organism in his parents' garage, are greatly enhanced by the fact that all the findings outlined above were openly published, together with full accounts of the materials and methods used, in journals that anyone can get hold of. Some believe that the journals involved were irresponsible to publish such findings or irresponsible, at least, to publish full accounts of the materials and methods used.

Michael Selgelid of the Hastings Centre,[35] for example, claims this amounts to giving terrorist organisations a manual for the production of a biological weapon.[36] He calls for the censorship of any scientific papers that might pose a threat to security.

But to suggest that scientists do not publicise their findings is to strike at the very heart of science. To suggest that they do not publish full details of the materials and methods used to achieve a result has the same effect. How after all can a finding be replicated if other scientists do not have access to such information?

In response to this problem the editors of *Science, Nature* and *The Proceedings of the National Academy of Sciences*, together with the American Society for Microbiology, published a joint statement in which they said:

'On occasion an editor may conclude that the potential harm of publication outweighs the potential societal benefit ... under such circumstances, the paper should be modified or not published.'[37]

But some, for example Ian Ramshaw, one of the authors of the mousepox publication, argue that it is already too late for censorship. The dangerous information is already in the public domain and it is not obvious that anything could now be published that would make it worse.

Another problem with withholding publication of papers with security implications is that the findings being publicised are often the very findings that are needed if we are to respond appropriately to the threat of biological weapons, or indeed to naturally occurring viruses.

Recent events illustrated this when the powers that be became so afraid of the H1N1 strain of bird flu that a pandemic was declared. This led to many countries greatly accelerating their attempts to find, produce and stockpile an effective vaccine. Clearly achieving such an aim depends on a solid understanding of past pandemics and their causative agents.[38]

In pursuit of this a team of microbiologists, this time from the Centers for Disease Control and Prevention in the United States, synthesised the strain of 'Spanish' flu that was responsible for a pandemic that killed between 50 and 100 million people in 1918–19. This was achieved by reverse genetics from an archived sample of the lung tissue of a woman who died in 1918.[39] Having succeeded in synthesising this virus the team published their findings detailing, of course, the materials and methods they used. This success was described by Craig Venter as 'the first true Jurassic Park scenario'.[40]

Should the journal that published their results be censured for having published them? If so how are other scientists supposed to build on those results and – with luck – produce an effective vaccine to defend against the certainty of another epidemic?

Box 16.7 Activity: Group discussion

Publication is the life blood of science, no journal should refuse to publish any findings for security reasons.

Participants should be allowed to choose their own sides unless there is reason to think that only one side is adequately represented. In this case sides can be allocated.

It might be argued that the way to deal with this problem is not to ban, but to restrict publication of security sensitive findings. Perhaps information about the findings could be disseminated only to a relatively small – though international – audience of scientists on a 'need to know' basis?

Lone operators

But even this wouldn't necessarily prevent such findings falling into the hands of those who might use them for hostile purposes. Tucker and Zilinskas consider the possibility of a 'lone operator' developing and using a bioweapon.[41]

This person would be a professional biologist with all the training he needs for his nefarious task. He would have access to sophisticated laboratory facilities, to the raw materials he would need and to information restricted in the manner considered above. Nothing he does would be likely to trigger the interest of the authorities because everything he does could reasonably be considered to be part of the tasks he performs for his perfectly standard scientific day job.

If such a person had a grudge of some kind, against authority, against people generally, or even against a particular person, or if he had a determination to prove his superiority, such a person could be extremely dangerous. That such people exist is proven by the activities of Theodore Kaczynski, the so-called 'Unabomber'.

Box 16.8 Factual information: Theodore Kaczinski

The Unabomber, so called because he bombed *uni*versities and *ai*rlines, was dubbed a 'domestic terrorist' by the Federal Bureau of Investigation. He was the target of one of their costliest ever investigations.

From 1978 to 1995 the Unabomber planted 16 bombs, killing three people and injuring 23. In 1995 he wrote to the *New York Times* to say he would stop if they published a 'manifesto', in which he argued that his bombings were necessary if the world was to pay attention to the erosion of human freedom caused by modern technology.

As a result of the publication of this document a man came forward saying he recognised the style and sentiments as those of his brother Theodore John Kaczinski.

Kaczinski was born in Illinois. He went to Harvard and then did a PhD in mathematics at the University of Michigan. At 25 he was made an assistant professor at the University of California, Berkeley, but resigned 2 years later to live in a remote cabin without electricity or running water. With the aim of becoming self-sufficient he taught himself survival skills.

In 1998 Kaczinski was sentenced to life in prison with no possibility of parole after avoiding the death penalty by pleading guilty.[42]

Restricting publication of security sensitive findings, even if it would make life harder for the terrorist organisation or the biohacker, would have no impact at all on the lone operator.

Dual use dilemmas

In discussing such issues we are facing an example of the so-called 'dual use dilemma'.[43] These dilemmas arise when the same scientific work can be used for good and for evil. The difficulty posed by such dilemmas is how we can reap the benefits promised by such work whilst avoiding the evils posed by misuse.

> ### Box 16.9 Activity: Brainstorm
>
> How many examples of 'dual use' research can participants list?

One such difficulty is clearly that of whether and how the publication of scientific results should be censored. Another is the question of whether there is any scientific research that should simply be banned as too dangerous. In 1975, at a conference in Asilomar on genetic engineering,[44] then in its infancy, delegates voted to accept at least a moratorium on the carrying out of certain research pending discussion of new biosafety regulations.

Of course a moratorium – a temporary ban – is not the same as a permanent ban. But delegates to this conference were prepared at least temporarily to put safety considerations before scientific freedom. Is there any research, however, the implications of which justify a permanent ban?

As we saw in Chapter 8, many countries imposed a ban on human reproductive cloning research after the announcement of the birth of Dolly. Box 8.1 on page 117 summarises the sudden imposition of international legislation banning reproductive cloning that followed this announcement.

There are people who would argue that research that could produce nuclear weapons should be banned. Some of these people would point to the grievous loss of life in Hiroshima and Nagasaki as reason for banning it. Still others insist that the promise of a reliable and sustainable source of energy justifies the research. Their opponents then point to Chernobyl, Three Mile Island and Fukushima, only to have their claims rejected by those who claim that such accidents can be avoided by proper and enforced regulation.

The person who discovered nuclear chain reaction, Leo Szilard,[45] realising its implications, was worried enough to suggest that the research at least be kept secret. But even such secrecy would not have been of much use when a similar discovery was made in France. Clearly any ban, either on publication or on research itself, would have to be international in scope. It would, of course, suffer from all the problems of compliance we considered above.

It is certainly the case that the threat of global warming makes the development and use of nuclear power, as a sustainable source of clean power, far more attractive than it once was. We shall be discussing this in Chapter 21.[46] The developed world is now looking at nuclear power very differently from the way it looked at it 40 years ago. But had research into nuclear power been banned after, say, the Chernobyl disaster in 1990, consider how far behind we would now be.

> ### Box 16.10 Activity: Paired discussion
>
> Let us imagine that it would be possible effectively to police an international ban on certain types of research. Would it ever be justifiable?

The regulation of research

International legislation regulating scientific research is probably vital even if it is not, in practice, very effective. At least it sends a clear message about the values to which everyone is expected to adhere by the international community. It also permits the imposing of sanctions or other measures on those found to be in breach of such legislation.

But with respect to research that has implications for public health and/or the environment there are two other sorts of regulation that need to be considered. These are self-regulation by scientists, and regulation by the law within a state. It is hardly to be questioned with respect to research of the kind we have been discussing – research that generates the 'dual use' dilemma – that both sorts of regulation will be needed. The interesting question is how the two should be balanced.

Self-regulation of research

Clearly scientists would prefer to be self-regulated as far as possible because this is less likely to impinge on their freedom to carry out their research as they wish. To this end scientists are likely to claim that research should be regulated mainly by science itself, with the state playing a role only in supporting self-governance and ensuring compliance.

In support of this Tucker and Zilinskas claim that the self-governance guidelines on recombinant DNA research issued at Asilomar in 1975 have:

'functioned reasonably well to protect scientists and the public from potential hazards while allowing science to advance relatively unhindered.'[47]

These guidelines were adapted and adopted by the National Institute of Health (NIH) in the United States in 1976. The NIH also established a Recombinant DNA Advisory Committee to develop biosafety guidelines and a process of institutional oversight.[48]

These guidelines depend on a rigorous risk assessment, several levels of biocontainment[49] and the requirement that any host microbe that receives foreign DNA should have features that prevent survival and replication outside the laboratory. Until the NIH guidelines and oversight processes were in place scientists observed a self-imposed ban on work involving the insertion of toxin genes and virulence factors into bacteria.

Not everyone, however, would agree that these guidelines, which rely so heavily on self-regulation, are the success suggested by Tucker and Zilinskas. The ETC Group, for example, argue that the guidelines were developed by 'a handpicked group of elite scientists' and designed to pre-empt government regulation and public debate. As they put it:

'By appearing voluntarily to relinquish some recombinant DNA experiments (if only for a brief period of time) the Asilomar scientists took the heat out of a rising storm of debate and avoided public participation in the issues.'[50]

Certainly there was little or no public consultation on whether self-regulation was a good thing.

But perhaps this doesn't matter given that no accidental release of a genetically modified organism has ever been reported in the United States. Tucker and Zilinskas recognise that this doesn't necessarily mean that there has never been an accidental release, but if there has, they point out, 'the effects were so unremarkable as to remain undetected'.[51]

In Europe, however, things have turned out very differently. The UK followed the United States' lead in allowing scientists to regulate their own research into the new methods of genetic engineering. There was as little public consultation in the UK as there was in the United States. Scientists were allowed to get on with their research whilst the public carried on in blissful ignorance of what they were doing. But this approach backfired badly.

When the public learned that genetic engineering was not only being carried out, but that genetically modified (GM) ingredients were becoming commonplace in food, there was an uproar. Most of this uproar was driven by ignorance, but whatever its cause it is the fact of the uproar that is important.[52] We shall be discussing this in depth in Chapter 17. Here we need only note that the result of this uproar is that the once-thriving GM industry in the UK is now all but moribund.

The self-regulation that has (supposedly) worked so well in the States has, in the UK, resulted in millions of pounds being lost, careers being destroyed and manufacturers, restaurants and retail outlets having to go to great lengths to reassure customers that they do not use GM ingredients in their products. Research in the UK has virtually ground to a halt for lack of funding (because governmental support vanished as it became clear that public support had vanished) and commercial organisations no longer think it worth their while to operate in the UK.

It is important to note that none of this is the result of any failure in the self-regulatory regime. In the UK the regime of self-regulation was arguably working as well as it was working in the United States. But once public confidence was lost, this quickly became irrelevant. The fact is that the regulation of research must not just work it must also be *believed* to work by the public.

That the same problem could arise in the US with respect to synthetic biology is considered by Tucker and Zilinskas who remark:

'One can imagine the impact of a news report that a team of scientists has created an entirely new life form that is busily replicating itself in the laboratory.'[53]

One might also imagine the public response to learning more about garage biology and the biosecurity implications of synthesising viruses. Might public discovery of the biosecurity issues in the US have the same effect that the public discovery of biosafety issues has had in Europe? This is definitely something that most scientists would want to avoid.

Box 16.11 Activity: Scrutinising proposals for self-regulation

Despite the risks of self-regulation a new regime of self-regulation was proposed as recently as 2006 at the Second International Conference on Synthetic Biology. The proposal argued that four steps should be taken with respect to self-governance in synthetic biology:[54]

1. the improvement of screening software for oligonucleotide orders and 'a community pledge' no longer to buy from companies that do not properly screen orders for oligonucleotides, together with liaison between companies to ensure that dangerous sequences cannot be split over several orders;
2. the development of an ethics advisory committee and a hotline set up to provide free and confidential advice on ethics;
3. a website where scientists can report potential accidents and biosecurity threats, together with the creation of a professional society responsible for convening an advisory board and a code of conduct;
4. scientists should develop only 'inherently safe' organisms that cannot survive or propagate in nature, and that embody a barcode that identifies their creator.

Participants should be divided into four groups, representing:

- the public;
- science;
- the government;
- commercial interests.

Each group should be asked to read and reflect on these proposals and then report to the group as a whole their responses to them. The whole group should then be asked to discuss whether the implementation of these proposals, supplemented by institutional oversight, is likely to avoid a repeat of the response of the European public to GM.

It should be noted that those putting forward the proposals claimed that adopting them did not preclude additional, more formal, regulations.

One of the main worries about self-regulation is that it depends so heavily on the willingness of scientists to adhere to it. But scientists can only adhere to a voluntary regulatory regime if they know and care about it.

But there is good evidence to suggest that many scientists are not even aware of the biosecurity issues generated by synthetic biology never mind the proposals made to deal with them.

Alexander Kelle of Bradford University in the UK interviewed 20 practitioners about their awareness of biosecurity issues and discovered a widespread lack of awareness'.[55] Even those scientists who were 'in principle aware of the unfolding biosecurity discourse', in that they had heard of some of the important reports in this areas, showed at best only a very superficial understanding of the contents of these reports. Another study, based on responses from 1,600 practitioners, during 60 seminars in 8 countries, suggests that life scientists generally are unaware that their work might contribute to any security threat and have 'no knowledge of the debates within and concerns of the security community'.[56] It would seem that few of the life scientists responding even knew of the legally binding regulatory instruments such as the BWC.

At the very least it would seem that a self-regulatory regime would have to start by initiating a major campaign to make scientists aware of the issues and concerned about how to tackle them.

Box 16.12 Activity: Small group discussion

Participants should be put in groups of four and asked to brainstorm on:

(i)   the importance of professional awareness of biosecurity issues;
(ii) possible ways of engaging the profession in debate on such issues;
(iii) the barriers to engaging the profession;
(iv) ways in which these barriers might be overcome

Each group should appoint a spokesperson to report back to the group as a whole, which should then discuss the questions as a whole group.

Another major difficulty is the fact that when a self-regulatory regime is required to be international in scope it requires scientists from very different cultures and backgrounds to act upon the same principles. This will sometimes bring scientists into conflict with their governments, and not all governments, it must be said, are equally respectful of scientific freedom. Even if all scientists world-wide, furthermore, were to honour a voluntary pledge to order only from oligo companies that screen, would this mean that all oligo companies *would* screen all their orders? Or would commercial considerations recommend a different approach?

A final difficulty for reliance on self-regulation, pointed out by Michael Selgelid, is that assessing biosecurity risks depends to some – possibly major – extent on knowledge of facts that scientists can't be expected to have. How is it possible, for example, to assess the possible security implications of publishing the mousepox study described above, in the absence of some understanding of the capabilities of organisations such as al-Qaeda? But such understanding is often classified. Scientists can't get hold of it *even in principle*. As Selgelid puts it:

'The scientific community is systematically denied information that is absolutely essential to estimate security risks.'[57]

State regulation of research

It might seem in the end that some sort of state regulation is necessary if we are to maximise our chances of avoiding the intentional misuse of biotechnology. But now a host of other concerns come into play. Whereas scientists might be biased towards scientific freedom (of research and publication) despite security issues, the state might be biased in the other direction.

Science does not want to find itself over-regulated, even for reasons as important as biosecurity. Over-regulation might smother the research at its inception, either by making funding difficult, and/or by making the research unattractive to those who want to work without interference or red tape. Most scientists would believe it imperative to avoid regulation of the sort that the UK imposed on GM research in the final decade of the twentieth century.

The trick, therefore, will be to avoid the two evils of over- and under-regulation. Clearly this will be accomplished only if scientists work with the state to construct a regulatory regime acceptable to all. A suggestion about how that might be achieved is described in Box 16.13: do you think it will work?

Box 16.13 **Factual information: A proposal for compromise**

Michael Selgelid suggests that a balance can only be achieved between the competing interests of science and the state if decisions about regulation for biosecurity purposes are handled by 'an individual or group embodying both kinds of values'. To this end he suggests a panel comprising equal numbers of:

- civilian scientists;
- government scientists;
- civilian security experts;
- government experts.

These experts could, he argues, be nominated by various interested groups, and each group should have some veto power over the nominations of other groups' members.

The important thing, says Selgelid, is that the reference of problematic cases to this panel should be obligatory, and the decisions of the panel should be binding.[58]

It seems clear, however, that over-regulation will be avoided only if the state is confident that the public is unlikely to react to discovering about research in the way that the British public, and later the European public, reacted to learning about GM research. To the extent the state is worried about public reaction heavy-handed regulation is inevitable. One only has to consider the regulations in force for human reproductive cloning to see this.

Much of the public panic and fear occasioned by GM was, as we shall see in Chapter 17, the result of ignorance. The only source of information the public had about genetic engineering prior to discovering that so much of their food contained GM ingredients was from science fiction. Once the panic and fear had started the facts became irrelevant. In the next chapter we shall consider the GM debacle and what it told us about the importance of scientifically informed public debate.

Summary

In this chapter we have considered how biotechnological advances might be used for hostile purposes. In particular we have:

- considered the international regulations governing biological and chemical warfare and the effectiveness of such regulations;

- the possibility that terrorist groups might start to engage in biological and/or chemical warfare;

- synthetic biology and its potential misuse by:
  - terrorist organisations;
  - trained individuals;
  - bio-hackers and garage biologists.

- open resource wetware and its potential for misuse;

- the lack of regulations regarding the screening of oligonucleotides;

- whether scientific publications with security implications should be censored and if so how;

- the nature of dual use dilemmas;

- governmental versus self-regulation of science;

- the importance of public understanding.

Questions to stimulate reflection

To what extent do you think international regulations regarding biological and chemical warfare are likely to be effective?

Do you think synthetic biology should be regulated by the state or by scientists or by some combination of the two?

What is a 'dual use dilemma'? How many dual use dilemmas can you think of?

Do you think that information of potential use to terrorists and other hostile people should not be openly published on the web or are the security implications outweighed by the benefits to science?

How might the activities of the 'lone-operator' or the 'garage biologist' be detected and prevented (or at least rendered harmless)?

Should scientific publication of sensitive information be subject to censorship? If so who should the censors be?

How can scientists get the public onside with respect to research that could have security implications?

Additional activities

Here is a topic guide written by Kedra Hildebrand, a teaching assistant, and Karen Adams, a faculty advisor, as a topic guide to a model UN debate on biological warfare: http://www.cas.umt.edu/mun/documents/GA1%2009%20topic%20Strengthening_Enforcing_Convention_on_Biological_Weapons.pdf. Use it to stimulate a discussion of the future of warfare.

Consider this policy statement on publishing where there are security implications from the Society for General Microbiology: http://www.sgm.ac.uk/pubs/policy.cfm. Do you agree with it? Give reasons for your answer.

Research the advice given by your government for dealing with the threat of biological terrorism. Does it make you feel safer?

Organise a debate on the publication of scientific papers with security implications.

Use this BBC discussion of biological warfare to start your own discussion: http://www.bbc.co.uk/history/worldwars/coldwar/pox_weapon_01.shtml.

Notes

1 http://www.guardian.co.uk/world/2002/may/26/september11.terrorism1.
2 http://www.who.int/mediacentre/factsheets/fs103/en/. The World Health Organization on the Ebola virus.
3 http://www.ncbi.nlm.nih.gov/pubmed/18712585.
4 http://www.wired.com/wiredscience/2010/05/scientists-create-first-self-replicating-synthetic-life/.

5 http://www.brad.ac.uk/acad/sbtwc/. Everything you need to know about biological warfare from the Bradford University Centre for Peace Studies.

6 http://www.selectagents.gov/.

7 http://www.australiagroup.net/en/index.html.

8 http://www.armscontrol.org/factsheets/bwc.

9 http://www.telegraph.co.uk/news/obituaries/1363752/Vladimir-Pasechnik.html. Obituary for Vladimir Pasechnik.

10 David Kelly, The Trilateral Agreement. In *Verification Yearbook* 2002, pp. 94–96.

11 http://bwm.bwpp.org/bwm/pub/index.jsp. The BioWeapons Prevention Project database on compliance.

12 http://news.bbc.co.uk/1/hi/in_depth/world/2001/war_on_terror/default.stm. BBC website on al-Qaeda. http://www.abc.net.au/rn/talks/bbing/stories/s48674.htm.

13 http://www.inthenews.co.uk/news/science/biological-weapons-greatest-terror-threat-uk-$1231187.htm.

14 Tucker, J.B. and Zilinskas, R. (2006) The promise and perils of synthetic biology. *The New Atlantis,* http://www.thenewatlantis.com/publications/the-promise-and-perils-of-synthetic-biology.

15 http://www.timesonline.co.uk/tol/news/world/asia/article4418867.ece. A report on the death of al-Qaeda's biological and chemical weapons 'expert'.

16 http://syntheticbiology.org/FAQ.html. Everything you might want to know about synthetic biology.

17 http://www.parliament.uk/documents/post/postpn298.pdf. A Postnote on synthetic biology from the UK parliament.

18 http://biobricks.org/. The Biobricks Foundation.

19 http://www.syntheticgenomics.com/pdf/Choetal.pdf. An article on the ethical issues associated with creating a minimal organism.

20 CIA, 'The Darker Bioweapons Future', November 3 2003 at http://www.fas.org/irp/cia/product/bw1103.pdf.

21 Cello, J., Paul, A.V. and Wimmer, E. Chemical synthesis of poliovirus cDNA: generation of infectious virus in the absence of natural template. Originally published in *Science Express* on 11 July 2002; *Science* 9 August 2002: **297**(5583): 1016–1018.

22 http://poliomyelitus.comxa.com/. A website about polio.

23 http://www.msnbc.msn.com/id/41626296/ns/health-infectious_diseases/.

24 http://www.precaution.org/lib/05/poliovirus_baked_from_scratch.020712.pdf.

25 http://www.bbc.co.uk/worldservice/sci_tech/highlights/010117_mousepox.shtml. A BBC report on the mousepox superstrain.

26 http://www.britannica.com/EBchecked/topic/141309/cowpox. The *Encyclopaedia Britannica* on cowpox.

27 http://www.bt.cdc.gov/agent/smallpox/overview/disease-facts.asp. Information about smallpox from the Centers for Disease Control and Prevention.

28 http://www.wired.com/wired/archive/13.05/view.html?pg=2. An article on garage biology from Wired.com.

29 http://diybio.org/. The website for diybio.

30 http://www.biopunk.org/.

31 http://openwetware.org/images/3/3d/SB_Primer_100707.pdf. A draft of the primer.

32 http://www.guardian.co.uk/science/2006/jun/23/weaponstechnology.guardianweekly. Randerson's article.

33 http://news.bbc.co.uk/go/pr/fr/-/1/hi/uk/2949356.stm.

34 Randerson (2006).
35 http://www.thehastingscenter.org/.
36 Selgelid, M. (2007) A tale of two studies: ethics, bioterrorism and the censorship of science. A Hastings Centre Report 37, no. 3.
37 Statement on Scientific Publication and Security, February 2003.
38 http://www.who.int/csr/disease/swineflu/frequently_asked_questions/vaccine_preparedness/en/index.html. The World Health Organization on the H1N1 vaccine.
39 Trumpey, T. M., Basler, C. F., Aguilar, P. V. *et al.* (2005) Characterisation of the reconstructed 1918 Spanish influenza pandemic virus. *Science*, **310**: 77–80.
40 http://www.nytimes.com/2006/01/29/magazine/29flu.html.
41 Tucker and Zilinskas (2006), p. 17.
42 http://en.wikipedia.org/wiki/Ted_Kaczynski.
43 http://www.parliament.uk/documents/post/postpn340.pdf. A Postnote on the Dual Use Dilemma from the UK Parliament.
44 http://www.nature.com/nature/journal/v455/n7211/full/455290a.html. A *Nature* report on the development of the agreement.
45 http://www.britannica.com/EBchecked/topic/579362/Leo-Szilard. The *Encyclopaedia Britannica* on Leo Szilard.
46 http://www.bbc.co.uk/climate/adaptation/nuclear_power.shtml. The BBC on nuclear energy as a source of clean power.
47 Tucker and Zilinskas (2006), p. 18.
48 http://www.cdc.gov/biosafety/.
49 http://www.answers.com/topic/biocontainment-laboratories.
50 Extreme Genetic Engineering: An Introduction to Synthetic Biology, The ETG Group, January 2007, http://www.etcgroup.org/upload/publication/602/01/synbioreportweb.pdf.
51 Tucker and Zilinskas (2006), p. 9.
52 http://www.parliament.uk/documents/post/postpn211.pdf. A Postnote on GM food in the UK.
53 Tucker and Zilinskas (2006), p. 18.
54 Maurer, S.M., Lucas, K.V. and Terrell, S. (2006) From understanding to action: community-based options for improving safety and security in synthetic biology, http://gspp.berkeley.edu/iths/UC%20White%20Paper.pdf.
55 Kelle, A. (2007) Synthetic biology and biosecurity awareness in Europe. Synbiosafe/Bradford Science and Technology Report No. 9, University of Bradford, http://www.brad.ac.uk/acad/sbtwc/ST_Reports/ST_Report_No_9.pdf.
56 M.R. Dando, contributing to a round table discussion of bioethics at a conference, as reported by Alexander Kelle.
57 Selgelid (2007), p. 41.
58 Selgelid (2007), pp. 41–42.

Further reading and useful websites

Gross, M. (2006) *Bioethics and Armed Conflict: Moral Dilemmas of Medicine and War (Basic Bioethics)*. Cambridge, MA: MIT Press
Schamoo, A. and Resnik, D. (2009) *Responsible Conduct of Research*. Oxford: Oxford University Press.

Wadsworth, W. D. (2003) *Biological Warfare (Opposing Viewpoints Series)*. Farmington Hills, MI: Gale Research.

http://debatepedia.idebate.org/en/index.php/Debate:_Artificial_life. Debatepedia on synthetic life.
http://www.youtube.com/watch?v=UF1y7loIU9o. A video from the Hastings Centre about the ethics of synthetic biology.

Section 5
Our duties to each other

Food and energy security: GM food, biofuel and the media

Objectives

In reading this chapter you will:

- learn about the growing population, the shortage of land and the prospect of a world food crisis;
- learn about the interaction of food and energy security;
- reflect on the means by which a food crisis might be averted;
- consider the pros and cons of using GM technology to alleviate a food crisis;
- consider the importance of politics, the media and the public perception of a technology.

We have already looked at genetic engineering in the context of human enhancement. In this chapter we shall look at the same technology in the context of our attempts to secure, for everyone in the world, food and energy security by the genetic modification of plants and animals.[1]

Genetic modification, food and energy security

Many people believe that it is only by using the technology of genetic modification that the global community will be able to solve the current food crisis.

'Food crisis? What food crisis?' you might say, as you butter another slice of toast. If you live in the west you might be forgiven for not realising there is a food crisis, for thinking, indeed, that the only food crisis around is the obesity crisis.[2]

You'll know, of course, that large parts of the world are starving: news reports on famine in Africa will have been the wallpaper of your childhood television viewing. The starvation continues. But the current food crisis is different. It is a matter (in part) of the price of food being so high that many simply can't afford it.

In the three years between 2005 and 2008 prices of staple foods rose by 80%. In 2008 they rose 55%. In the UK in 2009 they rose 59%.[3]

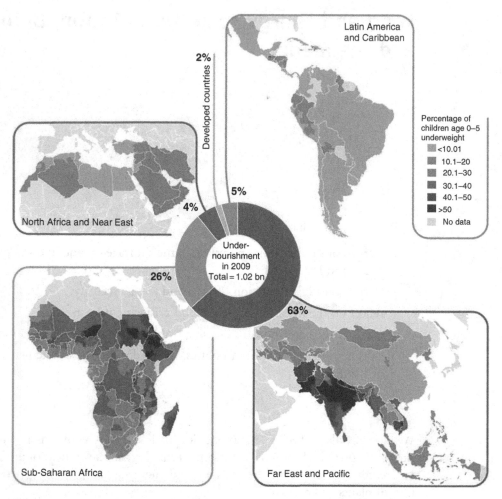

Figure 17.1 In 2009, more than 1 billion people went undernourished – their food intake regularly providing less than minimum energy requirements – not because there isn't enough food, but because people are too poor to buy it. Reprinted with permission from Macmillan Publishers Ltd: 'Food: The growing problem' *Nature*, **466**, 546–547, © 2010.

You may have noticed that your own food bill has been increasing. Possibly you've had to supplement meat with pulses? Your plight is as nothing to those for whom rising food prices make the difference between survival and starvation.

In India two-thirds of the population – hundreds of millions of people – manage on less than $2 per day.[4] Eight million children under five have severe, life-threatening, malnutrition.[5] Price rises mean that the tens of millions with chronic malnutrition will probably join them. In Egypt food prices have soared. They are expected to rise further since Russia imposed an export ban after fire devastated their wheat harvest during the summer of 2010.[6] Poor families, many of whom spend 80% of household income on food, can no longer eat three meals a day. In Thailand in 2008 rice, the staple diet, was double the price it was in 2007, one-fifth of the Thai population are not getting enough to eat.[7]

The UN's World Food Programme provides food aid to 70 million people annually. In 2008 its budget fell short of its needs by $750 million thanks to the rise in the cost of basic foodstuffs. They are cutting their programme and reducing their rations. The head of the UN World Food Programme has described the situation as 'a silent tsunami, that knows no borders, sweeping the world'.[8]

Once prices have risen other factors kick in: panic, hoarding and speculation. Food exporters, for example, start to sit on their holdings: why sell rice at $750 a tonne, when by waiting for a few weeks, you'll get $1000 a tonne?

This all leads to civil unrest. In Cameroon 24 people were killed and 1,600 arrested during food riots.[9] In Indonesia 10,000 people demonstrated outside the presidential palace after soya prices rose 125% during 2008.[10] In Egypt seven people were killed or died from exhaustion in queues for bread.[11] In Pakistan thousands of troops were deployed to guard trucks carrying wheat and flour. In total 33 countries across the world faced destabilising unrest during 2008. 2010 and 2011 have not been much better, especially in areas like Russia and Pakistan where events such as the summer fires[12] and the devastating floods have badly hit food supplies.[13]

This sort of unrest prompts frightened governments to intervene. The president of the Ivory Coast, for example, cut taxes on rice, sugar, milk, fish, flour and oils, and cancelled customs duties on imported staple foods.[14] Other governments are providing emergency food aid to the poorest, and introducing high penalties for food hoarding. China is imposing price controls, and many other countries are raising wages, lowering prices or banning exports: anything to alleviate the situation within their borders. The global recession is likely to undermine many of these initiatives and contribute to global unrest.[15]

Box 17.1 Activity: Role play

Participants should be divided into groups of four. Each person should then take one of the following roles:

- parent of hungry children;
- one of her children;
- official responsible for food distribution;
- police official charged with guarding food.

Each group should write and perform a 5-minute play for the rest of the group.

The rise in world food prices is partly the result of rises in other prices, mainly fuel and fertiliser, and of climate change which has led to water shortages in some areas, flooding in others (see Chapter 21).

It is also a function of a growing population. In 1798 Thomas Malthus, the political economist, argued that:

'the power of population is indefinitely greater than the power in the earth to produce subsistence for man.'[16]

The world's population is currently 6.8 billion. It will be 9 billion by 2050.[17] All these people will need feeding. They'll need feeding, furthermore, on the basis of less agricultural land than we currently have: the land cleared to provide homes for these people will become unavailable for growing crops.

Box 17.2 Factual information: The global food crisis

At the 1996 World Food Summit[18] 'food security' was defined as:

'when all people, at all times, have physical and economic access to sufficient safe and nutritious food to meet their dietary needs and food preferences for an active and healthy life.'[19]

Food security has four components:

(i)   food availability (production, distribution and exchange);
(ii) food access (affordability, allocation and preference);
(iii) food utilisation (nutritional value, social value, food safety);
(iv) food stability (seasonal and interannual variation in supply).

The current global food crisis is not a matter of lack of food. If we divide the number of calories generated by current global food output by the number of people worldwide, the result is 2,500 calories per day per person: more than enough to sustain health, never mind life.[20]

But this food is not distributed evenly. The developed countries have too much food, whilst the developing countries have too little. If we could even out the distribution of food there would not currently be a food crisis.

By 2050, however, the growing population and global warming make it likely that food shortages will greatly exacerbate the food crisis.

Energy security and biofuels

Three-quarters of the recent increase in world food prices, the World Bank estimates,[21] can be laid at the door of our attempts to achieve a reliable (and preferably domestic) supply of cheap, clean energy.[22]

The extraordinary growth seen by the developed world over the last century or so has been supported by the burning of fossil fuel. But fossil fuel is running out. It consists in deposits of once-living organisms, which take centuries to form. The supply is finite. The International Panel on Climate Change estimates we have between 5,000 and 18,000 billion barrels of oil left. But a group of Swedish scientists from Uppsala University think this is an over-estimate. In their view we have only 3,500 billion barrels left.[23] We use 23 billion barrels of fossil fuel a year. It has been estimated that oil supplies hit their peak in 2010, gas shortly afterwards.[24]

The little that is left, furthermore, is not under the control of those who, arguably, rely on it most: the west. The restless political situation, especially in the oil-rich

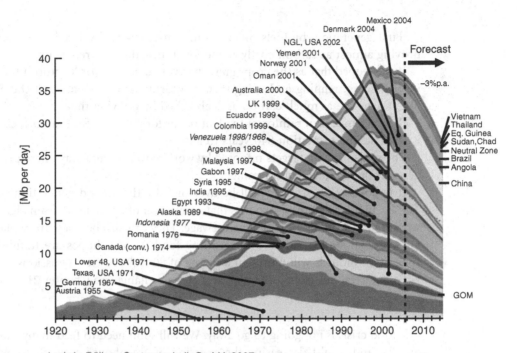

Ludwig-Bōlkow-Systemtechnik GmbH, 2007
Source: IHS 2006; PEMEX, petrobras; NPD, DTI, ENS(Dk), NEB, RRC, US-EIA, January 2007
Forecast: LBST estimate, 25 January 2007

Figure 17.2 A forecast of oil production in regions that have passed their peak. Dates next to country names indicate the year of peak production. From Zittel, W. and Schindler, J. (2007) Crude Oil: The Supply Outlook. Report to the Energy Watch Group, October 2007, EWG-Series No 3/2007 (www.energywatchgroup.org).

Middle East, makes those in the west nervous that even before the fossil fuel runs out, we might lose access to it.

This, together with climate change which we'll be discussing in Chapter 21, makes it imperative we find an alternative supply of energy. One possible solution began to be implemented almost as soon as we realised energy security was under threat: biofuels. These fuels – bio-ethanol and bio-diesel – fuelled the first cars ever made.[25] They may yet be the saving of civilisation.

In this hope vast tracts of land – 8 million hectares worldwide – have been switched from growing crops for food, to growing crops for fuel production. Tens of thousands of farmers, attracted by generous subsidies, have turned land over to the production of fuel.[26] The developed world's need for fuel seems to be trumping the need of those in the developing world for food.

Box 17.3 **Factual information: Biofuels and global warming**

The UK now requires 2.5% of the fuel sold in petrol stations to be biofuel. 60% of new cars, meanwhile, run on a fuel mix containing 85% ethanol.

'First generation' biofuels, made from maize, soy and oilseed rape, however, are proving almost as carbon costly as the fossil fuels they are replacing.

It was hoped that as the crops grew they would absorb (or 'capture') the CO_2 used in producing, refining and using them. Unfortunately, it seems that these processes might generate as much carbon as is absorbed by growing them.

Burning an area of rainforest to plant palms for palm oil, for example, emits carbon it will take the plantation 840 years to absorb.

The well-meaning targets imposed by world governments may, therefore, currently be *contributing* to global warming.

It is hoped this problem will be overcome by the second generation of biofuels. These will be made using enzymes that convert cellulose material from algae, manure, straw, food waste and possibly even sewage. They can also be made from plants grown on marginal land unsuitable for growing food. If such hopes are fulfilled the new generation biofuels will represent a saving of 80–90% in CO_2 emissions.[27]

For more about global warming and climate change see Chapter 21.

The food crisis is not going to go away. We will soon need to feed many more people, on less land, whilst decreasing the emission of greenhouse gases that contribute to global warming. What are the options for dealing with this problem?

The options

The options are few:

(i)   we eat less meat or find replacements such as 'in vitro meat';
(ii)   we switch to organic farming methods;
(iii) we improve conventional agricultural practice;
(iv)   we use genetic technology.

These options could – to some extent – be implemented in tandem. Let's look at them.

Eating less meat and in vitro meat

Americans eat 123 kg of meat a year, Britons 74 kg, Indians 3 kg.[28] If everyone started to eat like the United States it would take only 11 years to exhaust the global reserves of petroleum. If Americans were to become vegetarians, on the other hand, oil imports could be cut by 60%.

It takes 10 times as much land to produce food for the average American diet than it would for a vegetarian diet. An acre of land can produce 20,000 pounds of potatoes, but only 165 pounds of beef. In the United States 260 million acres of forest have been destroyed for use as agricultural land to support meat-eating (over 1 acre per person). One hundred times more water is used in producing meat than in producing wheat. To feed an American for a day 4,000 gallons of water are used. (It's 1,200 for vegetarians and 300 for vegans.)[29]

Livestock produces 20 times more waste than humans. This gets into rivers and lakes increasing nitrates, phosphates, ammonia and bacteria, and decreasing oxygen, thereby killing plants and animals. Around 85% of topsoil loss, in fact, is directly associated with raising livestock. The USDA says crop productivity is down 70% as a result of topsoil loss. It takes nature 500 years to build an inch of topsoil. Livestock farming generates more greenhouse gases than emissions from all the world's cars, boats, planes and trains put together.[30]

It is clear that eating less meat would make a major contribution to alleviating the problem of food security.

But maybe biotechnology could help by producing 'in vitro', or cultured, meat.[31] There are two methods for producing such meat, both of which have the potential for large scale meat production:

(i)   cells are grown in large flat sheets on thin membranes. This produces 'sheets' of meat which would be grown and stretched, then removed from the membranes and stacked to increase thickness;

(ii) muscle cells are grown on small three-dimensional beads that stretch with small changes in temperature. The mature cells are harvested and turned into a processed meat, like nuggets or hamburgers.[32]

The result tastes like beef, poultry, pork, lamb or fish, and has the same nutrients and the same texture as meat from a living animal.[33]

A big problem that would face such a response to the food crisis would be to overcome the 'yuk' factor.[34] Such a response cannot, of course, be the final response to such technology, as we saw in Chapter 6, pages 76–79. In this case, however, it is likely to be the first response of many people.

It should, however, be noted that this technology has one major advantage: no animal is harmed in the production of it. It is, in the words of PETA (People for the Ethical Treatment of Animals[35]) a 'victimless meat'. For this reason in 2008, PETA offered a $1 million prize for the first person to come up with a method of producing commercially viable quantities of it.[36] The meat, it is required, must be chicken and it must have the same taste and texture as meat from a living bird.

The journalist, Carol Midgley, responds to those who say they could never eat such a product with this riposte:

'How can it possibly be more disgusting than, say, eating chickens that have ulcerated backsides from sitting for weeks in their own excrement, bodies five times their natural size, with leg abscesses the size of 50p pieces and end their lives strung upside down with their heads hacked off?'[37]

Perhaps in vitro meat is the answer to all our woes?

Box 17.4 Activity: Conducting an opinion poll

Participants should work together to produce a questionnaire to gather information from friends, family and fellow students about attitudes to eating in vitro meat. This questionnaire might be accompanied by an information sheet about in vitro meat.

Participants should then discuss the contribution in vitro meat might make to averting the global food crisis.

Organic farming

Organic farming techniques include:

- crop rotation;
- a prohibition on chemical pesticide and synthetic fertiliser use, antibiotics and food additives;
- no genetically modified organisms;
- use of livestock manure for fertiliser and feed produced on the farm;
- choice of species that are resistant to disease and adapted to local conditions;
- raising livestock in free-range conditions and feeding them with organic food.

It is argued that such methods are 'in harmony with nature', that they produce healthier food and that they do not contribute to climate change.[38]

That such methods are more 'natural' is not necessarily a recommendation, as we saw in Chapter 6, pages 72–76. Something's being natural is neither necessary nor sufficient for making it good.

Organic food is not obviously healthier either.[39] According to the UK's Food Standards Agency, for example, organic food has no nutritional advantage over conventionally produced food.[40] Its report was written by The Nutrition and Public Health Intervention Research Unit at the London School of Hygiene and Tropical Medicine[41] and based on evidence published over the past 50 years of the different nutrient levels found in crops and livestock from organic and non-organic farming methods. Critics of the report have argued that it failed to consider fertiliser and pesticide residues in food.[42] It might be argued, however, that as regulations regarding such residues are so strict this wasn't necessary.[43]

The claim that organic farming does not contribute to climate change is also not entirely true: the ploughing involved in crop rotation releases a great deal of CO_2 into the atmosphere.[44] It is undoubtedly the case, however, that the refusal to use chemical fertilisers and pesticides is beneficial for the environment.

The biggest objection to the idea that organic farming might solve the food crisis, however, lies in the claim that the yield produced by organic farming is far lower than that produced by conventional farming methods. For example, organic farmers will get approximately 4 tonnes of wheat from a hectare whilst conventional farming methods get approximately 9 tonnes. This makes it difficult to see how organic farming could be a solution to the food crisis.

This, however, might be changing.[45] A recent UN analysis of 114 projects in 24 African countries found that yields had more than doubled where organic or near-organic practices had been used. That increase in yield jumped to 128% in east Africa.[46] Perhaps the future *is* organic?

Improving conventional agriculture

Modern agriculture started in the 1960s when a 'green revolution' was brought about by Nobel Peace Prize winner Norman Borlaug's new short-stemmed wheat varieties.[47] These nearly doubled yields in India and Pakistan. Billions of people lived who would otherwise have starved thanks to the work of Borlaug, who died in 2010. Today three-quarters of the world's cultivated land is sown to high yield grain crops and oilseeds.

Unfortunately, the increase in yields was brought about partly by high use of nitrate fertilisers, pesticides, monoculture, diesel fuel and heavy machinery. This has led to environmental damage that will undoubtedly hamper our ability to respond to the food crisis.[48]

For example, plants take up only about half of the nitrogen fertiliser used, the rest produce a toxic run-off that contaminates aquifers, rivers and the sea.[49] This produces huge blooms of algae that take the oxygen out of the water suffocating fish and other marine life. Such 'dead zones', according to the UN, will deplete fish stocks already depleted by overfishing and add to the food crisis.[50] The monoculture beloved of modern agriculture has contributed significantly, furthermore, to the loss of biodiversity we shall be discussing in Chapter 21.

Grain crops put nothing back into the soil, leaving it exhausted.[51] This means the land must be left fallow for periods, which weakens the structure of the soil so it becomes unstable and easily eroded. It is estimated that modern agricultural techniques have led to the degradation of 1.9 billion hectares of farmland, that the world's soils are eroding at a faster rate than any time in history, and that the weight of soil washing downstream in rivers is 4 tonnes a year for every human being on the planet. As Graham Harvey puts it:

'For all our technology, civilisation continues to depend on a few centimetres of topsoil.'[52]

Clearly this cannot continue. Would it be possible, though, to reap the benefits of modern agricultural methods without paying these environmental costs?

> **Box 17.6 Activity: Research and essay writing**
>
> Conduct some research into the 'green revolution' and its impact on the environment. Write a short (1,500 word) essay in response to the following statement:
>
> 'The green revolution has been an environmental disaster. Discuss.'

One thing that would help, according to Graham Harvey, is if we stopped feeding cattle on grain and instead put them out to pasture. Cows are ruminants and, arguably, this would suit them better and make their meat healthier. It would certainly suit the land better. Perennial grasses maintain their root system; need only the sun not fertilisers for growth and trap CO_2 in the soil. This move, however, is unlikely on its own to solve our problems, not least as countries like China and India express their new affluence in the adoption of western-style diets (see Box 17.7).

Box 17.7 Factual information: Meat-eating in China

On the 24 June 2008 *China Daily* featured self-employed 'garment seller' Qiao Sheng, from Qianqiao Town in Anhui Province.[53]

Qiao was brought up on salted vegetables, made without oil. He is proud of having made enough money to be able to provide his five children with meat every day.

In 2008 each person in China ate 5% more meat, 10% more milk and used 8% more cooking oil than they did in 2003.

A similar story is true of India, where the growing middle class also demands more and better food for their children.

As it takes 7–8 kg of grain to produce 1 kg of meat an increase in the demand for milk and meat means that grain that would previously have fed the poor is instead feeding the growing livestock herds of India and China.

In recent years conventional farming has been trying to mend its ways. The name of the game is sustainable agriculture.[54] This embraces some of the principles of the organic methods including the encouragement of healthy soil by rotating crops, ideally with minimal tilling, planting fields with different crops year after year, avoiding monoculture, and integrating croplands with livestock grazing. It also involves minimising the use of pesticides by nurturing the presence of organisms that control crop-destroying pests.

It is possible, of course, that mitigating modern methods of farming by such principles will reduce yields. Although such farming methods – it is hoped – will not damage the planet in the way previous methods did, they will not obviously, therefore, help us feed the growing population. For that, it is argued, we need to turn to biotechnology: specifically, we need to turn to genetic engineering.

Genetic technology

Many people believe food security will be achieved only by supplementing modern agricultural techniques with genetic engineering.[55] This technology, it is claimed, will increase plant yields, animal produce and the nutritional value of food, whilst decreasing the amount of land needed and minimising damage to the environment.[56]

By means of GM techniques we should be able, relatively quickly, to produce strains of plants that will be resistant to pests, diseases and drought. This will immediately increase yields in a world in which as much as half the global crop can be lost to these three evils. It will also reduce our carbon footprint and avoid environmental damage because we will be able to reduce our use of fertilisers, pesticides and water, and where use of such products is unavoidable, use more environmentally friendly versions.[57]

Transgenic animals will also contribute to food security. For example, cows engineered to resist mastitis,[58] an infection of cows' milk glands, could save the US dairy industry $2 billion a year and greatly improve milk production.

Those who support the use of this technology argue that it is not, in nature, different from the technique of selective breeding that farmers have used for 10,000 years.[59] It was by means of selective breeding that Borlaug increased yields so dramatically in the 1960s. But selective breeding is slow and hit and miss. Genetic modification promises to achieve the same ends as selective breeding but in a much more targeted way, and much more efficiently. It will, it is hoped, bring about a second green revolution.[60]

Box 17.8 Case study: Potato cyst nematode

Nematodes (*Globodera rostochiensis* and *G. pallida*) are microscopic worms that invade the roots of potato plants and inject a substance that causes the plant to create a unique cell from which the nematode feeds via a specialised tube, stunting root growth and depriving the potato plant of essential nutrients. This leads to lower quality, smaller crops.

Nematodes cost farmers in the UK £65 million a year in pesticides and crop losses. The cost worldwide is more like £60 billion.

Nematodes are currently treated with toxic chemicals such as astelone, which do not enter the food chain, but are expensive to apply and can make soil sterile, killing other living organisms within it.

A team from the Leeds University Centre for Plant Science has discovered that a protein that occurs naturally in rice and maize can be added to the roots of potato plants so that when the worms eat it their digestion is affected to the extent they can't breed.[61]

GM technology also holds out the promise of increasing the nutritional value of food. Perhaps one day, for example, it will be possible to deliver the day's nutrients in a single meal. We have already, for example, produced milk with a protein content 13% higher than usual.[62]

This technology would have obvious applications in the developing world. Golden rice, for example, was first produced in 1999 by means of the insertion of daffodil and bacterial genes coding for an enzyme involved in the synthesis of beta-carotene (a precursor of vitamin A) into the rice genome.[63] This 'poster child' of GM foods promises to provide the recommended daily allowance of vitamin A in the daily 100–200 g of rice eaten by children in countries like India, Vietnam or Bangladesh.

Were golden rice to be made available in the 118 countries of the world in which there is a vitamin A deficiency, it might save up to 500,000 children each year from losing their sight. Given that half of these children die within 6 months of going blind, the use of golden rice would also save many lives.

But the technology also has application in the west. In the UK, for example, 70% of the population does not eat the oily fish that would give them the recommended daily amount of omega three fatty acids needed for health. This could be remedied if crops were modified with genes from the algae that is the source of the omega three content of fish, and of animals fed on fish meal.[64]

By increasing the nutritional value of food and so reducing the amount of food needed for life and health GM technology could enable us not only to increase yields, but to make the food we produce go further. This explains why GM technology has been embraced enthusiastically in many parts of the world. By the end of 2009, for example, GM crops were grown commercially on 134 million hectares across 25 countries, involving 14 million farmers. The United States is the leading adopter of GM technology followed by Brazil, Argentina, India, Canada and China.

Box 17.9 Factual information: The BioCassava Plus Project

Over 250 million sub-Saharan Africans rely on cassava as their major source of calories, but a cassava-based diet does not provide complete nutrition. BioCassava Plus aims to reduce malnutrition by delivering more nutritious, higher yielding and more marketable cultivars of cassava.

The improved traits promised include: enhanced bio-available levels of zinc, iron, protein, vitamin A, vitamin E and reduced quantities of toxic cyanogenic glycosides, improved post-harvest durability and improved resistance against viral diseases.

Field and human feeding trials will be conducted in close collaboration with African scientists to demonstrate efficacy.

BioCassava Plus has six major objectives:

1. To increase by six-fold the content and bioavailability of zinc and iron in cassava tubers and demonstrate its viability in the field and efficacy in humans.
2. To increase by four-fold the protein content of cassava tubers and demonstrate its viability in the field and efficacy in humans.
3. To increase by 10-fold the vitamin A and E content of cassava tubers and demonstrate its viability in the field and efficacy in humans.
4. To decrease by 10-fold the cyanogen content in cassava tubers and demonstrate its resistance in the field.
5. To delay the rapid post-harvest physiological deterioration of cassava tubers and demonstrate its resistance in the field.
6. To develop virus-resistant cassava varieties and demonstrate its resistance in the field.

The first field trials of the transgenic cassava were started in Nigeria in late 2009.[65]

Many people, however, are unhappy about the use of genetically modified crops. This is especially true in Europe. In the EU GM crops are grown in just six countries (in 2010). This is because public opinion in Europe is largely anti-GM.

Some worry simply that it is 'unnatural'. There is undoubtedly truth in this. Even if genetic engineering is very similar in nature to selective breeding no selective breeder could hope to breed chickens with the GFP gene from jellyfish. As we saw in Chapter 6, pages 72–76, however, if we worry about a technology's being unnatural we might not benefit from all that science has to offer. There are, however, five other worries:

(i)   GM will not live up to its promises;
(ii)   GM food might harm human health;
(iii)   GM food might damage the environment;
(iv)   GM food generates unacceptable monopolies.

It has been suggested that these worries ensure that in Europe food made from GM ingredients will never be accepted by the public. Let's look at each of these problems.

Over-hype

One of the objections to the idea that GM technology will help alleviate food crises is that the promises made on its behalf are over-hyped. Studies at the universities of Kansas and Nebraska,[66] for example, found that GM soya produced approximately 10% less food than its conventional equivalent. Although it was discovered this deficiency could be made up by adding extra manganese, even then the GM crop produced only as much, not more, soya as its conventional counterpart.

Two explanations have been put forward for these results. The first is that the genetic changes as the soya was modified actually *depress* productivity, the other that whilst we experiment with GM conventional crops are improving. The supplier of the grain used in the Kansas study, Monsanto, argued, however, that the seed used to produce the crop had not been engineered to increase yields but only to be herbicide resistant. The herbicide-tolerant trait, however, is associated with decreased yield, especially when water supply is limited.

In 2007 a UN-sponsored review, involving more than 400 scientists and chaired by one of the UK's former Chief Scientists, professor Bob Watson, concluded that the benefits of GM are 'variable': in some areas there are increases in yield, in others, decreases.[67]

It is important, therefore, to remember that despite the significant advances and successes of genetic technology, genetic engineering is still a young discipline. It would be a shame to rely on genetic miracles if these miracles are not forthcoming. This is not, however, a reason to reject GM technology as *one* of the means by which we might hope to tackle the world food crisis. Even if genetic technology has only a limited role in tackling the world food crisis, it might still play that role. This cannot be a reason comprehensively to reject GM technology.

Human health

Another worry is that in genetically modifying food we are taking risks with human health.

In Chapter 6, pages 79–85, we considered the nature of risk in regard to the precautionary principle. We saw there that in assessing risk we must take into account the risk of *not* adopting a technology. One risk we would run, in eschewing GM technology, would be the risk of failing to solve the world food crisis.

There is some evidence, however, that GM food can be harmful. In 2005 Dr Irina Ermakova, a leading scientist at the Institute of Higher Nervous Activity and Neurophysiology of the Russian Academy of Sciences fed female rats food to which flour from soy beans modified to be resistant to the pesticide Roundup™ had been added. The rats were then allowed to become pregnant. During their pregnancy the feeding regime continued. A total of 55.6% of the offspring of these rats died within 3 weeks, and 36% were significantly stunted – weighing less than 20 g after 2 weeks. In contrast only 9% of the offspring of rats fed non-GM soy died and 6.7% were stunted.[68]

In another study, researchers at Australia's CSIRO took the gene for a protein capable of killing pea weevil pests from the common bean and transferred it into the pea. Some mice were given injections of the protein, whilst others had the protein put into their airways. The injected mice showed a hypersensitive skin response, while the airway-exposed mice developed airway inflammation and mild lung damage.[69]

On the other hand, this sort of thing can happen with conventionally grown food too. If you modify celery plants by selective breeding to add psoralens, for example, the plants will repel pests much more effectively. But they'll also give mice cancer and human beings skin rashes.[70]

It should be noted also that the evidence for the dangers of these foodstuffs were all picked up because modified foodstuffs are required to undergo strict screening procedures. No food, GM or not, gets onto our tables without having undergone very stringent testing.[71] It seems unlikely that a GM variety harmful to human health would survive this screening process. Should the evidence outlined above be taken as evidence for the dangers of any sort of modification (conventional and genetic) or for the success of the regulations on screening?

It is also important to note that the first commercial crops were grown in the United States in 1995. They have been using GM food for approximately 16 years. This is a very large field trial. It seems inconceivable that in a country as litigious as the United States, where 200 million people have been eating GM foodstuffs for so long there would not have been lawsuits launched against suppliers of GM foods if a health hazard had been identified. No such lawsuits have been launched. It is difficult not to conclude that GM food, when put through the screening procedures required of food, poses little or no risk to human health.[72]

Box 17.10 Activity: Paired reflection

In pairs discuss to what extent you believe fears about health might put people off using GM food. Do they put *you* off?

Environmental damage

The third worry is that genetically modified organisms might damage the environment.[73] One concern that has been expressed is that herbicide-tolerant crops might encourage even greater uses of herbicides than so far used.[74] Other worries involve the fear that such crops will 'escape' into the wild by pollinating related species, and that selective pressures will result in weeds that are themselves tolerant to herbicides, mandating the use of different, and possibly more damaging, herbicides.[75]

In the United States in 2006, for example, a herbicide resistant grass designed to improve golf courses and domestic lawns was found three miles outside its test site in Oregon.[76] Some had grown from seeds produced by GM plants, others had hybridised as a result of the pollination of a non-GM plant by the GM strain. The grass, *Agrostis stolonifera* or creeping bentgrass, is a perennial grass with many relatives in the wild (making pollination easier). Its escape was blamed on human error.

The advent of glyphosate-resistant crops, furthermore, has led to a dramatic increase in the use of glyphosate as a weedkiller. This has in turn led to many common weeds – ragweed, waterhemp, goosegrass – evolving a resistance to glyphosate. A recent study in Missouri, which tested waterhemp from 144 locations across the state, found 58% of the populations were resistant to glyphosate.[77] The glyphosate-resistant giant ragweed has also been found to have at least moderate resistance to other herbicides.

Crops genetically modified to be resistant to insect pests generate similar worries regarding insecticides and resistance. There are also, however, additional worries. The use of this technology means that there is less food available for birds and other forms of wildlife that rely on insects for their survival.[78] It is also possible that such GM plants could have an adverse effect on beneficial insects that prey on the insects to which the crops are resistant. For example, a transgenic potato expressing the snow-drop lectin gene for aphid resistance caused an adverse effect on ladybirds, which prey on aphids.[79] This could increase the loss of biodiversity that we shall be discussing in Chapter 21.

Finally, genetically engineering plants to resist viruses often takes the form of introducing a form of the virus into the plants as a sort of vaccine. If such plants were to pollinate near relatives there is always the possibility of a hybrid virus that could cause more damage than the original virus.[80]

One way of dealing with such worries is to insist on strict bio-containment in at least initial testing of GM varieties. If such plants are initially tested in laboratories or closed greenhouses this would minimise the possibility of genetic pollution of the environment. Eventually, however, plants would have to be sown in open ground.[81]

Box 17.11 Activity: Group discussion

Participants should discuss how concerns about the environmental impact of GM technology should be taken into account in the government's thinking about the use of GM technology.

In particular should governments:

(i)   ban the use of GM technology because of such worries?
(ii) ignore such worries?
(iii) regulate the use of GM technology to alleviate such worries?

Participants choosing (iii) should be invited to outline the sort of regulation they envisage.

Another suggested solution has been the introduction of a 'terminator' gene. GURT, gene use restriction technology, ensures that a plant will make a lethal protein late in seed development, ensuring that the seed can't be germinated without the application of a specific chemical stimulus. This would make it impossible for a GM plant to 'pollute' the environment. This might alleviate some of our worries about a GM plants escaping into the environment.[82] But it introduces other problems...

Unacceptable monopolies

The effect of using terminator technology would be to make farmers dependent on whichever agrochemical company provided the chemical stimulus that facilitates germination of a crop. The seed would be useless without this stimulus.[83]

In Chapter 18 we shall be discussing the ethical implications of allowing the patenting of biological processes and products. Since the development of GM technology, however, companies have been taking out such patents. This has resulted in a handful of giant companies holding enormous power when it comes to global crop production.

One such company, Monsanto, which commercialised the world's first biotech crop in 1996, has become a 'hate object' to many of the world's environmental organisations.[84] It has recently been accused by its nearest rival, DuPont, of having acquired a monopoly on pest- and herbicide-resistant soybean and corn and of using that monopoly to coerce seed dealers, farmers and others into a reliance on Monsanto products. As DuPont put it:

'The ag-biotech trait market is firmly in the grip of a single supplier, acting as a bottleneck to competition and choice. This threatens the global aim of doubling the world's food supply by 2050.'[85]

DuPont estimates that Monsanto has 98% of the US soybean market and 79% of the corn market.

There are companies other than Monsanto, of course, (and including DuPont) that have bought patents on GM processes and products. It is difficult not to feel uncomfortable at the recognition that global agriculture is in the hands of such a relatively small, and hugely powerful, group of major corporations.[86]

On the other hand, a lot of the profits made by these giant corporations are fuelling the research and development that will, it is hoped, help to solve the world food crisis. Monsanto's annual research budget alone, for example, is US$1.2 billion.[87] This is larger than the US government's total spend on agricultural science ($1.1 billion in

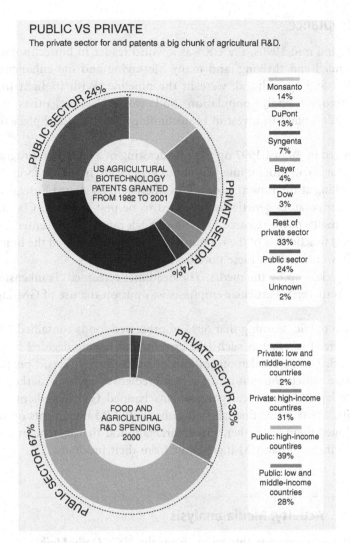

Figure 17.3 Public versus private: agricultural R&D. Reprinted by permission from Macmillan Publishers Ltd. Gilbert, N. (2010) Food: Inside the hothouses of industry. *Nature*, **466**, 548–551.

2007). The chart above gives some idea of power that is in the hands of these conglomerates.

Box 17.12 Activity: Research and presentation

Participants should be divided into two groups. One group should be asked to construct and present a case *against* giant agro-chemical companies like Monsanto, the other should construct and present the case *for* such companies.

Once each side has presented their case, the issue should be opened for group discussion.

Public acceptance

In the early and mid 1990s, the UK was a world leader in biotechnology. Research was well-funded and thriving, and many life-saving and life-enhancing products, both medical and agricultural, were in the pipeline. With its light touch regulation, technology-friendly population and world-class scientists, Britain was deemed the ideal place to invest in biotechnology, and the ideal place for scientists to work.

This changed in August 1997 on the broadcasting of a television programme called *World in Action*. The programme was about genetically modified food. It featured a scientist working at the Rowett Institute in Aberdeen. Dr Arpad Pusztai was working on rats fed on potatoes genetically modified to be pest-resistant. Claiming that the preliminary results of his research had shown such rats to have stunted organ growth and depressed functioning of the immune system, Pusztai uttered the immortal words 'I personally would not eat these potatoes'.[88]

This was picked up by the media. The headlines screamed 'Frankenstein Foods',[89] and 'Eat at Your Peril'. Particular emphasis was put on the use of GM ingredients in babyfood.[90]

The British public, learning that 60% of processed foods contained GM, and that foodstuffs weren't labelled as such (the government having decided it wasn't necessary), revolted. There were demonstrations outside supermarkets,[91] people boycotted those fast food outlets thought to use GM ingredients[92] and the market for prepared babyfood collapsed. Soon local governments banned GM ingredients from use in school meals,[93] restaurants first labelled dishes with GM ingredients on their menus, then abandoned them altogether, supermarkets found that to remain competitive it was essential they too ban GM ingredients from their products.

Box 17.13 Activity: Media analysis

Print out and photocopy this article from the UK's *Daily Mail*:

http://www.dailymail.co.uk/sciencetech/article-505561/Alert-march-grey-goo-nanotechnology-Frankenfoods.html.

Give participants a copy then, dividing them into small groups, ask them (in the case of questions marked '*' after they have had time to conduct some research) to answer the following questions:

1. What role is played by the word 'Frankenfood' in this article?
2. Make explicit the analogy between nanotechnology and GM food and why it is drawn by the author (for an explanation of 'analogy' see Chapter 11, Box 11.5)?
3. Do you think the analogy is a good one?
4. What about the analogy between thalidomide and nanotechnology?

5. The views of various 'experts' are quoted. Do they support the writer's case? Say why (not)?
6. *What is the mention of 'grey goo' about? (search for it online if necessary)
7. *Check out the *Which?* report mentioned. Has the article added its own 'spin' or is it an accurate report?
8. *Check out the Defra report and see if it has been 'spun'.
9. What is the view of nanotechnology that *Daily Mail* readers are likely to form as the result of this article?

This activity might be followed by a whole group discussion on the article.

The government was caught on the hop. Having been extremely pro-GM food, it first tried to resist the onslaught, but soon gave in. It quickly put together a set of requirements on the labelling of GM food, then it underwrote in law the originally self-imposed ban on unlabelled GM ingredients in restaurants and retail outlets.[94] Noting that the 13 member committee charged with granting licences for GM crops consisted mainly of people likely to sympathise with the GM industry, it replaced 10 members with people more likely to be hostile.

You might wonder about the scientist who started all this. Pusztai was in fact retired. He was working for the Rowett Institute on a freelance basis. The results that were leaked to the press came from experiments that had no proper controls. Shortly after triggering the GM panic, Pusztai was disciplined by the Rowett Institute who said that his findings had been tentative, they had not been peer-reviewed and that in talking about them publicly he had been irresponsible. The press reported that he had been dismissed from his post, but as he didn't *have* a post this was not true.[95]

Even so the media scented a conspiracy on discovering the Institute was funded in part by Monsanto and the flames, if anything, were fanned. Pusztai's results were later condemned by a group of internationally renowned scientists.[96] They said his methodology was inadequate and his arguments bad. But by then there was no chance of putting the genie back in the bottle.[97]

Environmental activists noted that before GM ingredients get into food they first have to be grown as crops. Pointing out that between 1996 and 1998 the area planted with GM crops worldwide had increased from 2 million to 28 million hectares they held out the vision of environmental disaster. What if these GM crops were to spread their new genes to wild varieties of the same plant? What would be the effect of introducing these new elements into a fragile ecosystem?[98]

The authorities tried to insist such 'genetic pollution' was improbable, but then pollen from a GM crop grown in Oxfordshire was found 3 miles away and honey on sale in a supermarket was found to be 'contaminated'. Soon activists wearing decontamination suits (to make a point that GM crops are dangerous to handle), many politicised only by the GM panic, were ripping up fields of GM crops.[99] The media were having a field day.

In 2010 Britain is no longer a world leader in GM technology. Hostile regulation makes it uneconomical to grow GM crops commercially and all the major agro-chemical companies have left the UK. In 2004 the only company that had succeeded in gaining a licence to grow GM maize commercially in Britain, the German company BayerCropScience, withdrew.[100] Noting its inability, despite its licence, to clear all the regulatory hurdles, Bayer said it was simply losing too much money.

Bayer are far from the only losers: it has been estimated that British farmers have lost up to £600 million in revenue as a result of the GM debacle.

It has also become difficult to grow crops for research purposes. This is because by EU regulations field trials have to be publicised. In 2008, for example, Leeds University planted 400 GM potato plants on a field near Tadcaster. A map reference to the site was posted on the website of the Department for the Environment, Food and Rural Affairs and within 2 weeks activists had uprooted the lot.

Box 17.14 Activity: Creative writing

In small groups participants should choose one of the following uses of bio-technology and write an article about it for a popular newspaper:

(i)   the use of artificial sperm or the use of eggs from aborted foetuses (Chapter 10, page 159);

(ii) the development of an artificial womb (Chapter 10, page 159);

(iii) the possibility of genetic enhancement creating a new species (Chapter 14, page 256);

(iv) the use of synthetic biology to create an organism unknown in nature (Chapter 16);

(v)   the use of synthetic biology by a 'garage biologist' (Chapter 16);

(vi) in vitro meat;

(vii) the seeding of clouds to avert global warming (Chapter 21).

Participants might also be asked to read the section 'It's disgusting' in Chapter 6, pages 76, 79.

It is only very recently, as our understanding of the looming food crisis has grown, that the UK government has started to take a stand for the reinvigoration of the GM industry in Britain.[101] In 2010 permission was finally given to the Sainsbury Laboratory in Norwich to run a field trial of GM potatoes.[102]

Even if this trial is allowed to continue, however, and is successful, genetic technology is far from rehabilitated: a recent survey showed 90% of the British public were still against GM food, and, as journalist David Aaronovitch notes, 'GM-Free' is still a badge of quality throughout the UK.[103] But there are some signs that moves are afoot that might result in this hostility abating: Tesco, one of the UK's largest supermarket chains, recently reviewed its 'no GM' policy[104] and a couple of other supermarket chains have tentatively followed suit.

Public perception worldwide

It is not just in Britain, however, that the public is hostile to GM foods. In 2002 Zambia rejected 27,000 tonnes of GM food donated by the US government, despite the fact that one-quarter of Zambia's 10.4 million people were starving.[105] When this caused riots, Zambia's agriculture minister accused western donors of 'promoting food riots in order to force Zambia to accept GM maize'. President Levy Mwanawasa of Zambia said:

'Simply because my people are hungry that is no reason to give them poison, to give them food that is intrinsically dangerous to their health.'[106]

It is difficult to see where President Mwanawasa got the idea that GM food is 'intrinsically dangerous to health' unless he caught it from the activists in the Europe.[107]

This idea prompted David King, a former UK Chief Scientist, to claim that Africa's ills are 'largely down to western do-gooders' who oppose GM food in favour of organic food.[108] 'Organic food', King argues 'is a luxury Africa cannot afford. Modern agricultural technology is the only way to solve their problems'. Lord Krebs, the former Chairman of Britain's Food Standards Agency said, in a 2009 debate:

'The moral tragedy of the whole GM debacle is the fact that European prissiness about genetic modification has affected its adoption in Africa.'[109]

It should not be forgotten that it is not currently, and in the future is unlikely to be only, food shortages that result in food crises. The political situation in Africa and other countries in the developing world is often not conducive to the fair distribution of food, whether imported, home grown or provided as food aid.

The infrastructure in many such countries is also far from helpful: you can only distribute food efficiently if the roads are good, there is transport to carry the food, carrying the food around is safe, and officials who distribute the food are not corrupt. In some countries none of these conditions is satisfied.[110]

> **Box 17.15 Activity: Debate**
>
> Participants should be asked to debate the following motion:
>
> *This house believes that GM technology is the best solution to the global food crisis.*

It seems clear that, unless the public image of GM undergoes a radical change, the idea that GM technology might help us solve the world food crisis is a forlorn one.[111]

Summary

In this chapter we have considered the use of GM technology as a means of averting or alleviating a global food crisis. In particular we have:

- learned about food security and its four components;
- reflected on energy security and the use of land for growing crops for biofuels instead of food;
- considered the factors contributing to a global food crisis, including population growth, urbanisation, climate change and change of land use;
- learned about the ways in which a global food crisis might be averted or alleviated;
- mused on whether the 'yuk' response to in vitro meat is reasonable;
- considered the pros and cons of using GM technology to alleviate the food crisis;
- learned about why GM technology is rejected by many in the UK and in Europe;
- noted the importance of politics, the media and the public perception of GM technology.

Questions to stimulate reflection

Do you think we will ever achieve food security or was Malthus right?

Could diverting land to grow crops for fuel be justified in a world where there isn't enough food?

If there is enough food being grown to give every human being 2500 calories why are so many people starving?

How might a government respond to food riots caused by a staple food's being too expensive?

Will organic farming provide us with a solution to the global food crisis? If not why not?

Why have modern farming techniques been so disastrous for the environment?

Could conventional farming techniques be modified in such a way as to help alleviate or avert the food crisis consistently with reducing the carbon emissions that will otherwise contribute to climate change?

What are the main benefits of GM technology in dealing with a food crisis?

What are the main difficulties with relying on GM technology as a response to the world food crisis?

Why is the public perception of GM technology in the UK so poor? Could this poor perception be spreading to other parts of the world?

What role has been played by the media in the poor European perception of GM technology?

What might be done to rehabilitate GM technology in the eyes of the public? What role might scientists play in this?

Is it reasonable for a government to try to rehabilitate a technology in the eyes of the public, as opposed to merely responding to the will of the public?

Additional activities

Contact your local supermarket and ask them if they have a policy regarding GM food and/or GM ingredients in food.

See what percentage of restaurants in your vicinity make explicit the fact they don't use GM ingredients. Contact one and ask their reasons for their policy.

Find out who does the catering for the building in which you work or are studying. Approach the manager and ask the policy on GM foods.

Conduct an opinion poll amongst friends and family: how many people would countenance eating food with GM ingredients?

In pairs find an article in the newspaper about a biotechnological advance and decide whether the article is a reasonable representation of the technology. Give reasons for your answer.

Check out the archive of your local newspaper and see how they reported on the GM food crisis. Do you think their reporting was fair?

Look at the section on GM technology on the 'senseaboutscience' website: http://www.senseaboutscience.org.uk/index.php/site/project/16/.

Look also at this website from the Natural Law Party who have a campaign to ban GM food: http://www.btinternet.com/~nlpwessex/Documents/gmoquote.htm.

Notes

1 http://www.bionetonline.org/english/content/ff_cont3.htm. Four examples of genetically engineered crops from Bionet.org.
2 http://news.bbc.co.uk/1/hi/health/7404268.stm. The BBC on links between obesity and the food crisis.
3 http://www.supermarket.co.uk/news/2010/Aug/staple-food-prices-up-59-per-cent-in-three-years-97424050.html.
4 http://www.thaindian.com/newsportal/world-news/900-mn-indians-live-on-less-than-2-a-day_10059330.html.
5 http://www.pediatriconcall.com/nutrition/malnutrition.asp.
6 http://latimesblogs.latimes.com/babylonbeyond/2010/08/egypt-fears-of-a-crisis-after-russias-wheat-export-ban.html.
7 http://www.irinnews.org/Report.aspx?ReportId=77608.

8 http://news.bbc.co.uk/1/hi/in_depth/7361945.stm. A BBC report on global food shortages.

9 http://www.rnw.nl/africa/article/cameroon-food-prices-changing-eating-habits. An update on food distribution in Cameroon 2 years after the riots.

10 http://www.biofuelsdigest.com/blog2/2008/01/16/indonesian-food-riots-spread-force-government-to-declare-emergency-as-rising-soybean-prices-fuel-unrest/.

11 http://www.youtube.com/watch?v=xhI-FSKgTfs. A You Tube video of food queues in Egypt.

12 http://speakingofmedicine.plos.org/2010/08/12/russian-fires-could-result-in-a-global-disaster%E2%80%94another-food-crisis/.

13 http://news.sky.com/skynews/Home/World-News/Pakistan-Floods-Threaten-Deadly-Food-Crisis-As-Asif-Ali-Zardari-Awaits-Talks-With-David-Cameron/Article/201008115676590?f=rss.

14 http://news.bbc.co.uk/1/hi/world/africa/7325733.stm.

15 http://news.bbc.co.uk/1/hi/in_depth/world/2008/costoffood/default.stm. A BBC report on the recession and the food crisis.

16 Malthus, T.R. (1798) An Essay on the Principle of Population.

17 http://www.worldmapper.org/display.php?selected=11.

18 http://www.ipu.org/splz-e/food.htm.

19 http://www.who.int/trade/glossary/story028/en/.

20 http://www.stanford.edu/group/FRI/indonesia/documents/foodpolicy/chapt1.fm.html.

21 An unpublished report written for the World Bank and reported in the *Guardian* at: http://www.guardian.co.uk/environment/2008/jul/03/biofuels.renewableenergy.

22 http://news.bbc.co.uk/1/hi/world/europe/7435439.stm. A BBC report on the impact of biofuels on food production.

23 *New Scientist*, 2 October 2003.

24 http://www.independent.co.uk/news/science/world-oil-supplies-are-set-to-run-out-faster-than-expected-warn-scientists-453068.html.

25 http://biofuel.org.uk/history-of-biofuels.html.

26 http://www.geographyteachingtoday.org.uk/ks3-resources/resource/you-are-what-you-eat/biofuels-exploiting-farmland-and-the-natural-environment/. A GCSE teaching resource for land-use change.

27 http://www.bbc.co.uk/bloom/actions/biofuels.shtml.

28 http://www.guardian.co.uk/lifeandstyle/2010/jul/18/vegetarianism-save-planet-environment. A *Guardian* article listing 10 ways going vegetarian can help save the planet.

29 In this chapter I have used pounds and acres rather than the usual SI units, but the old-fashioned measures give nice round numbers for discussion so I have left them in!

30 The *Guardian* on whether vegetarianism will save the planet: http://www.guardian.co.uk/lifeandstyle/wordofmouth/2010/feb/24/vegetarianism-save-planet-safran-foer.

31 http://www.timesonline.co.uk/tol/life_and_style/health/features/article3894871.ece. A *Times* article on in vitro meat.

32 *Tissue Engineering*, 29 June 2005.

33 http://www.guardian.co.uk/environment/2010/aug/16/artificial-meat-food-royal-society.

34 http://www.hplusmagazine.com/articles/bio/eight-ways-vitro-meat-will-change-our-lives.

35 http://www.peta.org.uk/. The PETA website.

36 http://thebovine.wordpress.com/2010/02/08/vat-grown-meat-getting-closer-to-reality-as-peta-offers-million-dollar-prize-for-commercially-viable-test-tube-meat/.

37 *Times*, 9 May 2008. Is in vitro meat the future?

38 http://news.bbc.co.uk/1/hi/sci/tech/2017094.stm.

39 http://news.bbc.co.uk/1/hi/health/8174482.stm. A BBC report on the health benefits of organic food.

40 http://www.food.gov.uk/foodindustry/farmingfood/organicfood/.

41 Dangour, A. D., Lock, K., Hayter, A. *et al.* (2009) Nutrition-related health effects of organic foods: a systematic review. *American Journal of Clinical Nutrition*, 29 July.

42 http://www.soilassociation.org/News/NewsItem/tabid/91/smid/463/ArticleID/97/reftab/57/t/Soil-Association-response-to-the-Food-Standards-Agency-s-Organic-Review/Default.aspx.

43 http://www.senseaboutscience.org.uk/index.php/site/other/384. A 'senseaboutscience' report on the debate about organic food.

44 http://library.wur.nl/WebQuery/wurpubs/338840.

45 http://www.independent.co.uk/news/world/africa/organic-farming-could-feed-africa-968641.html.

46 UNCTAD/UNEP (2008) *Organic Agriculture and Food Security in Africa*. New York: UNCTAD/UNEP.

47 http://news.bbc.co.uk/1/hi/in_depth/6496585.stm.

48 http://www.global-greenhouse-warming.com/agriculture-and-climate-change.html.

49 http://www.vision.org/visionmedia/article.aspx?id=21824.

50 http://science.howstuffworks.com/environmental/earth/oceanography/dead-zone.htm. A Howstuffworks report on 'dead zones'.

51 http://www.telegraph.co.uk/earth/agriculture/farming/6828878/Britain-facing-food-crisis-as-worlds-soil-vanishes-in-60-years.html. The *Telegraph* on the loss of soil.

52 Harvey, G. (2008) *The Carbon Fields: How Our Countryside Can Save Britain*. Carlsbad, CA: Grassroots.

53 http://www.chinadaily.com.cn/china/2008-06/24/content_6790223.htm.

54 http://defrafarmingandfoodscience.csl.gov.uk/.

55 http://www.guardian.co.uk/science/blog/2009/jan/23/gm-crops-genetically-modified-food-crisis. A *Guardian* report of a debate on whether GM technology could sole the world food crisis.

56 http://www.guardian.co.uk/environment/gm. The *Guardian* resources on GM technology.

57 http://www.timesonline.co.uk/tol/news/science/article7023718.ece.

58 http://www.uvm.edu/~uvmpr/?Page=article.php&id=1617.

59 http://www.nature.com/nature/debates/gmfoods/gmfoods_frameset.html. A *Nature* debate on the pros and cons of genetic modification.

60 http://www.nerc.ac.uk/research/issues/geneticmodification/selective.asp. A Natural Environment Research Council account of genetic modification.

61 http://www.leeds.ac.uk/news/article/339/new_research_to_decode_the_genetic_secrets_of_prolific_potato_pest.

62 http://www.lifescientist.com.au/article/48780/nz_team_creates_high-protein_gm_milk/.

63 http://www.goldenrice.org/. The Golden Rice Project website.

64 http://www.newscientist.com/article/dn18049-us-fda-says-omega3-oils-from-gm-soya-are-safe-to-eat.html.

65 http://biocassavaplus.org/.

66 Gordon, B. (2007) Manganese nutrition of glyphosate: resistant and conventional soybeans. *Better Crops*, Vol. **91**(4), 12–13.

67 IAASTD (2008) Agriculture at a crossroads: synthesis report (v. 7). Science and Technology International Assessment of Agricultural Knowledge.

68 http://www.independent.co.uk/environment/gm-new-study-shows-unborn-babies-could-be-harmed-522109.html.

69 http://www.newscientist.com/article/dn8347-gm-pea-causes-allergic-damage-in-mice.html.

70 http://www.informaworld.com/smpp/content~db=all~content=a907625853.

71 http://www.food.gov.uk/safereating/. The Food Standards Agency guidelines on food safety.

72 http://www.newstatesman.com/environment/2010/01/nuclear-power-lynas-greens. http://www.sciencemuseum.org.uk/antenna/futurefoods/debate/debateGM_CIPsafety. asp. The Science Museum: resources on the safety of GM food.

73 http://www.sciencemuseum.org.uk/antenna/futurefoods/debate/debateGM_CIPenv.asp. The Science Museum on GM and the environment.

74 http://www.telegraph.co.uk/earth/earthnews/3349308/Prince-Charles-warns-GM-crops-risk-causing-the-biggest-ever-environmental-disaster.html. The Prince of Wales' worries about GM and the environment.

75 http://www.dailymail.co.uk/news/article-1244824/Fears-grow-study-shows-genetically-modified-crops-cause-liver-kidney-damage.html.

76 http://www.timesonline.co.uk/tol/news/world/us_and_americas/article604820.ece.

77 http://extension.missouri.edu/p/IPM1030.

78 http://www.actionbioscience.org/biotech/sakko.html.

79 Nuffield Council on Bioethics (1999) *Genetically Modified Crops: The Ethical and Social Issues.*

80 http://www.independent.co.uk/news/science/gm-researchers-created-virus-as-dangerous-as-tb-678799.html.

81 http://www.gmo-compass.org/eng/news/stories/458.issue_contradictory_results_biosafety_studies.html.

82 http://www.globalissues.org/article/194/terminator-technology.

83 http://news.bbc.co.uk/1/hi/sci/tech/465222.stm.

84 http://news.bbc.co.uk/1/hi/talking_point/468270.stm. A BBC report on a debate between Greenpeace and Monsanto.

85 http://www.reuters.com/article/idUSN087196620100108.

86 http://www.bbc.co.uk/news/10136310. A report from the BBC on GM seeds in India.

87 http://www.monsanto.co.uk/.

88 http://openlearn.open.ac.uk/mod/oucontent/view.php?id=398604&section=3.1. An Open University resource on GM food and the 'Pusztai Affair'.

89 http://www.bbc.co.uk/dna/h2g2/A156511&clip=1. A BBC report on 'Frankenstein Food'.

90 http://www.edie.net/news/news_story.asp?id=1541.

91 http://news.bbc.co.uk/1/hi/england/bristol/3596383.stm.

92 http://www.greenpeace.org.uk/media/press-releases/mcdonalds-to-ban-meat-milk-and-eggs-from-gm-fed-animals.

93 http://www.cardiff.gov.uk/content.asp?Parent_Directory_id=2865&nav=2869, 3047,3065,4732#6. Cardiff Council's food policy statement including the banning of GM ingredients.

94 http://news.bbc.co.uk/1/hi/uk_politics/298731.stm.

95 http://www.healthwatch-uk.org/awardwinners/bernarddixon.html.

96 http://news.bbc.co.uk/1/hi/sci/tech/346651.stm.

97 http://www.guardian.co.uk/education/2008/jan/15/academicexperts. highereducationprofile. A 2008 *Guardian* interview with an 'unrepentant' Pusztai.

98 http://news.bbc.co.uk/1/hi/sci/tech/371353.stm.

99 http://news.bbc.co.uk/1/hi/uk/397633.stm.

100 http://news.bbc.co.uk/1/hi/sci/tech/3584763.stm.

101 http://www.guardian.co.uk/environment/2010/jan/06/gm-food-revolution-government-scientist.

102 http://www.bbc.co.uk/news/10254905.

103 http://www.timesonline.co.uk/tol/comment/columnists/david_aaronovitch/article7036900.ece.

104 http://www.foodmanufacture.co.uk/Business-News/Tesco-boss-prepares-for-GM-u-turn.

105 http://news.bbc.co.uk/1/hi/world/africa/2371675.stm.

106 http://news.bbc.co.uk/1/hi/world/europe/3826261.stm.

107 http://www.scidev.net/en/agriculture-and-environment/opinions/taking-on-biotechnology-the-african-way.html.

108 http://www.guardian.co.uk/science/blog/2009/jan/23/gm-crops-genetically-modified-food-crisis.

109 http://www.foodmanufacture.co.uk/Business-News/Tesco-boss-prepares-for-GM-u-turn.

110 http://www.foe.co.uk/resource/media_briefing/food_crisis.pdf.

111 http://news.bbc.co.uk/1/hi/sci/tech/474978.stm. A BBC report on the 'Pusztai Affair'. http://newsforums.bbc.co.uk/nol/thread.jspa?forumID=7490&start=30&edition=1&ttl=20100825124528.

Further reading and useful websites

Allan, S. (2002) *Media, Risk & Science (Issues in Cultural and Media Studies)*. Maidenhead, UK: Open University Press.

Ingram, J., Erickson, P. and Liverman, D. (2010) *Food Security and Global Environmental Change*. Oxford: Earthscan Ltd.

Rosillo-Carre, F. and Johnson, F. (2010) *Food versus Fuel: An informed introduction to biofuels*. London: Zed Books.

http://www.ncl.ac.uk/peals/research/completedprojects/gmjury.htm. A website from PEALS (Policy, Ethics and the Life Sciences, describing its Citizens' Jury on GM crops).

http://www.citizenshipfoundation.org.uk/main/page.php?199. A debate resource from the UK's Citizenship Foundation.

http://www.foodsecurity.ac.uk/. Useful information from Global Food Security.

18

Bio-ownership: who owns the stuff of life?

Objectives

In reading this chapter you will:

- learn about Henrietta Lacks and her singular contribution to science;
- reflect on whether Lacks had a moral right to share in the profits generated by her cells;
- consider John Moore and the need for fully informed consent;
- reflect on the notion of informed consent for specific and commercial uses of tissue;
- examine a UK scandal to reflect further on consent to specific uses of tissue;
- consider the notions of biopiracy and bioprospecting in the context of the Biodiversity Convention;
- learn about the recent history of patenting DNA and other biological resources;
- reflect on whether the 'stuff of life' should be patentable at all.

In the eighteenth century surgeons were trained by the Company of Barber Surgeons[1] who were alone allowed legal access to the corpses of criminals executed by the state. The many private schools of anatomy made do with the services of grave-robbers or those, like Burke and Hare,[2] who murdered their victims to provide fresh corpses.

The authorities turned a blind eye to the activities of the grave-robbers (though not the murderers) because of their service to society. In those days, anyway, the notion of 'informed', 'genuine' or 'appropriate' consent was unknown.

HeLa cells

This was still pretty much the case in 1951. In October of that year a 31-year-old mother of five named Henrietta Lacks died of cervical cancer in the 'coloured ward' of Johns Hopkins University in Baltimore. In the same hospital Dr George Gey[3] had been trying – and failing – for 20 years to grow human cells in the laboratory for use in medical research. Gey was given tissue samples from every patient with cervical cancer. Cells from Henrietta Lacks, therefore, soon came his way.

Her cells survived. They didn't only survive, furthermore, they reproduced an entire generation every 24 hours. This was the first time ever that human cells had grown and reproduced outside the human body.

They have done so ever since: more than 50 million tonnes of Henrietta's cells – known as HeLa ('hee-lah') cells – have been grown since she died. Over 60 000 scientific papers have acknowledged their use (with 10 new studies being added every day).[4] Millions of dollars have been made on the back of them. Thousands of scientific careers have flourished and hundreds of millions of patients have benefited from the use of them. In 2009 there were 11,000 patents involving them waiting to be processed.

With their help the polio vaccine was produced, IVF techniques discovered and drugs for herpes, flu and leukaemia, Parkinson's disease and haemophilia developed. Chemotherapy and the breast cancer drug tamoxifen came about because of them. They were the first cells ever cloned and contained the first genes ever mapped.

Despite being cancerous, the HeLa cells divided, generated energy, 'communicated', produced proteins, expressed and regulated genes. They were vulnerable to hormones and toxins and they could be frozen and irradiated.[5] Thirty years after Henrietta's death her cells were instrumental in production of a vaccine for the cervical cancer that killed her, earning German virologist Harald zur Hausen a Nobel Prize.

Box 18.1 Factual information: Henrietta Lacks: a real person

Mary Kubicek, George Gey's research assistant, was asked to extract more cells from Henrietta Lacks whilst she lay in the autopsy room. Averting her gaze from Henrietta's face Mary noticed her toenails were covered in chipped red varnish. 'I nearly fainted,' she said 'I thought "Oh Jeez, she's a real person." I started to imagine her sitting in her bathroom painting those toenails and it hit me for the first time that those cells we'd been working with all this time and sending all over the world came from a live woman.' Skloot, R. (2010) *The Immortal Life of Henrietta Lacks*. London: Macmillan, pp. 90–91.

The cells of Henrietta Lacks are immortal and beyond value. But what, you might ask, became of Henrietta Lacks herself and her five children, left motherless so young? What happened to Henrietta's young husband, left with so many children for whom, singlehandedly, to care?

At this point the story becomes embarrassing. Until April 2010 Henrietta lay in an unmarked grave in Virginia. One of her children, Ellie, died aged 15, in the Hospital for the Negro Insane of Maryland. Her other children – still living – are unable to afford health insurance.

Over the years the family heard dribs and drabs of news about their mother's cells. But the author of a recent best-seller about the life of Henrietta Lacks,[6] Rebecca Skloot,[7] claims they lived in a 'mist of fear, anger and misconception', mindful of the stories they had heard about 'night doctors', white people who kidnapped black people for medical experiments. It was only in 2009 that two of her surviving children were finally taken into a laboratory to see HeLa cells for the first time. Henrietta's daughter Deborah says:

'Truth be told, I cannot get mad at science, because it helps people live, and I'd be a mess without it. But I won't lie I would like some health insurance so I don't got to pay all that money every month for drugs my mother's cells probably helped to make.'[8]

The Lacks family's grievances do not turn only upon the fact that so much money was made from their mother's cells without any of it coming to them.

They are angry also because in 1976 they gave blood samples to the geneticist Victor McKusick,[9] believing they were being tested for cancer. McKusick then published a paper 'Genetic characteristics of the HeLa cell' in which he listed 43 genetic markers in their DNA, enabling HeLa cells to be identified in any lab sample. This paper discussed Henrietta by name and described her family as 'husband', 'child one', 'child two', etc., thereby breaching the confidentiality that today is taken so seriously.

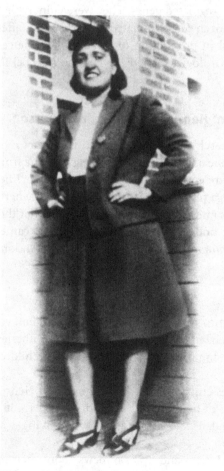

Figure 18.1 Henrietta Lacks, after whom HeLa cells are named, standing outside her home in Baltimore, United States. © Obstetrics & Gynaecology/Science Photo Library.

This wasn't the only violation of the Lacks' privacy. In 1986 a journalist, Michael Gold, published a book called *A Conspiracy of Cells: One Woman's Immortal Legacy and the Medical Scandal it Caused*.[10] In his book Gold described in gruesome detail Henrietta Lacks' autopsy. It transpired that he had been given access to Henrietta Lacks, medical records. No one in the Lacks family had given – or been asked for – their permission to release them.

It is important to note that the only unique element in this sorry tale is the extraordinary value, to scientific research and therefore to humanity, of Henrietta Lacks' cells. That no one secured her consent or that of her family to the use of those cells, or to the release of her medical records, was not unusual at the time. Nor was it unusual that no one should have explained what they were doing or why. The doctor–patient relationship was different then: doctors were omniscient, paternal and God-like, patients were respectful and obedient.

It is interesting, though, to ask whether Henrietta Lacks, or her family, were morally entitled to share in the profits made from Henrietta Lacks' cells. We might also ask whether, if they were, this has implications for the rest of us who give bio-specimens that are used in research.

The 'Mo cell line'

One answer was given to this question in 1988 after a long and tortuous legal process instituted by patient John Moore against the Regents of the University of California.[11] In 1976 Moore had been diagnosed with hairy cell leukaemia. His spleen, usually about 0.5 lb in weight, weighed 14 lbs. With Moore's consent it was removed.

Moore's doctor, David Golde,[12] had seen before Moore's operation that Moore's blood was unusual. It contained a rare type of T-lymphocyte that produced an unusually large amount of lymphokine protein which regulates the immune system. After Moore's splenectomy Dr Golde took tissue from his spleen and in 1979 he and his research associate Shirley Quan replicated John Moore's cells in the same sort of immortal cell-line that had been made from Henrietta Lacks' cells. They applied for a patent on the 'Mo cell line' in 1979. The patent was granted in 1984.

The cell line was used to produce several products, most notably granulocyte–macrophage colony-stimulating factor, a substance that helps to make white blood cells and that was then being tested for use in AIDS. Golde, Quan and the University of California entered into an agreement with Genetic Institute and Sandoz Pharma-ceuticals. The value of the Mo cell line was estimated at several billion dollars.

Over the intervening years John Moore had, at the request of Dr Golde, returned several times to the UCLA Medical Centre where further bio-samples were taken from him. But he was suspicious. Several times he asked whether there was any financial benefit to be gained from his tissue. He received no answer. In 1983, however, he was asked to sign a form that, he was assured, was a formality. The form asked him to waive all his rights, and those of his heirs, to any product that might be developed from his tissue. Moore refused to sign and consulted a lawyer who discovered the patents taken out on products made from John Moore's cells.

Moore sued the university. He claimed that the university's use of his cells constituted a 'conversion'[13] (where property belonging to one person is wrongfully disposed of or converted to the use of another, to the detriment of its rightful owner). He also claimed that he had not given his informed consent to the university's use of his cells. And he claimed that Dr Golde had breached his fiduciary duty (his duty to act for the benefit of Moore as his patient).

The Supreme Court of California rejected his claim of conversion on the grounds that Moore's tissue had not belonged to him at the time that the university, in the persons of Golde and Quan, had used it. In signing the consent form before his splenectomy, they ruled, Moore had relinquished ownership of his tissue. As he did not own it, it could not have been converted by Golde and Quan.[14] According to the Supreme Court of California, therefore, in signing a form consenting to an operation Moore had given up any right he might have had to a say over, or to a profit from, the use of tissue removed in that operation.[15]

It might immediately be objected that if Moore didn't explicitly consent to the use of his tissue for commercial purposes, it was morally wrong of his doctor to use that tissue for such purposes. Such a claim suggests that it is morally improper of a doctor to use tissue for

(i) *any* purpose other than that for which explicit consent has been given;

or

(ii) any *commercial* purposes without explicit consent to such a use.

Let's consider the implications of both these claims.

(i) Consent for specific uses

Let us assume that Henrietta Lacks or her family would have consented to the use of her cells to find a vaccine for cervical cancer. Her cells were used for this purpose. They have also been used, however, to research the effects of zero gravity in space, and the mating habits of mosquitoes.[16] It would have been impossible to predict, in 1951, that Lacks' cells might have had such uses. It would have been impossible, therefore, to have obtained her specific consent, or that of her family, to their use for such purposes or for many of the other myriad purposes to which they have been put.

If the law, or professional codes of conduct, were to require such specific consents this could seriously hamper scientific research, much of which depends on accessing tissue held in store to be used as and when a research project is conceived or a new technique becomes available.

It might be suggested that researchers could always go back to those whose samples are stored, or their families, and ask for explicit consent to a different use of their tissue. This would require full details of samples and who gave them to be kept on file and up to date. It would also involve the time and effort spent by administrators in contacting families and asking for their consent each time a new use for their tissue was found. This would be a huge and costly administrative burden, especially if anonymity had been assured.

But perhaps it would be worth it? That doctors and scientists should seek permission to use tissue is extremely important to people. According to Skloots, who has interviewed many people who have sued researchers over the use of their tissue, 'Over and over again they say "if they had just asked us, we'd have said "yes"'.

One response to this difficulty is for consent forms to include a section for 'open' consent, where people consent to their tissue being used for *any* purpose (or perhaps any non-commercial purpose). Many people are happy to sign for open use, because they altruistically want to help research that might help others.

Box 18.2 Activity: Small group discussion

In small groups participants should be asked to discuss the pros and cons of requiring that consent forms mention specific uses for which tissue may be retained.

Having done so they should report back to the group, after which the discussion can be opened to the group as a whole.

(ii) Consent for commercial use

The Supreme Court of California rejected John Moore's claim that the university wrongfully 'converted' his tissue. But they accepted his claim that Dr Golde had breached his fiduciary duty to Moore. A 'fiduciary duty' obtains when one person has a moral or legal obligation to act in the best interests of another.

Dr Golde, the court argued, had a fiduciary duty to secure John Moore's *fully informed* consent to the taking of his tissue. When he failed to disclose to Moore that he had a financial interest in Moore's tissue he breached that duty. In order to obtain fully informed consent, the court argued, Dr Golde should have disclosed even 'personal interests unrelated to the patient's health, whether research or economic, that may affect his or her judgements'.

This ruling leaves unclear the exact nature of a medic's fiduciary duty. If a doctor has a small number of shares in a pharmaceutical company that may end up benefiting from research involving the patient's sample, does this count as a financial interest in the sample? What if at the time of taking a patient's tissue a doctor has no thought of a commercial use? Does this mean he can't later use it for commercial purposes (at least without getting back to the patient)? Many people would happily consent to the use of tissue for medical research, would they be as happy to see it used for commercial benefit?

The aim of the big pharmaceuticals, after all, is not directly to benefit humanity. It is to benefit their shareholders. Usually they will successfully benefit shareholders only if they benefit humanity. But this will not always be the case. Why, anyway, should a patient donate their tissue for the benefit of shareholders, even if a side effect of this is a benefit to humanity? Why shouldn't they derive some personal benefit from their tissue? Is it morally acceptable that neither Henrietta Lacks nor John Moore made a penny from their tissue whilst others made millions? Perhaps samples should be taken only on the understanding that if they prove commercially valuable, the patient will get a share?

One difficulty would again be administrative. When huge profits are made, this is rarely on the back of the tissue of one individual. It is far more often the case that numerous individuals have contributed tissue leading to a profitable advance. Imagine having to track all these individuals. Imagine having to work out, in the case of each individual, their rightful share of the proceeds. Might this be so expensive that it would deter companies from conducting the research and development needed to make such huge advances?

Another difficulty would be that such a clause would draw patients' attention to the possibility of making money from tissue. Could this prompt mistrust of doctors, a sense that the doctor wants to profit from them rather than help them get better? Might this result in unseemly bargaining in which patients hold out for a better 'price' for their tissue? What would be the 'rightful' share in a medical advance of one person who gave blood that, along with the blood of hundreds of others, was used to produce it? Should the open clause in consent forms be understood to include consent to commercial uses, or does this violate a fiduciary duty to the patient?

Box 18.3 Activity: Role play

Participants should be asked, in fours, to role play an interaction between a doctor asking for consent to take a sample, a patient aware of the possibility of money's being made from such samples, the partner of that patient and a hospital administrator.

Participants should have 20 minutes to prepare their role play.

Such considerations raise an interesting question. What if medics were to come across a person whose biospecimens, like those of Henrietta Lacks or John Moore, would be extremely valuable for medical research and potentially therefore for humanity, but who refused to consent to their use for any purpose but their own healthcare? Should medics resign themselves to this? Or do they have a duty to put pressure on this person? If the latter what form might this pressure take? Would it be morally permissible, for example, for the medic to take such a person to court in the hope of compelling him to give tissue? Would it be permissible to make his treatment dependent on his consenting to the use of his tissue?

How in this situation could the right of this person to be treated as an end in himself be squared with any desire we might have to produce the greatest happiness of the greatest number? (See the discussion of deontology and Kant in Chapter 4.)

> **Box 18.4 Activity: Brainstorm**
>
> The group should be asked to brainstorm their views on what should happen in the case of a person whose cells are potentially as valuable as those of Henrietta Lacks, but who refuses to consent to their being used for any purpose other than his own well-being.

Alder Hey Hospital scandal

In the UK consent for specific uses (though not commercial uses) *is* now required from those who give biospecimens for research purposes. That this is the case is arguably the direct result of a major scandal involving the retention of body parts.

In 1999 it was discovered that, stockpiled at the Alder Hey Hospital in Liverpool,[17] were literally thousands of organs taken from the bodies of babies and children who, between 1988 and 1996, had died at the hospital. The parents of the children had consented to post-mortems, but not to the retention of organs. When they discovered the organs of their children might have been kept by the hospital the switchboards were jammed by worried parents, according to the BBC, demanding to know if their child was involved.[18]

Annette Grimes discovered that the baby she had buried 40 years before was without his heart, lungs and oesophagus. Janet Dacombe held three funerals for her son James as Alder Hey returned his organs one by one. The 11-month-old son of Paula O'Leary had had his heart and 36 other body parts taken following his death from a brain haemorrhage in 1981.

At the final enquiry – the Redfern Enquiry[19] – in 2001 it was stated that 2080 organs, from 800 children, were retained together with 3,575 aborted or stillborn foetuses. It was only in January 2010 that a final burial service was held at Liverpool's Allerton Cemetery for the tissue samples, organs and foetuses that had not been claimed by relatives. A memorial garden was dedicated at the same time.[20]

As a result of the Alder Hey scandal an enquiry, led by the UK's Chief Medical Officer Liam Donaldson, was launched into the use of children's organs. It reported that 105,000 organs were retained at hospitals and medical schools throughout England. It recommended major changes in the law to ensure informed consent to the removal of organs and tissue during post-mortem.

At the centre of the scandal was Professor Dick van Velzen, a Dutch pathologist, an expert on cot death and Senior Pathologist at Alder Hey from 1988–95.[21] According to the Redfern Enquiry report he 'systematically ordered the unethical and illegal stripping of every organ from every child who had a post-mortem'. His excuse was that the hospital had not allowed him the time and the resources to conduct post-mortems properly. He kept the organs hoping one day to complete them to his satisfaction. As he put it 'children are too precious to die without using every scrap of information which could help the next child'.[22] Notwithstanding this he was struck off the medical register in 2005.[23] According to the *British Medical Journal*, van Velzen's actions led directly to the 2004 Human Tissue Act.[24]

This act makes consent fundamental to the use and storage of human tissue. It is overseen by the Human Tissue Authority (HTA) which will issue licences to institutions, such as schools of anatomy and museums that store human tissue.[25] The act makes the following actions illegal:

- removing, storing or using human tissue without consent;
- taking and testing DNA without consent;
- organ trafficking;
- storing tissue or organs for a purpose not stated.[26]

As the Act came into force Peter Furness, Vice-president of the Royal College of Pathologists,[27] said that although there were good points about the Act, the licensing would be expensive, time-consuming, complicated and over-bureaucratic. The Act has now been in force for some years. Many believe that the stringency of its conditions, and in particular its requirement that tissue and organs can be stored only for stated purposes, are a significant barrier to medical research.

Box 18.5 Factual information: A view on the Human Tissue Act 2004

On the 9 July 2010 the new coalition government in the UK launched a website on which they invited members of the public to nominate laws and regulations that should be repealed as unnecessary.

The following posting was made on 1 July:

'*Repeal the Human Tissue Act 2004*

The HTA was introduced, no doubt with excellent intentions, as a response to the Alder Hey organ retention scandal. However, as with most legislation introduced as a knee-jerk reaction to something, it has had seriously adverse unintended consequences.

The HTA is a complete nightmare for most people engaged in legitimate clinical research. Even taking a single blood sample is regulated by the HTA, and researchers and ethics committees waste huge amounts of time trying to determine whether clearly harmless procedures are compliant with the HTA.

Repealing the act won't lead to a repeat of the Alder Hey scandal. The medical profession are well aware of the issues in organ retention, and their professional standards won't let something like that happen again. Repealing the act will, however, greatly reduce one of the burdens on legitimate clinical research, which is such an important part of the progress in medicine that lets us find cures for diseases.'

This reply was made 15 minutes later:

'As a medical student, I agree wholeheartedly with comment above. At my medical school we perform cadaveric dissection. The HTA adds an extra layer of bureaucracy for our course organisers to deal with and engenders an atmosphere during dissection that is less about respect for the subjects and more of fear of breaking the law.

Repeated, insistent warnings from the first day of our course have added little beyond unnecessary scaremongering, as a culture of respect and dignity already is already strong within the body of medical students, staff and academics.'[28]

It has been argued by Dr Michael Fitzpatrick[29] that in responding thus to the Alder Hey scandal the government conflated two attitudes to the human body that, for the sake of medical progress, need to be kept separate. The first is the 'popular perception' of the body, the second the 'approach of medical science'.

The former, claims Fitzpatrick, extends our 'narcissistic obsession with the living body into a morbid preoccupation with the dead body'. It dwells on the symbolic associations of the organs, seeing them as an integral part of the body which is itself seen as an important part of what makes a person. This attitude is perfectly proper, argues Fitzpatrick, in the funeral parlour, a public place where a dead body is treated with ritualised respect, and sympathy and compassion are vital.

Box 18.6 Factual information: Gunther von Hagens

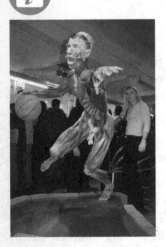

Von Hagens[30] is an anatomist who has become (in)famous for the process of 'plastinating' human bodies. First he removes the fat and body fluids from a corpse, then he replaces them with plastic. He then exhibits these bodies in various life-like poses (see Figure 18.2).

Von Hagens' exhibitions are controversial. Sometimes he courts controversy by the poses in which he arranges his bodies (e.g. for an exhibition in Berlin he arranged two bodies as if they were making love), but often it is simply because it is thought he is not properly respectful to the human body. In 2002 he performed the first public autopsy to be held in the UK for 170 years.

Figure 18.2 Plastination of a baseball player in action. © Photolibrary.com.

The medical approach to the body, says Fitzpatrick, is quite different. This sees the body as an integrated biological system, the organs part of the whole without wider significance, viewed dispassionately in terms of their function. In the discreet and concealed world of the pathology laboratory, argues Fitzpatrick, this detached and objective view is the appropriate attitude to take to the human body. The world of the pathologist has always been concealed, says Fitzpatrick, precisely *because* most people find it distasteful, not because anything goes on there that is improper.

Fitzpatrick is almost certainly right to think a surfeit of the popular perception of the body would hamper the activities of those who must dissect it. Could Fitzpatrick also be right to claim that in responding as it did to the Alder Hey scandal the government in effect insisted that the attitude appropriate to the funeral parlour be applied to the pathology lab?

> ## Box 18.7 Activity: Creative writing
>
> Participants should be asked to write a short (1,000-word) essay describing a day in the life of a pathologist who is required to adopt the 'attitude of the funeral parlour' to the dissection of human bodies.
>
> The best contribution might be read out to stimulate a discussion in which people should be asked to comment on the extent to which the 'attitude of the funeral parlour' *is* appropriate in the laboratory (for example, is it acceptable for medical students to play 'catch' with human organs?).

Bioprospecting and biopiracy

Whole communities can also feel wronged when someone takes from them something they believe rightfully to be theirs. Like John Moore, these communities are not averse to pursuing their perceived rights through the courts (see Box 18.8).

Box 18.8 Factual information: The Mexican yellow bean patent

Mexican farmers had been exporting the *mayocaba* yellow bean to the US for years when Larry Proctor, a farmer from Colorado, bought some, grew them, harvested them then grew another generation. At this point, through his company POD-NERS, he patented *mayocaba* as the 'Enola Bean' (after his wife), being awarded patent number 5,894,079 in April 1999.

POD-NERS then sent a letter to every importer of Mexican beans in the United States warning them that royalties would have to be paid if they sold this bean in the United States.

Many merely stopped importing the bean. The Agricultural Association of Rio Fuerte in Sinaloa Mexico saw a 90% drop in export sales of beans. The effects would have been felt by up to 22,000 Mexican farmers.

In December 2000 the International Center for Tropical Agriculture (CIAT) challenged POD-NERS patent, claiming it violated Mexico's sovereign rights over its genetic resources as recognised by the Convention on Biological Diversity.

In 2009 the US Court of Appeal ruled POD-NERS patent invalid, not because the bean had been wrongfully misappropriated, but because it did not meet the criteria that patented products must have a 'non-obvious' step in their production: Larry Procter, the court argued, only did what anyone else would have done with the bean.

POD-NERS, however, had held their patent for 10 years – half the term of a normal patent – before the patent was revoked.[31]

Dr Conrad Gorinsky,[32] an ethnobiologist of Guyanese descent, spent months with the Wapishana Tribe[33] of the Amazon, learning their ways. This tribe have long used gratings from the nut of the greenheart tree (*Ocotea rodiaei*) to stop haemorrhages, prevent infection and to provoke abortion. After leaving the forest, Gorinsky patented active bisbenzylisoquinoline alkaloids that he had isolated from the greenheart tree and named rupununine (after the village in which he grew up), claiming they could be used to treat cancer and possibly AIDs.[34]

The Wapishana believe that Gorinsky has stolen knowledge that has long been theirs, and that he is using that knowledge for personal profit. In effect their claim is that Gorinsky is a biopirate, one who commercially develops genetic resources and/or native knowledge without compensating those who actually found or developed such resources.

'Biopiracy' is a recent term. It is often contrasted with the term 'bioprospecting'.[35] Both involve the activity of travelling to a region, taking biosamples, then taking these biosamples to another country to produce some benefit. Some believe the two terms are interchangeable. Others believe that biopiracy is morally unacceptable, whilst bioprospecting is morally acceptable.

Bioprospecting (to use the less pejorative term) has a long and – until recently – respectable history. Charles Darwin, for example, went bioprospecting when he set off in the *Beagle*. He simply took whatever interested him and brought it home. Was Darwin a biopirate?[36] The efforts of the Victorian botanists largely stocked the Royal Botanic Gardens in Kew, near London.[37] Many of us have in our gardens plants that arrived in our land thanks to the efforts of people who might now be termed biopirates. These people did not, of course, think they were doing anything wrong. Nor were they by the standards of their day. It is undoubtedly the case furthermore that their efforts hugely increased the sum of human understanding and in many cases led to medical breakthroughs.

But nor does Dr Gorinsky believe he did anything wrong. He claims that the Amazon is like a library and the tribal people are the librarians. This library, he believes, is being destroyed (by burning and logging see Chapter 21) and the librarians 'massacred'. He sees himself as the saviour of the knowledge he patented.[38] Gorinsky claims he is being labelled a biopirate only because the 1993 Convention on Biological Diversity,[39] signed at the Earth Summit of Rio Janeiro,[40] 'effectively nationalised plant resources'. This, he says, gave control to governments who are now 'in league with' the big pharmaceuticals, getting cheap drugs in return for giving big pharma the run of the forest. All this, he argues, is with the protection of the Biodiversity Convention and the support of western environmentalists. The Biodiversity Convention and the anti-piracy laws it embraces, according to Gorinsky, are 'not being used to protect the people of the forest and their knowledge', he says, 'but to destroy them'.

It is true that at the 1993 Biodiversity Convention the sovereign rights of a country over the plants and other biological materials[41] found within its borders was recognised for the first time. Until then such resources had been deemed the common heritage of humanity. The point of recognising such rights, however, was to enable countries to pass new laws making it an offence to take biological resources and/or understanding without permission. Now any individual or organisation wanting to make use of the biological resources belonging to a given country must negotiate with the government of that country an agreed compensation for access to such resources. These negotiations produce 'Access and Benefits Sharing Agreements' (ABAs).[42] ABAs are underpinned by the notion of informed consent. A country consents to the use of its resources but only in exchange for compensation it deems acceptable. Such compensation might include support for conservation, education and research, contributions to equipment and materials, assistance to indigenous and local communities, up-front fees, milestone payments and royalties. It is by means of such ABAs that the signatories to the Biodiversity Convention hope to achieve their stated objectives:

'the conservation of biological diversity, the sustainable use of its components and the fair and equitable sharing of the benefits arising out of the utilisation of genetic resources, including by appropriate access to genetic resources and by appropriate transfer of relevant technologies, taking into account all rights over those resources and to technologies, and by appropriate funding.'[43]

The agreement underpinning the Biodiversity Convention undoubtedly generates a legal tool that enables biodiversity rich countries to insist on compensation for the use of their natural resources, and to punish those who 'poach' resources without permission.

On the other hand, this agreement equally undoubtedly facilitates the view that 'every gene and property of every plant and animal down to the smallest microbe is potentially patentable and thus available for commercial ownership and profit'.[44] The only boundaries, according to John Vidal, writing for the *Guardian* newspaper in the UK,[45] are provided by people's understanding of 'the fiendishly complicated patent laws'. Companies with large legal budgets for patent lawyers, he points out, often understand them best. So, he might have added, do governments.

Assuming we can be certain that governments in biodiversity rich countries will not sell too cheaply their biological resources, and that they will make sure that those within their borders benefit fairly from their bargains, the Biodiversity Convention has secured justice of some kind for these nations and their citizens, consistently with permitting the sort of bioprospecting that helps science to advance. The price of securing this justice, however, is acceptance of the idea that biological resources are not the common heritage of humanity, but rather the sovereign property of governments and those to whom governments allow access.

> ### Box 18.9 Activity: Debate
>
> *This house believes that the 1993 Biodiversity Convention is destroying rather than protecting the people of the forest and their knowledge.*
>
> Participants should be given time to prepare, then organised into teams 'for' and 'against' the motion. Some participants might find themselves arguing against their preferred stance, and should see it as practice in playing devil's advocate.

Ownership of the 'stuff of life'

The idea that biological resources are the common heritage of humanity has taken a severe knocking over the last three decades. This can be traced to a legal battle that was fought in US courts between 1972 and 1980 by a genetic engineer, Ananda Chakrabarty,[46] who worked for General Electric. In 1972 Chakrabarty applied for a patent[47] to cover a genetically modified bacterium (*Pseudomonas* sp.) capable of breaking down crude oil and therefore of potential for use in bioremediation. Chakrabarty's application was first turned down on the basis that the bacterium was a product of nature. This ruling was overturned by the patent appeal court, whereupon Sidney Diamond, the US commissioner for patents and trademarks, appealed to the Supreme Court to overturn the new ruling. In 1980 the US Supreme Court found in favour of Chakrabarty by five votes to four on the grounds that the bacterium had been genetically modified making it 'the work of man' rather than a product of nature and so unpatentable.[48]

Box 18.10 Factual information: Patents

When a patent is granted to an inventor he is thereby granted the exclusive right to benefit from his invention for a set period of time (usually 20 years). He might set up business for himself, or he may, for a fee, license others to use his invention.

Patents can be granted for products, processes or uses of products/processes. They will be granted only if the invention for which the patent is applied is (i) novel, (ii) non-obvious, (iii) useful, (iv) not contrary to morality or public order.

It is a condition of applying for a patent that the inventor describe his invention in full. This description is a matter of public record and ensures that technological information about the invention is available to other inventors.

The most important part of the application for a patent is the 'claim' made by the inventor. This describes the invention and will be used in determining whether an infringement of the patent has occurred.

Patents have two benefits:

(i) they reward inventors for their ingenuity and investment;
(ii) they ensure technological information is in the public domain.

If patents were not available inventors would have to rely on secrecy to protect their investment and profit from their invention. This would not be conducive to the public good.[49]

Some years later, in 1990, the mapping of the human genome started. The Human Genome Project (HGP) was a publicly funded venture that made its findings freely available to anyone with access to the internet.[50] Simultaneously, however, a private company, Celera Genomics[51] owned by Craig Venter, was also sequencing the genome. It incorporated into its own database the information made public by the HGP.[52] It also applied for patents on genes as it sequenced them.

It might be thought that as genes are clearly *not* inventions, Celera's application would have been turned down flat. But this wasn't the case. Celera argued that in isolating these genes it was adding value to them in such a way as to make them patentable. This argument was accepted. Suddenly DNA itself – albeit isolated or purified DNA – was amongst the biological resources that could be patented.

This prompted an explosion of patent applications. Organisations weren't even waiting until they knew what a gene did, or until they had some commercial application for it, before patenting it: they would patent it as soon as they had isolated it. This meant that other companies who actually did the work to develop a diagnostic test or therapy involving the gene would have to pay high fees to a company who had done nothing but isolate the gene, a process that, as sequencing became computerised, became easier and easier. Soon it wasn't even whole genes for which patents were applied. Patents were issued for partial gene sequences (expressed sequence tags)[53] and for single base-pair differences (known as SNPs)[54] that can act as markers for particular conditions. It wasn't just human DNA that was being patented, furthermore, it was plant and animal genes and partial gene sequences. The techniques of genetic engineering, on the model of Chakrabarty's transgenic bacterium, were also patented.

Box 18.11 Activity: Brainstorm

In order to be patentable an invention must be 'novel', not occurring in nature. This clause has been deemed to be satisfied in the case of a gene sequence by the isolation of that gene for its normal context. Can participants think of ways in which the following could be made novel on this model:

- water
- gravity
- the human eye
- grass

Participants might be asked to conduct a search of existing patents to see if any of their suggested 'inventions' have already been patented. The website of the UK Patent Office is: http://www.ipo.gov.uk/types/patent.htm.

The patenting fever wasn't confined to the private sector. Governments soon acted to enable universities to start 'spin out' companies which patented the discoveries they made as they made them.[55] Universities made a lot of money in this way, as did individual academics. By 2000 patents were being applied for at extraordinary rates. GeneWatch UK logged 126,672 patents granted or pending on whole or partial human genes in October 2000, and one month later, 161,195. This represents an increase of 27%, or about 34,500 in one month.[56] This continued throughout the 1990s and the 2000s. By 2010 it was estimated that 20% of the human genome was privately owned by some company. Some of these patents, furthermore, were extremely broad. A company who isolated a gene would, for example, patent every possible use of that gene, in effect taking ownership of that gene and everything anyone did with it for the next 20 years.

This did not happen without protest. Throughout this time organisations and individuals had been trying to make the case against the patenting of 'the stuff of life'. Common objections included:

(i)   the criteria required of an invention, particularly the 'novelty' and the 'non-obviousness criteria', are not properly met by many of the products and processes being patented;

(ii) the costs associated with research on patented genes were deterring research, not least because single gene sequences were being patented in several different ways, requiring the payment of multiple royalties;

(iii) costs also increased because of the need to search for patents before embarking on research and occasionally because of legal battles;

(iv) healthcare was being affected as costs were passed onto the consumer, so diagnostic tests and therapies increased significantly in price;

(v)   patent filings are replacing journal articles as the places for disclosure of the fruits of research.[57]

The idea that people – and indeed countries – are being priced out of the market for healthcare is considered in Chapter 19, pages 375–385 where we consider the effects of drug patents on the sick of the developing world.

It seemed likely that sooner or later there would be a backlash against the 'private appropriation of genetic commons'.[58] In 2010 indications of this started appearing. Two rulings were made, both of which might prove to be the sort of landmark in the case *against* patents that the diamond and Chakrabarty ruling was in the case *for* patents. These rulings were the decision made in the case of the Association for Molecular Pathology *et al.* v. The United States Patent and Trademark Office *et al.*,[59] and that made in the case of Monsanto v. Cefetra.[60] Let's look at these two rulings.

The Patents on *BRCA1* and *2*

In 1994, using $22 million of private venture capital, grants from various public bodies, and the results of publicly funded research on the hereditary disposition to breast cancer, Myriad Genetics[61] identified the nucleotide sequences composing the *BRCA1* gene. It patented this, together with the *BRCA2* gene,[62] and used them to develop BRAC*Analysis*, a genetic test for the mutations associated with an increased risk of breast cancer. The test was launched in 1996. In 2009 it accounted for most of Myriad's $326 million pa revenue from molecular diagnostics.[63] The test is now extremely expensive – $3,150 per test – and not, therefore accessible to many women, although Myriad points out that 90% of those tested are covered by insurance, and that it permits researchers to use the test without charge. This is true, but it did not permit researchers to inform the women on whom the tests were used of the results. Were it not for the patent, of course, other, less expensive, and perhaps more sensitive or specific tests could be developed. With the patent, this is impossible. When Myriad applied for European patents comparable to those it held in the United States, some of its applications were rejected and the claims on others were limited. Even then Myriad's patents gave it an effective monopoly on testing for breast cancer.

In March 2010, however, a US Federal District Court Judge, Robert Sweet, invalidated some of the patents that had been granted to Myriad in the United States.[64] He claimed that it is a condition of being patentable that a product have 'markedly different characteristics' from what is found in nature. He pointed out that it is possible to use a sequence of purified DNA reliably to detect mutations in the DNA of a patient only if the nucleotide sequence of the purified DNA remained constant. This very fact, he argued, ensures that the process of purification (or isolation) will not on its own justify the claim that purified DNA is 'novel'. On such grounds Judge Sweet invalidated the product patents granted to Myriad on the DNA sequences themselves.

Turning to the patents on Myriad's use of these sequences, Judge Sweet pointed out that Myriad's patent covered the process of comparing the patient's DNA with purified DNA. The process of comparison, argued Judge Sweet, is an 'abstract mental process'. As such, he argued, it is not patentable because it involves no 'transformative step'. In this ruling Judge Sweet relied on a precedent that had been set in a case before the Supreme Court: *In re Bilski*.[65] This case involves not the use of DNA, but the use of methods of hedging risk in commodities trading. In that case the judge had also ruled that a transformative step was needed for a use to be patentable.

In March 2011 the US Department of Justice upheld Judge Sweet's ruling.[66] This could unleash a storm of legislation intent on invalidating many of the patents granted over the last two decades. Any product patent based purely on isolating or purifying a gene, and any process or use patent based solely on an 'abstract mental process' could be overturned, dramatically changing the landscape for genetics in the 2010s.

> ### Box 18.12 Activity: Web research
>
> Find out whether the ruling in the Bilski case was overturned, and if it was whether this led to an appeal in the Myriad case.
>
> Use this, and the results of putting 'Patenting the Stuff of Life' into a search engine, to construct a 'for' and 'against' case for patenting an isolated gene sequence.

The patents on 'Round-up ready' traits

Monsanto has a patent, in both the United States and Europe, on a trait of soybeans that make them resistant to the herbicide glyphosate. This trait allows farmers to use the herbicide to kill weeds without affecting their crop of soybeans. Argentina does not recognise Monsanto's patent, however, so Monsanto asserts the rights it believes it has under its patents to sue anyone who imports, from Argentina, soybeans grown from its seeds. In 2006 Monsanto did exactly this when it sued a Dutch company for importing soymeal from Argentina.

In July 2010, however, Advocate General Paolo Mengozzi of the European Court of Justice threw out Monsanto's claim.[67] His grounds for doing so were that the trait patented by Monsanto was not performing the function of resisting glyphosate in the soymeal brought from Argentina to the Netherlands. In effect Advocate General Mengozzi's ruling made it a condition of Monsanto's 'use' patent that the trait actually be capable of being used in the manner described in the patent in the context in which a claimed infringement was supposedly occurring. This means that even if the DNA of the soybean could be extracted from the meal and *then* used to confer resistance to glyphosate, it was not, whilst in the meal, performing that function.

Again this ruling has significant implications. As the European Court of Justice is the highest court of appeal, this ruling will not be overturned. Again this will have significant implications for the usefulness of patents on DNA.

> ### Box 18.13 Activity: Small group presentations
>
> Participants should be divided into small groups and asked to prepare a presentation giving the 'for' and the 'against' in the case of patenting DNA. Box 18.10 will help them on the nature of patents.

That patenting fever isn't over yet, however, was firmly demonstrated in May 2010 when Craig Venter applied for a patent for the methods he used to create Synthia, the organism he created from scratch using the techniques of synthetic biology (see Box 16.3). Importantly, the patent for which Venter has applied does not cover merely Synthia itself. It covers *the methods used to create Synthia*.[68] According to Professor John Sulston, one of the leaders of the publically funded Human Genome Project, if this patent were granted Venter would effectively have the monopoly over the techniques of synthetic biology.[69] Perhaps given the way things are currently going on the possibility of patenting the 'stuff of life' Venter's patent will be denied, or at least, its claim restricted ... but we must watch this space.

Box 18.14 Activity: Group discussion

After performing an internet search about Synthia and/or looking at Box 21.18, participants should, as a group, discuss the patent that might reasonably be granted to Venter as recognition of his development of the world's first 'built from scratch' organism. In particular the group should discuss whether Venter should be granted a patent over the method used to build Synthia.

Summary

In this chapter we have considered the ethical and social implications of bio-ownership. In particular we have:

- reflected on HeLa cells and the extent to which Henrietta Lacks had a moral right to compensation for their use;

- learned about the case of John Moore and the implications of the ruling on this for the notion of informed consent;

- reflected on the Alder Hey organ retention scandal, the Act to which it led and the consequences of this Act for scientific research using human tissue;

- asked whether it is important to medical science to take an attitude to the body other than that taken in 'ordinary life';

- considered the 1993 Biodiversity Convention, and the pros and cons of its granting of sovereign rights over biological resources to countries;

- acquired the concepts of 'biopiracy' and 'bioprospecting' and reflected on their application;

- learned about patenting, the different sorts of patent and the importance of the 'claim' made by a patent;

- looked at the explosion of patents on DNA triggered by the Diamond v. Chakrabarty case;
- considered the pros and cons of the patentability of the 'stuff of life';
- wondered whether this era of patenting genes is coming to a close.

Questions to stimulate reflection

Do you think Henrietta Lacks' family should be compensated for the use of her cells?

Should consent forms include mention of all the specific uses to which a sample might be put?

Should consent forms include a waiver to any claim on profits to be made on tissue samples taken?

Does an overly sentimental attitude to dead bodies inform the UK Human Tissue Act 2004?

Was Darwin a bioprospector or a biopirate? What's the difference?

Will the 1993 Biodiversity Convention protect indigenous peoples or facilitate their exploitation?

Is isolating a gene enough to make it an *invention* rather than a *discovery*?

Are patents on the whole a good thing because they reward creativity, or a bad thing because they increase the costs of medical research?

If an organisation owns a particular trait of a soybean seed does this mean it owns every product that can be made from that seed?

Additional activities

Read Rebecca Skloot's book *The Immortal Life of Henrietta Lacks* and use it to trigger a discussion of whether Johns Hopkins University have a duty of care towards Henrietta Lacks' family.

Write and prepare a play about Henrietta Lacks and her family.

Approach your local hospital or medical centre and ask them how they approach the issue of informed consent for the taking of bio-samples. See whether their forms contain an 'open' clause, or a clause covering possible commercial uses.

Do a websearch on the Alder Hey scandal. Find out more about the doctor at the centre of it (Professor van Velzen). Do you think he was wrongly hounded, as some have said, or that he received his just desserts?

Write a short story about Darwin as a biopirate.

Find out more about the 1993 Convention for Biodiversity. Ask yourself whether you think it is, on the whole, a good thing or a bad thing.

Find a current application for a patent on a DNA sequence. Take a close look at the claims being made in this patent. Ask whether these claims are justifiable given the investment made by the person or organisation applying for the patent.

Imagine you are a woman with a family history of breast cancer. You have become interested in having a test to see whether your genes confer an increased chance of your getting it. Consult the web to find out what you next steps might be and how much the test is likely to cost you.

Follow up court case on Myriad genetics and the BRCA genes or the application for the patent on Synthia.

Notes

1 http://www.bbc.co.uk/dna/h2g2/brunel/A885062.
2 http://www.scotshistoryonline.co.uk/burke.html.
3 http://www.pittmag.pitt.edu/mar2001/culture.html.
4 http://www.guardian.co.uk/world/2010/apr/04/henrietta-lacks-cancer-cells.
5 http://www.telegraph.co.uk/science/7845119/The-Immortal-Life-of-Henrietta-Lacks-a-bittersweet-legacy.html.
6 Skloot, R. (2010) *The Immortal Life of Henrietta Lacks*. London: Macmillan.
7 http://video.pbs.org/video/1494660650/. An interview with Rebecca Skloot.
8 Skloot (2010).
9 http://www.nytimes.com/2008/07/24/health/24mckusick.html. Obituary for Victor McKusick from the New York Times.
10 Gold, M. (1986) *A Conspiracy of Cells: One Woman's Immortal Legacy and the Medical Scandal it Caused*. New York: State University of New York Press.
11 http://forhealthfreedom.org/Publications/Informed/WhoOwns.html.
12 http://www.universityofcalifornia.edu/senate/inmemoriam/davidwgolde.htm. A tribute to Dr David Golde from the University of California
13 http://en.wikipedia.org/wiki/Conversion_(law).
14 Hartman, R.G. (1993) Beyond Moore: issues of law and policy impacting human cell and genetic research in the age of biotechnology. *Journal of Legal Medicine*, **14**(3):463–477.
15 http://ohsr.od.nih.gov/info/sheet6.html. NIH guidelines for obtaining informed consent.
16 http://magazine.jhu.edu/2010/06/immortal-cells-enduring-issues/.
17 http://www.alderhey.nhs.uk/.
18 http://news.bbc.co.uk/1/hi/1136723.stm.
19 http://news.bbc.co.uk/1/hi/uk_politics/1144454.stm.
20 http://news.bbc.co.uk/1/hi/england/merseyside/8486721.stm.
21 http://news.bbc.co.uk/1/hi/health/1154181.stm. A BBC interview with Dick van Velzen.
22 http://www.independent.co.uk/life-style/health-and-families/health-news/dutch-hospital-to-sack-alder-hey-doctor-soon-689827.html.
23 http://news.bbc.co.uk/1/hi/england/merseyside/4112232.stm.

24 http://www.bmj.com/cgi/content/full/330/7506/1464-a.
25 http://www.opsi.gov.uk/acts/acts2004/ukpga_20040030_en_1.
26 http://www.open2.net/historyandthearts/philosophy_ethics/practical-ethics.html. An EthicsBites podcast about the problems of obtaining informed consent.
27 http://www.rcpath.org/resources/pdf/faq_hta-sep07.pdf. Q&A on the Human Tissue Act 2004 from the Royal College of Pathologists.
28 http://yourfreedom.hmg.gov.uk/repealing-unnecessary-laws/human-tissue-act.
29 http://www.spiked-online.com/Printable/000000005482.htm.
30 http://www.bodyworlds.com/en/gunther_von_hagens/life_in_science.html.
31 http://ipsnews.net/news.asp?idnews=42449.
32 http://www.williams.edu/go/native/hero_or_pirate.htm.
33 http://www.native-languages.org/wapishana.htm.
34 http://www.guardian.co.uk/science/2000/nov/15/genetics2.
35 http://www.kahea.org/gmo/pdf/bioprospecting_people.pdf.
36 http://www.actionbioscience.org/biodiversity/gollin.html.
37 http://www.kew.org/.
38 http://www.flutrackers.com/forum/showthread.php?t=8594.
39 http://www.iisd.ca/biodiv/cbdintro.html.
40 http://www.un.org/esa/earthsummit/.
41 http://www.springerlink.com/content/uv6mq62u520653l7/.
42 http://www.ukabc.org/ukabc6.htm.
43 http://www.cbd.int/.
44 http://www.guardian.co.uk/science/2000/nov/15/genetics2.
45 http://www.guardian.co.uk/science/2000/nov/15/genetics2.
46 http://www.uic.edu/depts/mcmi/faculty/chakrabarty/index.htm.
47 http://www.ornl.gov/sci/techresources/Human_Genome/elsi/patents.shtml. Everything about patents from the Human Genome Project.
48 http://www.answerbag.com/q_view/1995649.
49 http://academic.regis.edu/kgleason/Lectures/Bioethics%20Case%20Studies%201.ppt. A presentation on patents.
Harris, T. (2001) How Patents Work. HowStuffWorks.com. http://www.howstuffworks.com/patent.htm.
50 Lander, E. S., Linton, L. M., Birren, B. *et al.* (2001) Initial sequencing and analysis of the human genome. *Nature*, **409**(6822), 860–921.
51 https://www.celera.com/.
52 Venter, J.C., Adams, M.D., Myers, E.W. *et al.* (2001) The sequence of the human genome. *Science*, **291**(5507), 1298–1302.
53 http://www.ncbi.nlm.nih.gov/About/primer/est.html.
54 http://www.ncbi.nlm.nih.gov/About/primer/snps.html.
55 http://www.telegraph.co.uk/finance/yourbusiness/6860386/Tracking-50-top-university-spin-out-companies.html.
56 http://www.genewatch.org/uploads/f03c6d66a9b354535738483c1c3d49e4/Patenting_Genes_A4_Version.pdf.
57 Human Genome Project Information: http://www.ornl.gov/sci/techresources/Human_Genome/elsi/patents.shtml.
58 The Nuffield Council for Bioethics (2002) The ethics of patenting DNA: a discussion paper.
59 http://richarddawkins.net/articles/5418-the-gene-patents-case-association-for-molecular-pathology-et-al-v-united-states-patent-and-trademark-office-et-al.

60 http://www.eplawpatentblog.com/eplaw/2010/03/eu-monsanto-v-cefetra.html.

61 http://www.myriad.com/.

62 http://www.cancer.gov/cancertopics/factsheet/Risk/BRCA.

63 Kesselheim, A. and Mello, M. (2010) Gene patenting: is the pendulum swinging back? *New England Journal of Medicine*, **362**,1855–1858.

64 http://www.project-syndicate.org/commentary/dickenson2/English.

65 http://www.wlf.org/publishing/publication_detail.asp?id=2108.

66 http://www.genomicslawreport.com/index.php/tag/supreme-court/.

67 http://ec.europa.eu/avservices/services/showShotlist.do?out=PDF&lg=En&filmRef=69030.

68 http://www.etcgroup.org/en/node/665.

69 http://topnews.net.nz/content/24439-scientists-venter-and-sulston-odds-again-over-synthia-patenting.

Further reading and useful websites

Gold, E. (1996) *Body Parts: Property Rights and the Ownership of Human Biological Materials*. Washington DC: Georgetown University Press

Koepsell, D. (2009) *Who Owns You? The Corporate Gold Rush to Patent Your Genes (Blackwell Public Philosophy Series)*. Oxford: Wiley Blackwell.

Robinson, D. (2010) *Confronting Biopiracy*. Oxford: Earthscan Ltd.

http://www.beep.ac.uk/content/162.0.html. A useful case study from the Bioethics Education Project.

http://www.idebate.org/debatabase/topic_details.php?topicID=32. Debating guide on gene patenting.

http://www.nuffieldbioethics.org/go/ourwork/humanbody/introduction. The Nuffield Council for Bioethics on human bodies used for research.

http://www.ornl.gov/sci/techresources/Human_Genome/elsi/patents.shtml. Everything about patents from the Human Genome Project.

Human justice: the developed and developing worlds

Objectives

In reading this chapter you will:

- learn about the international regulations governing experiments involving human subjects;
- examine the cultural difficulties involved in obtaining 'informed consent';
- reflect on whether the standard of care for subjects during clinical trials should relate to international or local standards;
- reflect on the nature of intellectual property, and in particular patents;
- examine the tension between the protection of intellectual property and public health in the developing world;
- learn about the serious shortage of human organs and tissue, for transplantation and research;
- consider the black market in human organs and tissue, and especially the trade between the rich in the developed world and the poor in the developing world;
- ask yourself whether the trade in human organs and tissue should be legalised.

There are many things we could learn if we could freely experiment on human beings. Imagine the good that could be done with the knowledge that we acquired. But unless we think the end justifies any means whatsoever it is unacceptable to conduct experiments on human beings except in accordance with the strictest ethical standards.

Unfortunately we know that an action's being morally unacceptable does not prevent its being performed. In the case of experimentation on human beings the Nazi doctors Josef Mengele, Herta Oberhauser and Carl Clauberg cared not a jot for morality.[1] Mengele conducted experiments without anaesthetic on twins as young as five. In pursuit of a better understanding of the wounds German soldiers were sustaining Oberhauser deliberately inflicted wounds on conscious subjects, then rubbed wood, sawdust, rusty nails, dirt and slivers of glass into them. Clauberg's interest was in reproduction. He stood his 'patients' between two X-ray machines aimed at their sexual organs. The radiation burns they received rendered them unfit for work so they were gassed.

These and many other Nazi doctors conducted experiments of the most hideous brutality between 1933 and 1945. After the Allied victory 23 of these doctors were brought to trial in Nuremberg.[2] Fifteen defendants were found guilty, seven hanged and eight imprisoned for life. Despite international efforts to find him, Josef Mengele escaped. He lived freely for 35 years in Paraguay and Brazil and died of a stroke in 1979.[3]

The world was so horrified by the activities of the Nazi doctors that the Nuremberg Code was devised to govern all future experimentation on human subjects. You will find the first principle of the Nuremberg code in Box 19.1.

Box 19.1 Factual information: The Nuremberg Code: Principle One

'The voluntary consent of the human subject is absolutely essential. This means that the person involved should have legal capacity to give consent; should be so situated as to be able to exercise free power of choice, without the intervention of any element of force, fraud, deceit, duress, overreaching, or other ulterior form of constraint or coercion; and should have sufficient knowledge and comprehension of the elements of the subject matter involved as to enable him to make an understanding and enlightened decision. This latter element requires that before the acceptance of an affirmative decision by the experimental subject there should be made known to him the nature, duration and purpose of the experiment; the method and means by which it is to be conducted; all inconveniences and hazards reasonably to be expected; and the effects upon his health or person which may possibly come from his participation in the experiment.

The duty and responsibility for ascertaining the quality of the consent rests upon each individual who initiates, directs, or engages in the experiment. It is a personal duty and responsibility which may not be delegated to another with impunity.'[4]

In 1964 The Helsinki Declaration was adopted at the 18th World Medical Assembly.[5] This affirmed and extended the Nuremberg Code. It has been amended several times since and is viewed as the most important guidance on the ethics of research relating to healthcare.

Amazingly, though, despite international outrage at the actions of the Nazi doctors, the principles of the Nuremberg Code and the Helsinki Declaration were comprehensively ignored by those running the infamous Tuskegee syphilis study.[6] This started in 1932, but continued for 40 years until, in 1972, it was exposed by a newspaper.[7] The study involved 600 black men, 399 of whom had syphilis. The men were told they had 'bad blood'. They agreed to be examined and 'treated' in exchange for free medical exams, meals and burial insurance.

At no point were the men actually treated for their condition, even after 1947 when penicillin became available. In 1940 the researchers actually prevented 50 of the men from being treated by the military draft boards.[8]

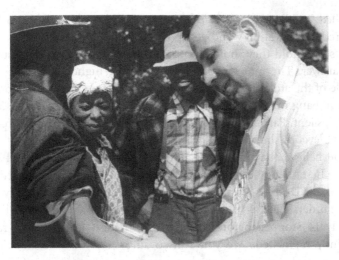

Figure 19.1 The Tuskegee syphilis study. Credit: The US National Archives and Records Administration (www.archives.gov).

It is interesting to speculate on the thinking of the researchers conducting this study. Could they have been unaware of the Nuremberg trial? Were they oblivious to the relevance of the Nuremberg Code? Did they think it didn't apply to them? Did they think *their* study subjects – black people – didn't count? What could possibly be the explanation of their failure to see that their study was completely unacceptable?

> ## Box 19.2 **Activity: Web-wandering and paired reflection**
>
> Enter 'Tuskegee syphilis study' into a search engine to discover the facts about this study. Then with a partner reflect on the mind-set of the researchers involved.
>
> Do you think they knew but didn't care that their actions were morally despicable?
>
> Could they have convinced themselves that in the case of their study the end justified the means?
>
> Do you think the end could ever justify the means used by these researchers and by the Nazi doctors?

You might think that you would never be guilty of the same sort of moral laxity. But are you sure? In 1961 a psychologist called Stanley Milgram became interested in obedience to authority when he heard the Nazi war criminal Adolf Eichmann defend himself by saying he was 'following orders'.[9] Milgram advertised for 40 men to earn $4.50 for an hour of work. He sat his subjects in front of a 'shock generator' with switches labelled 'mild' 'moderate' and 'severe shock', and upwards to 'XXX'. The shocks appeared to start at 30 V and go up to 450 V in 15 V steps.

The subjects were told they should administer a shock every time a 'student' gave an incorrect answer. The more incorrect answers the higher the voltage. An actor played the role of the student. As shocks were administered he would complain of a heart condition, bang on the wall and demand to be released. After the 300 V mark the 'student' fell silent. Participants were told to treat this as an incorrect response and deliver the next level of shock.

Most people believe that Milgram's participants would have pulled out at the halfway mark. In fact no fewer than 26 participants (65%) delivered the most severe shock of all. Despite becoming 'agitated', 'distraught' and 'angry' they continued to obey orders such as 'please continue' or 'it is absolutely essential that you continue'. Only 14 stopped before reaching the highest levels. These results have been consistently replicated. Are you still so sure that *you* wouldn't do anything unethical?

> ### Box 19.3 Activity: Group discussion
>
> As a group discuss Milgram's experiment, the results it demonstrates and what we learn from this about the need
>
> (i) for people to take *personal* moral responsibility for their actions;
> (ii) to monitor the ethical standards observed by those conducting research on human beings.

Guidance on experiments on human subjects

Facts such as these are behind the explosion, globally, of guidance and advice on the ethics of experimenting on human subjects. As well as the Nuremberg Code and the Helsinki Declaration there are also numerous guidelines or conventions governing the application of their principles in different contexts. In planning a clinical trial, for example, researchers or sponsors may have to refer to:

- international guidelines or conventions;
- European Union directives;
- national laws or guidelines;
- regulations or guidelines sponsored by the pharmaceutical industry;
- guidelines produced by funding agencies;
- institutional guidelines;
- guidelines relating to specific diseases;
- recommendations from advisory bodies.[10]

There are so many conditions that researchers and sponsors must satisfy that, understandably 'fatigue' can set in. Ethical review can start to look like a burden put upon science, rather than a set of constraints demanded by our desire to do the right thing by those who take personal risks to further the aims of science.

Another purpose of the guidance, of course, is to protect researchers from the threat of litigation. In 1974, a $10 million out-of-court settlement was reached on behalf of the participants in the Tuskegee Study. As part of it the US government promised lifetime medical and health benefits and burial services to all living participants, their wives, widows and offspring. In 2010, there are still 16 offspring currently benefiting from this settlement.

The Tuskegee settlement was made more than 36 years ago. People have since become more litigious. The drug company Merck is discovering this to its cost.[11] Its drug Vioxx, licensed in the late 1990s for pain relief, especially in arthritis, became one of the most prescribed drugs in history, taken by 80 million people worldwide. In 2004 it started to become clear that taking it was correlated with a significant increase in cardiovascular risk. In 2007 Merck was ordered to pay $4.85 billion to the 44,000 US claimants who could prove they had received at least 30 doses of the drug before health problems arose.[12]

This is not the end of it. A 2010 ruling by the Federal Court in Melbourne Australia ordered the company to pay £172,300 to Graeme Peterson, 59, who has been unable to work since a heart attack in 2003.[13] At least 600 other Australians are expected to follow suit, costing Merck an estimated $300 million. Lawyers in other countries, including the UK, have been watching with interest.[14]

If the plight of human subjects does not convince us of the importance of ethical review, therefore, we must also consider the huge potential cost of litigation, not to mention the reputation costs to organisations found to be conducting unethical experiments on human beings.[15]

> ### Box 19.4 Activity: Essay writing
>
> Consider the list of guidance that researchers and sponsors may need to refer to. Then write 1,000 words on the following topic:
>
> *The overly costly and time-consuming burden on scientific research posed by ethical review should be reduced*
>
> In your essay you should consider not only *whether* the burden of ethical review should be reduced, but also *how* it might be reduced consistently with protecting human subjects and the researchers against litigation.

Current research on humans

Despite the cost and complexities involved there is no possibility – yet – of avoiding experiments on human subjects. Computer simulations, research on human tissue and on animals can only take us so far. See Box 19.5 for an account of the test phases required to get approval for a new drug.

Box 19.5 Factual information: The drug testing process

In the laboratory stage drugs are tested by computer simulation, tissue tests and in vitro.[16]

Drugs are then tested on animals (we shall be discussing the moral acceptability of this in Chapter 20).

The drug must then be cleared for the three phases of human testing:

Phase One: tests for side effects and safety conducted on 15–30 healthy volunteers.

Phase Two: tests for side effects and effectiveness conducted on <100 volunteers with the condition targeted by the drug.

Phase Three: tests for full information about the drug conducted on 100–1,000s of volunteers with the condition.

If a drug successfully passes these three phases of human tests it will be licensed for use, but it still has to undergo a further phase of testing:

Phase Four: tests to monitor the long terms effects of the drug.

That such tests are necessary was demonstrated fairly recently by a drug trial conducted in the UK by Paraxel on behalf of the German drug company Te Genero. This trial, of TGN 1412, an anti-inflammatory drug for use in rheumatoid arthritis and leukaemia, went disastrously wrong. Six healthy young men were each paid £2000 to take part in the phase one trial held at Northwick Park Hospital. Payment of this money was grounded on guidelines that allow payment for 'reasonable expenses' but not as inducements.[17]

A short time after receiving his dose of the drug, the first subject complained of a severe headache. Shortly afterwards he removed his shirt complaining he was burning. Soon the other subjects were making similar complaints. All were vomiting. It soon became clear that all the subjects, except the two given placebos, had suffered a 'cytokine storm', a potentially fatal immune reaction. Within hours of treatment all their white blood cells had disappeared. None of the men died, but all now face an increased risk of cancer and auto-immune diseases such as multiple sclerosis, lupus and, ironically, rheumatoid arthritis.

Such disasters are rare. But naturally they are seized upon by the media. This influences beliefs about the dangers of participating in drug trials and makes it difficult for drug companies to recruit the volunteers they need. Even the sick can be reluctant to take part, as evidenced by the fact that of 333 trials on cancer patients conducted in the UK between 1971 and 2000 a fifth recruited fewer than 25% of the planned number of patients, half failed to reach the planned sample size, and only a fifth recruited at least 75% of the planned number.[18] Around 71% of cancer patients refuse to participate in clinical trials.

In recent years, however, pharmaceutical companies have found a way around this. It has become clear that if they hold clinical trials in the developing world, they will have no shortage of volunteers. Recognition of this has led to an industry in clinical trials in developing countries. An article in the *New England Journal of Medicine* states that approximately one third of the trials conducted by the 20 largest US-based pharmaceutical companies now take place in developing countries.[19]

Clinical trials in developing countries

India, a 'middle-income' country, is a particularly attractive place for clinical research. It has over 15,000 hospitals and more than half a million practising doctors, many of them trained in the UK or United States. Most speak English. As importantly India has a population of 1.1 billion people, many of them 'naïve' (such that they have never taken drugs). Many are also illiterate: even if the newspapers are available to them, they won't have read them.

As, or perhaps more, importantly costs in India are lower. A pharmaceutical company can save 50% of the cost of a trial by holding it in India. Conducting trials in India also reduces the time needed for research. Any time saved boosts profits by lengthening the time the company can sell its drug at a profit before the patent runs out. As each drug costs from $800,000 million to $1.2 billion to develop (from patenting to approval), the extra £100,000 million that can be squeezed from three months' extra time to sell the drug is useful. It is believed that by 2012 5% of clinical trials will be held in India and over 3 million Indians will be enrolled in them.[20]

It is not just India, of course, that provides a haven for those wishing to conduct clinical trials on a cost-effective basis. Countries in Africa, South America and South-East Asia provide similar benefits. Most low- and middle-income countries are

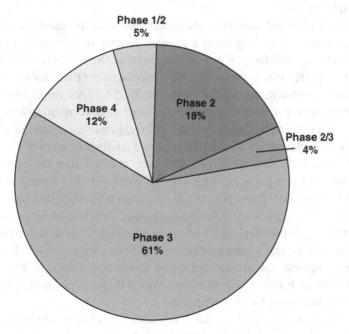

Figure 19.2 Clinical trials in India are on the rise. From Kermani, F. (2008) *Quick Guide to Clinical Trials.* Rockville, MD: BioPlan Associates, Inc., with permission.

keen to encourage pharmaceutical companies to conduct clinical trials within their borders, bringing benefits such as jobs, investments and public health.

There are, however, concerns about the eagerness with which 'Big Pharma' has embraced the opportunity to conduct clinical trials in the developing world. There is nothing questionable about a drug company wanting to take advantage of the benefits listed above. But there are other, less reputable, benefits.

We have already noted that many of the potential subjects in such countries are 'naïve' in never having taken drugs. It is unavoidable to note that many of them are also naïve in other, more chilling, ways. They may be illiterate, have little idea about clinical trials or ethical reviews and be very poor and so more susceptible to the free health care, expenses and other benefits offered. They are also unlikely to turn to litigation should things go wrong.[21]

In 2006 the BBC in the UK showed a documentary produced by Paul Kenyon who had travelled to India to follow up some of the patients who had taken part in clinical trials sponsored by some major drug companies.[22] Kenyon discovered disturbing evidence that many such trials were conducted in ways that would be deemed unacceptable in the sponsors' own countries.

Informed consent

Central to all guidance on experiments involving human beings is the requirement that subjects should give their free and informed consent to their participation. This, in the Kantian terminology we examined in Chapter 4, pages 37–42, ensures that such subjects are being treated as 'ends in themselves' as well as means to the ends of those conducting the research.[23]

The idea of *fully* informed consent is, of course, an unattainable ideal. No one, not even the researchers, knows *everything* about a research project. In particular no one knows everything about what will happen during the course of the research. Since 1995 it has therefore been suggested that consent should be *genuine* rather than 'fully informed'. The concept of genuine consent, introduced by the Nuffield Council on Bioethics, requires that researchers take care in detecting and eliminating lack of consent, and requires them to avoid 'coercion, deception, manipulation, deliberate mis-description of what is proposed and lack of disclosure about material facts and conflicts of interest'.[24]

Many of the subjects Kenyon filmed, however, claimed that they had had very little idea about what was going on. One subject, paralysed after having been injected with a drug, M4N, that later turned out not to have been properly tested on animals, said he thought he was being given an anaesthetic. Another, delighted to be given free drugs in a country with no entitlement to healthcare, had merely obeyed the man in a white coat. He had no idea he was taking part in the trial of an anti-psychotic drug.

These patients appear not to have consented in any meaningful way at all. It does not seem out of place, furthermore, to ask whether if they *had* given their consent that consent could in any sense be called 'genuine'.

It might be suggested – rightly – that it is difficult to obtain informed or genuine consent from people who are illiterate, uneducated, overawed by respect for doctors, perhaps only able to speak a language not used by those conducting the research and possibly, for cultural reasons, used to others determining their actions. It might also be pointed out – again rightly – that it is difficult to determine what will count as an 'inducement' for people who are extremely poor and have no access to healthcare.

But the centrality of the requirement of informed, or genuine, consent requires that these difficulties be overcome, not that they be ignored. That such subjects are unlikely even to consider, never mind be able to afford, litigation is a secondary consideration, though in our increasingly global world an important one.

Box 19.6 Activity: Small group exercise

In groups of three or four consider whether you believe that in the following cases genuine consent was, or could be, obtained from subjects by researchers:[25]

(i)   Parental consent was sought from mothers of semi-conscious children for these children to be given artesunate suppositories upon emergency admission to hospital in Malawi.
(ii)   In Kenya a consent form designed in English and translated into the local language contained mistranslations for several key terms.
(iii) In India the consent form for a trial of a rotavirus vaccine was 9 pages long and contained a great deal of technical information.
(iv)   In Mexico national regulations specify that consent is valid only if recorded on a form signed by the participant and two witnesses. The first witness is usually the researcher but, in the case of a woman, the second will often be a senior male relative.

In each case give reasons for the answers you give. If you think there are or might be difficulties in obtaining genuine consent consider how the difficulties might be overcome.

The problems of obtaining genuine consent are not restricted to research being conducted in the developing world. Some ethical difficulties involved in research in the developing world, however, do not arise in the developed world. One involves the standard of care offered to control groups.

Standards of care

Any scientifically respectable clinical trial of a new intervention must involve a control group who are not given the intervention. It is only by comparing the control group with those for whom the intervention has been used that the effects of an intervention can be measured. When a trial is being conducted in the developing world, however, the issue of the researchers' responsibility to those in the control group arises. What standard of care, if any, are those in the control group entitled to? Is it permissible, for example, for researchers to offer them no care beyond that which would persuade them to participate in the study? If more then what standard of care is it their duty to offer?

An answer to this is offered by the Helsinki Declaration which, in paragraph 32, states that:

'The benefits, risks, burdens and effectiveness of a new intervention must be tested against those of the best current proven intervention.'

This requirement, however, is ambiguous. Are researchers required to offer those in the control group the best current proven intervention available *globally*, or the best current proven intervention available *locally*?[26]

This ambiguity is important. If a study is required to give members of a control group the best current proven intervention globally for HIV/AIDS, for example, this would involve providing each person with the highly active anti-retroviral therapy (HAART) offered to those with HIV in the west. The cost of this could be huge. The cost of giving the control group the best current proven intervention *locally* could be much cheaper. It might be nothing at all.

This ambiguity became big news in 1997 when a paper appeared in *The New England Journal of Medicine* claiming that large-scale trials testing AZT for the prevention of perinatal transmission of HIV in the developing world were unethical.[27] Despite the fact that AZT had been the best proven therapeutic method since 1994 in the United States,[28] the authors pointed out, the trials were placebo controlled. They therefore violated the Helsinki Declaration, according to the authors.

It is clear that if we interpret paragraph 32 of the Helsinki Declaration as requiring the best current proven standard of care available *globally*, the authors of this paper were right. If, however, we interpret paragraph 32 as requiring only the best current proven therapy *locally*, the authors were not right. In 1997 there were no local means of preventing the transmission of HIV from pregnant women to their babies. By local standards women in the control group were no worse off than they would have been had the trials not taken place.

Lurie and Wolff, the authors of the paper, argued that even if the participants were no worse off such a trial would be unethical in the United States. Why therefore, they asked, should it be acceptable in the developing world? Isn't this a straightforward case of double standards: one standard for *us*, another standard for *them*?

Some suggest that requiring researchers to provide the best current proven therapy globally would ensure that trials that could be of particular benefit to those in the developing world couldn't take place. Any trial that tried to compare a possibly more effective therapy with the existing local therapy, for example, would be excluded on this interpretation of paragraph 32.

For this reason many statements of guidance on the application of the Helsinki Declaration[29] state that use of the best current local treatment might be acceptable in cases where an established effective intervention is not available or affordable locally. Many are uncomfortable with this, believing that it leaves the interpretation of paragraph 32 unacceptably vague and gives researchers and their sponsors too much discretion to interpret the ethical guidelines in a self-serving way.

Box 19.7 Activity: Group discussion

This house believes that it is wrong to accept double standards in clinical trials.

Participants might be left to argue for the side towards which they incline, or be allocated sides.

After the trial

Similar problems arise when we consider what happens after the trial finishes. If participants have been given free healthcare, for example, or a particular type of treatment during the trial is the study required to continue providing such benefits after the trial? If so, for how long? This could get expensive enough to deter sponsors preventing the trial from taking place at all.

This issue arises in particular with the question of whether it is morally acceptable to test, in a developing country, a drug that the developing country won't be able to afford. Is it acceptable, for example, to test drugs for HIV/AIDS in Africa and then market those drugs at prices few African countries can afford?

HAART became available in 1996. It is an effective antiretroviral combination therapy that delays the onset of AIDS. By 2000 its use had resulted in an 84% fall in the death rates for people with HIV in the developed world.[30] But it was costing the health authorities in countries using it $10–15,000 per person per year – *way* beyond the pockets of health ministries even in middle-income countries. The drug companies argued they were justified in charging such high prices because they had spent millions developing the drugs. If they were forced to keep prices low, they pointed out, they would not be able to develop new drugs. Everyone would lose.

Others argued that Big Pharma was putting profits before people. Their claims were particularly poignant because in sub-Saharan Africa HIV/AIDS had reached epidemic proportions. According to the UN Secretary-General Kofi Annan more people died of AIDS in Africa during 1999–2000 than in all the wars on the continent. Approximately 24 million Africans were infected with the virus in 2000, nearly all were expected to die before 2010. Around 6,000 Africans died every day in 2000 from AIDS and another 11,000 were infected.[31]

The tension between protecting the profits of the drug companies and the health of the poor came to a head in 2001. The Indian drug company Cipla[32] reverse-engineered the triple therapy antiretrovirals and produced a generic version.[33] This generic drug was bioequivalent to the branded drugs sold under patent by the big drug companies, but it cost only $350 per person per year. Cipla's act generated a price war that sent the price of AIDS drugs in the developing world plummeting.[34]

The pharmaceutical companies were outraged. Of course a pharmaceutical company prepared to reverse-engineer a drug would be able to sell the drug more cheaply: it had not incurred *any* of the *c.* $802 million cost of producing the drug. They had not paid the salaries of the scientists needed to develop the drug, or the $millions

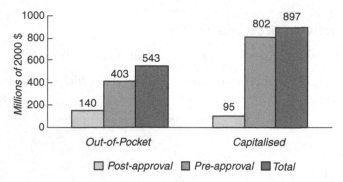

Figure 19.3 Out-of-pocket and capitalised total cost per approved new drug for new drugs and for improvements to existing drugs. Reprinted from DiMasi, J.A., Hansen, R.W. and Grabowski, H.G. (2003) The price of innovation: new estimates of drug development costs. *Journal of Health Economics*, **22**(2), with permission from Elsevier.

needed to test it for safety and efficacy. Nor had they risked the failure of the drug despite the $millions spent in development. Didn't Big Pharma have a point?[35]

It might be suggested, of course, that even if the major drug companies dropped their prices they would still make a profit because they would sell far more of the drug. But the big drug companies didn't see it this way. In 2001 39 of them attempted to prosecute the South African Government for making it easier in law to produce and import generic drugs in the hope of stemming the tide of AIDS deaths.

Their action backfired. It produced an international outcry.[36] A petition was produced that was signed by 300,000 people worldwide. It led to the formation of many high-profile pressure groups who kept the issue in international headlines for weeks. The big companies backed off.

Generic drugs are now the drugs of choice for the treatment of HIV/AIDS in the developing world. In Namibia and Rwanda in 2003 less than 1% of those with HIV/AIDS were treated with antiretrovirals. In 2007, the figures were 88% and 71%, respectively, thanks to the affordability of generic drugs. In 2008 UNAIDS claimed:

'The rapid growth in antiretroviral therapy coverage represents one of the great success stories in recent global health history. Less than 10 years ago, even as antiretroviral drugs were contributing to sharp declines in HIV mortality and morbidity in high income countries, it was widely assumed that these life-preserving medications would remain unaffordable and thus unavailable in low income countries, perhaps for decades.'[37]

There is, however, concern about whether this will continue. To see why let's consider the international trade agreements that affect the cost of pharmaceuticals.

TRIPS: Trade-related international property rights

When a drug company thinks it has found an effective new therapy it patents it under the TRIPS agreement.[38] This agreement, drawn up by the World Trade Organization (WTO) and binding on all member states, came into force in 1995. It brings all intellectual property rights under a common set of international rules and requires

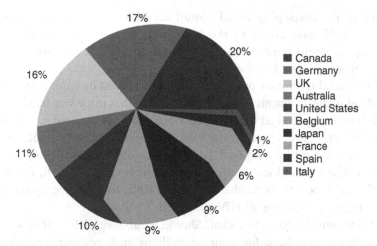

Figure 19.4 Generics as percentage of total market in 1999 (http://www.themedica.com/articles/2009/04/the-us-generic-drugs-industry.html).

each of its 148 member countries to protect the intellectual property of the others. TRIPS is not itself a law, it is rather enforced by the laws of each of its member countries. If a member fails to introduce laws enforcing TRIPS, however, the WTO can penalise it by means of trade sanctions.

When a pharmaceutical company patents a new drug under TRIPS its patent ensures that it is exclusively entitled to all the profits from the drug for the duration of the patent. Patents typically last 20 years.

When TRIPS was introduced most high-income countries already had intellectual property laws capable of enforcing TRIPS. But this was not the case in many developing countries. In recognition of the need for new legislation it was agreed that different countries would have different timescales by which to implement TRIPS. Developed countries were allowed 1 year (to 1996), developing countries were given 5 years (to 2000) and the least developed countries were given 11 years (to 2006).

When Cipla produced its generic version of the triple-therapy antiretroviral in 2001, India had not yet implemented TRIPS. This enabled Cipla to ignore the patents owned by three different companies to combine three different antiretrovirals into a single pill that was resistant to heat. This greatly simplified the therapeutic regime and made it more practical for use in countries without ready access to refrigeration. This increased the likelihood of the drug being used properly, minimising the chances of the virus becoming resistant.

In 2006, however, the TRIPS agreement kicked in for many of the countries – India, Brazil and Thailand – producing generic drugs. This had no effect on the 'first-line' AIDS drugs. These were already out of patent. But it had a major effect on the 'second-line' drugs. These drugs are needed when resistance to first-line drugs has set in (or a person is sensitive to first-line drugs). Up to 15% of HIV-positive people show viral resistance to first-line drugs within 4–5 years of starting their regime.

That many of the countries producing generic drugs are required to observe the patents on second-line drugs is having a huge effect on the price of second-line drugs.

Countries in the developing world cannot afford them. Once again people in the developed world have access to the best drugs money can buy, while people in the developing world must make do with second best, despite the fact that many of these drugs were tested in their countries.

What is needed is another price war of the sort started by Cipla's production of its generic drug in 2001. But given TRIPS how can such a price war be started?

This is happening at a bad time. The economic crisis in the west is prompting many countries to cut their aid budgets. In May 2010 Médecins Sans Frontières published a report entitled 'No time to quit: HIV/AIDS treatment gap widening in Africa'[39] to warn that major international funding institutions such as PEPFAR, the World Bank, UNITAID and donors to the Global Fund have, since 2008, been capping, reducing or withdrawing their spending on HIV treatment.[40]

Something must be done. But what? Should we abolish TRIPS? If so what incentive will drug companies have for pouring millions into research and development? Is there any way the effect of TRIPS on developing countries can be mitigated?[41]

> ### Box 19.8 Activity: Creative writing
>
> You are the public relations officer of a major pharmaceutical. Tomorrow your Chief Executive Officer will be interviewed on the radio about the price of your drugs in comparison with the price of generic versions.
>
> Write a briefing paper for your CEO, arming him with arguments he might use.

In 2001, during the first crisis, thought was given to the possibility of mitigating the impact of TRIPS. The DOHA Agreement[42] affirmed member countries' right to 'use in full' the flexibility offered by TRIPS for countries with a health emergency to secure access to generic drugs without danger of prosecution. It also allows countries to determine for themselves when they have a health emergency. Facing such a situation a country can secure one of two types of licence, both of which permit the import or manufacture of generic drugs, even in a country bound by TRIPS:

Voluntary licences can be issued by patent-holding companies on request. As such companies stand to lose a lot of money, however, negotiations can be long-winded and disagreeable and success depends on the willingness of the pharmaceutical to put health before profit.

Compulsory licences can be issued without the agreement of the patent-holder, by any country facing a 'health emergency'. The amount of the drug that can be manufactured or imported, however, is severely restricted, issuing compulsory licences is extremely complicated, and drug companies are not above placing trade restrictions on countries that take this route.

Though TRIPS has certain flexibilities the drawbacks of using them are not negligible. It seems inevitable, therefore, that the 2010s will herald the deaths, from treatable illnesses, of yet more millions of people in the developing world despite the fact that the drugs that would save their lives were tested in their countries.

> ### Box 19.9 Activity: Debate
>
> Participants should be divided into groups and required to argue on one or other side of the following motion:
>
> *This house believes that public health is more important that profit. The TRIPS agreement should be abolished.*
>
> Participants should be given time to prepare their arguments.
>
> Those arguing for the motion should be asked to consider how research and development should be rewarded if not with patents.
>
> Those arguing against the motion should be asked to consider how we might secure equity in healthcare for those in the developing world.

Let's now turn to another example of the way in which those in the developed world might be thought to exploit those in the developing world.

A trade in human organs and tissue

There are nearly 8,000 people in the UK on the waiting list for an organ transplant. In 2009 3,513 organ transplants were carried out with organs donated by 1,853 people, but about 1,000 people died whilst waiting for an organ. Clearly we need to increase the number of organs available for transplant. Instead, however, the supply is *decreasing*. Every advance in healthcare and every success in improving road safety reduces it further.

> ### Box 19.10 Activity: Small group work
>
> Three patients each need a heart transplant as quickly as possible. Unusually a heart is available for each, but budgetary considerations are such that only one of them can have the operation. The others, sadly, will die.
>
> The three patients are:
>
> - Daisy Simmonds, 5 years old. Daisy has a congenital heart defect and is currently very ill indeed, not least because in addition to her heart defect she has cystic fibrosis (which means she is unlikely to live past 30). Daisy's parents and her four brothers and sisters are distraught about Daisy's health.
> - James Trojan, 43 years old. James has not lived a healthy life (he is a heavy smoker, doesn't exercise and he is extremely fat, though not clinically obese),

and although he claims he will reform should he have the operation, his doctors are pessimistic. James is married, employed full time and has a child of 15.
- Hilary Playter, 61 years old. Hilary is a fit and active pensioner with an equally fit husband of 67, three children and six grandchildren, all of whom adore her.

Having appointed a spokesperson for your group decide who should have the operation and who should come second (in case the first person dies before the operation).

At the moment in the UK there is an 'opt-in' system for organ donation.[43] If you wish to donate your organs to others after death you can sign the NHS organ donation register. On 31 March 2009 16,124,871 people carried an organ donor card. Their family, though, can veto their donation. Some have suggested this should be disallowed. But doctors are ambivalent: imagine having to tell a traumatised family that you are taking the organs of their loved one – his heart, lungs, kidneys, pancreas and corneas – whether they like it or not.

Organ supply could be increased by an 'opt out' system.[44] This would assume consent to organ donation unless a person had actively opted out. In countries that have such systems there are many more transplants. But does this violate people's right to determine what happens to their own bodies? Some claim it amounts to theft. Should families have a say? In Spain medics take active steps to make sure families don't object. In Austria the consent of families is not sought. In the UK the issue is under debate.[45]

In the UK for some years it has been permissible for living family members to donate organs. But now there is no medical reason for living donors to be family members. Altruistic donation has recently been legalised. In 2009 there were 17. It seems unlikely, however, that altruistic donation will be the answer to our prayers.

The NHS is running a campaign in the hope of increasing the number of those on the organ donation register. We discussed in Chapter 10, page 168, a similar campaign hoping to increase the supply of donor gametes.

Box 19.11 Activity: Personal reflection/debate

Take a look at this website:

http://www.timesonline.co.uk/tol/life_and_style/health/article5151526.ece.

Then consider whether or not you think that the UK (or your own country) should move to a system of 'presumed consent'.

If you'd like to hold a debate on this topic, this topic guide from Debating Matters will help:

http://www.debatingmatters.com/topicguides/topicguide/organ_donation/.

Future supplies

Naturally biotechnology is working hard to find alternatives. Here are some ways in which it already helps, or hopes soon to help:

Artificial organs: Sujoy Gupta, a biomedical engineer at the Indian Institute of technology in Kharagpur, has developed an artificial heart – inspired by the anatomy of the cockroach – that could cost as little as £1,500.[46]

Reconditioned organs: in December 2009 James Finlayson, who suffers from cystic fibrosis, was given lungs, unusable when donated, but repaired by 'perfusion', where an oxygenated solution is pumped over them.[47]

Cloning spare parts: we saw in Chapters 7 and 8 that human clones could provide 'spare parts' for the nucleus donor. Current legislation prevents this technology from being used. This will not change anytime soon.[48]

Xenotransplantation: in the UK there is a moratorium on xenotransplantation, animal–human transplantation, for fear of porcine viruses being transferred to humans. In Mexico, experiments using pig islet cells have been conducted successfully.[49]

The future is looking quite good. But in the meantime people continue to die.

A black market in organs

As you can imagine, given the above, there is a thriving black market in human organs. Those who can afford organs simply buy them, sometimes from people in the west,[50] more usually from someone in the developing world. The World Health Organization estimates that one fifth of the 70,000 kidneys transplanted worldwide every year are bought on the black market. Only Iran has legalised the trade in human organs.

> ### Box 19.12 Activity: Web-wandering
> Wander around the web and see if you can find the going price for a kidney in your country. Would you sell your kidney for this?

Having a black market organ transplanted in the developing world can be dangerous. Twenty-nine patients at the Queen Elizabeth Hospital in Birmingham in 2002 had had black market kidneys transplanted abroad: 50% of these kidneys failed. Ten of the patients died.[51] It seems unlikely, however, that the black market in organs will disappear: if you are going to die you will want to explore every option. Some suggest, however, that legalising this trade would solve many of the problems we have discussed.

In Chapter 10, pages 164–166, we looked at the ethical issues associated with the 'commodification' of the human body. These arguments will also apply to the suggestion we legalise a trade in human organs. You might also look at pages 173–175 where we considered whether paying women from the developing world to be surrogate mothers amounts to exploitation.

The philosopher Janet Radcliffe-Richards rejects the idea that a legal trade in human organs would exploit those from the developing world. Interviewed by Nigel Warburton on Ethics-Bites she argues as follows for the legalisation of the trade in organs:

'There's no point, if you're trying to protect the exploited person, from just stopping what he regards as his best option. The person who enters into an exploitative relationship is getting something out of it. We want them to get *more* out of it.

We need to control the exchange: to have a minimum wage, or something. And you can't do this if it's illegal. Making it illegal just drives it underground so you can't protect the people involved.

If you ban the whole procedure because you want to stop the exploiters, then you're getting at the exploiters but you're not benefiting the exploited.'[52]

Imagine, for example, that we set up a global market licensing one body to buy and sell organs at a fair pre-determined price. Perhaps the operations of this body might even be subsidised by the developed world so organs could be offered *freely* to anyone who needs them (wherever they live)? Not only would this enable everyone in need, however poor, to secure an organ, it could also save the developed world a lot of money.

In the UK dialysis, for one patient for a year, costs an average of £30,800. There are 21,000 patients on dialysis. This amounts to 3% of the total NHS budget. A transplant, on the other hand, costs £17,000 per person, and the drugs needed thereafter cost £5,000 per person per year. In the second and subsequent year, therefore, the saving, per person, per transplant is £25,800. In 2008/9, when 2,497 kidney transplants were carried out, the NHS saved itself £50.3 million per year.[53]

Such a trade would allow the very poor to improve their lot by selling an organ, it would save many lives in the developed and the developing world, *and* it could save us money on healthcare. But where does out moral duty lie? Should we support a national or international market in human organs.[54] Or are the objections to such a trade too strong?[55]

Box 19.13 Activity: Essay writing

Conduct some research on how a global market in human organs might work. Then write 1,500 words arguing for or against such a market.

This concludes our consideration of the ethical and social issues generated by biotechnology and the relationships between the developed and the developing world.

Summary

In this chapter we have considered how biotechnological advances can affect relationships between the developed and developing world. In particular we have:

- considered the Nuremberg Code and the Helsinki Declaration and reflected on the perceived 'burden' of such codes on research involving human subjects;

- acknowledged the attractions of holding clinical trials in the developing world;

- looked at the importance of informed or genuine consent and the cultural difficulties that can arise in trying to secure it;

- considered whether it is morally permissible to offer a lower standard of care to control groups in clinical trials in the developing world;

- reflected on how the production of generic drugs revolutionised healthcare in the developed world during the 2000s;

- recognised the threat that the implementation of TRIPS poses to future health-care in the developing world;

- acknowledged that without TRIPS drug companies would find it harder to make the profit they need to fund research and development of new drugs;

- considered whether TRIPS is flexible enough to allow developing countries to deal with the new crisis in healthcare;

- reflected on the shortage of organs for transplants and the fact that this has resulted in a thriving black market;

- considered the arguments for and against legalising a national or international trade in human organs.

Questions to stimulate reflection

Do you think that too much emphasis is placed on ethical review of research involving human subjects?

Is it even possible, do you think, to secure genuine consent from someone in the developing world?

How, if at all, is it possible to avoid offering inducements for participation in clinical trials to a poor person in a country that lacks free healthcare?

If we do not have double standards in respect of the duty of care we owe to control groups, then many clinical trials that will be of benefit to those in the third world will not take place. Is this true?

What was it that revolutionised healthcare in the developed world during the 2000s? Why is it unlikely the same solution will pertain to the current healthcare crisis?

Why should a drug company spend $802 million developing a drug if it isn't allowed to patent that drug and make a profit?

Is it morally permissible to legalise an international trade in human organs? If not how else are we to increase the supply of such organs for transplant?

Additional activities

Use this topic guide from Debating Matters to organise a debate about whether it is fair to hold clinical trials in India: http://www.debatingmatters.com/topicguides/topicguide/clinical_trials_in_india/.

Approach your local university and ask for their policy on research on human subjects.

Imagine you were one of the people who obeyed orders during Milgram's experiments. Write 500 words on what you have learned.

Do some web-wandering: can you find a recent case of unethical research on human subjects?

Conduct some research on the cost of drug development. Compare the cost of developing a drug in a developed country and in a country of the developing world.

Write a story about a future in which organs are harvested from clones as a matter of course.

Approach your local hospital and ask them about their policy for organ transplants.

Notes

1　http://www.auschwitz.dk/doctors.htm.
2　http://nuremberg.law.harvard.edu/php/docs_swi.php?DI=1&text=overview. Resources on the Nuremberg Trials from Harvard University.
3　http://www.mengele.dk/.
4　http://www.cirp.org/library/ethics/nuremberg/.
5　http://www.wma.net/en/30publications/10policies/b3/index.html.
6　http://www.scribd.com/doc/20983187/IVMS-The-Tuskegee-Syphilis-Experiment.
7　http://www.cdc.gov/tuskegee/timeline.htm.
8　http://www.cdc.gov/tuskegee/timeline.htm.
9　http://www.experiment-resources.com/stanley-milgram-experiment.html.
10　http://www.nuffieldbioethics.org/fileLibrary/pdf/HRRDC_Follow-up_Discussion_Paper001.pdf, p. 4.
11　http://www.youtube.com/watch?v=k8IYKCkXXvY. A YouTube video of the questioning of Harvard's Dr Aaron Kesselheim on how the dangers of Vioxx would never have come to light without lawsuits filed by injured patients.
12　http://www.nytimes.com/2007/11/09/business/09merck.html.
13　http://www.pharmalot.com/2010/03/merck-loses-vioxx-case-in-australia/.

14 http://www.independent.co.uk/news/world/australasia/vioxx-ruling-gives-hope-for-payouts-to-british-lsquovictimsrsquo-1917042.html.
15 There is no intention to suggest that Merck was conducting experiments that were unethical.
16 www.clinicaltrials.gov/ct2//info/understand.
17 http://news.bbc.co.uk/1/hi/health/4808090.stm. A BBC Q&A on drug trials in the light of the TGN1412 disaster.
18 www.york.ac.uk//inst/crd//CRD_reports//crdreport31&32_summ.pdf.
19 http://content.nejm.org/cgi/content/full/360/8/816.
20 http://www.wired.com/wired/archive/14.03/indiadrug.html.
21 http://www.timesonline.co.uk/tol/news/world/asia/article4568717.ece. 49 babies die in Indian drug trial.
22 http://news.bbc.co.uk/1/hi/programmes/this_world/4924012.stm.
23 http://www.research.umn.edu/consent/. Tutorial on informed consent from the University of Minnesota.
24 http://www.nuffieldbioethics.org/fileLibrary/pdf/HRRDC_Follow-up_Discussion_Paper001.pdf.
25 Case studies adapted from http://www.nuffieldbioethics.org/fileLibrary/pdf/HRRDC_Follow-up_Discussion_Paper001.pdf.
26 http://news.bbc.co.uk/1/hi/health/736138.stm.
27 Lurie, P. and Wolfe, S. (1997) Unethical trials of interventions to reduce perinatal transmission of the human immunodeficiency virus in developing countries. *New England Journal of Medicine*, **337**, 853–856. http://content.nejm.org/cgi/content/short/337/12/853.
28 http://www.nih.gov/news/pr/nov96/niaid-27.htm.
29 e.g. CIOMS 2002, EGE 2003, NCOB 2002.
30 Porter, K., Babiker, A., Bhaskaran, K. *et al.* (2003) Determinants of survival following HIV-1 seroconversion after the introduction of HAART. *The Lancet*, **362**(9392), 1267–7124.
31 Brown, L.R. (2000) HIV epidemic restructuring Africa's population. *World Watch Issue Alert*, 31 October.
32 http://www.cipla.com/.
33 http://www.who.int/trade/glossary/story034/en/index.html.
34 http://www.avert.org/generic.htm.
35 http://news.bbc.co.uk/1/hi/health/medical_notes/a-b/537714.stm.
36 http://www.independent.co.uk/news/business/news/protest-in-britain-as-drug-companies-sue-south-african-government-694706.html.
37 http://data.unaids.org/pub/GlobalReport/2008/jc1510_2008_global_report_pp129_158_en.pdf, p. 136.
38 http://www.wto.org/english/tratop_e/trips_e/trips_e.htm#WhatAre.
39 http://allafrica.com/download/resource/main/main/idatcs/00020144:b44d98cae7f2989732ea70aaa0489f98.pdf.
40 http://www.healthgap.org/resources.htm. Information about funding from HealthGap.org.
41 http://www.bbc.co.uk/blogs/africahaveyoursay/2010/07/should-antiretrovirals-be-a-hu.shtml. A BBC Africa 'Have your Say' site on ARV drugs.
42 http://www.wto.org/english/thewto_e/minist_e/min01_e/mindecl_e.htm.
43 http://www.uktransplant.org.uk/ukt/how_to_become_a_donor/how_to_become_a_donor.jsp.
44 http://www.organdonation.nhs.uk/ukt/newsroom/statements_and_stances/statements/opt_in_or_out.jsp.
45 http://www.dh.gov.uk/en/Publicationsandstatistics/Publications/PublicationsPolicyAndGuidance/DH_090312.

46 http://www.timesonline.co.uk/tol/life_and_style/health/article6859344.ece. http://www.guardian.co.uk/science/2008/oct/28/artificial-human-heart-trial-2011. http://www.dailymail.co.uk/health/article-1306134/Artificial-corneas-restore-sight-partially- blind-patients-grown-lab.html?ito=feeds-newsxml.

47 http://news.patient.co.uk/newspaper.asp?ss=10&pc=10985.

48 http://science.howstuffworks.com/environmental/life/genetic/cloned-organ-transplant.htm.

49 http://www.newscientist.com/article/dn2722-pig-cell-transplants-cure-diabetes.html.

50 See: http://www.timesonline.co.uk/tol/life_and_style/health/article6850879.ece.

51 http://www.timesonline.co.uk/tol/news/uk/health/article731183.ece.

52 http://www.open2.net/ethicsbites/organ_transplants.html.

53 http://www.uktransplant.org.uk/ukt/newsroom/fact_sheets/cost_effectiveness_of_transplantation.jsp.

54 http://jme.bmj.com/content/29/3/142.full. The *Journal of Medical Ethics* on trade in human organs.

55 http://www.swissinfo.ch/eng/swiss_news/Cracking_down_on_organ_trafficking.html?cid= 24668630.

Further reading and useful websites

Goodwin, M. (2006) *Black Markets: The Supply and Demand of Body Parts.* Cambridge: Cambridge University Press.

Macklin, R. (2009) *Against Relativism: Cultural Diversity and the Search for Ethical Universals in Medicine.* Oxford: Oxford University Press.

Osewe, P. et al. (2008) *Improving Access to HIV/AIDS Medicines in Africa: Trade-related Aspects of Intellectual Property Rights Flexibilities: Assessment of Trade-related Utilization (Directions in Development).* New York: World Bank.

http://debatepedia.idebate.org/en/index.php/Debate:Human_Organs,_Sale_of. Debatepedia guide to a debate on trading human organs.

http://www.debatingmatters.com/topicguides/topicguide/Developing_Countries_and_clinical_ trials/. Debating Matters Topic Guide on clinical trials in developing countries.

http://www.idebate.org/debatabase/topic_details.php?topicID=24. Resources for a debate about generic AIDS drugs in developing countries.

Section 6
Our duties to nature

20 | Non-human animals: consciousness, rationality and animal rights

Objectives

In reading this chapter you will:

- ask whether animals are sentient and/or rational;
- consider whether deontologists would impose moral constraints on our use of animals;
- reflect on whether animals must be counted in the utilitarian calculus;
- consider whether animals have rights and if so what sort of rights they have;
- ask whether speciesism is comparable to racism and sexism;
- reflect on whether animals are good experimental models for human beings;
- reflect on how the moral status of animals impacts on our use of them for research purposes;
- consider how animal rights activism affects the public perception of the use of animals in scientific research.

Box 20.1 Factual information: The use of mice for research in the UK

From the 1970s until the 2000s there was a steady decline in the use of animals in research, possibly due to the activities of animal rights activists. The boom in genetic research reversed this decline.

Mice are particularly valuable for research because 99% of their 30,000 genes have direct counterparts in the human genome.

By 2003 there were already 3,000 GM strains of mice. It has been predicted there will be 300,000 by 2020.[1] Hundreds of mice are needed to produce each, though most of the mice are killed because they do not develop the needed mutation.

In the UK it is estimated that several million mice are used annually in genetic research. Some have suggested that mice are now little more than 'catalogue entries' like paperclips or biros to be routinely ordered for the proper functioning of the institution.[2]

The moral status of animals

You will almost certainly be familiar with this biblical passage:

'And God blessed them and said unto them, be fruitful and multiply, and replenish the earth and subdue it: and have dominion over the fish of the sea, and over the fowl of the air, and over every living thing that moveth over the earth.' Genesis 1:28

Until recently human animals have taken this exhortation at face value. We have assumed the right to use non-human animals for food, for clothing, for sport and recreation, for entertainment and for companionship. Many of the scientific advances that have made our lives so comfortable have been made at the expense of non-human animals.

Even if human animals do have 'dominion' over non-human animals this does not amount to a moral licence to treat them badly. Nowadays those who look to the Bible for guidance tend to rely on texts that emphasise stewardship rather than dominion.[3]

The words 'non-human animals' emphasise the fact we too are animals. Richard Dawkins illustrates this as follows:

'Imagine you are standing on the shore of the Indian Ocean in Southern Somalia, facing north. In your left hand you hold the right hand of your mother. In turn she holds the hand of her mother, your grandmother. Your grandmother holds her mother's hand, and so on. The chain wends its way up the beach, into the arid scrubland and westwards onto the Kenya border.'[4]

'How far do we have to go' asks Dawkins 'to reach the ancestor we have in common with the chimpanzees?' His answer is: under 300 miles. Our common ancestor stands well to the east of Mount Kenya. The daughter whose hand is gripped in her right hand is the one from whom we are descended. In her left hand is the hand of the daughter from whom the chimpanzees are descended.

The use of non-human animals cannot be justified, therefore, on the basis of the claim that they are animals and we are not. The use of 'non-human animal' and 'human animal' reminds us of this. Nevertheless for brevity's sake we shall use 'humans' and 'animals' on the basis of a commitment not to forget our animal nature. Our question is whether, consistent with this, it is morally acceptable to allow animals to suffer to achieve our ends.

Animal consciousness

The philosopher Descartes[5] (in)famously argued that animals do *not* suffer, that they are not conscious at all. In making this claim Descartes was not making an epistemological point, a point about how we *know* animals suffer, he was making a metaphysical claim to the effect that animals do *not* suffer. (For the distinction between epistemology and metaphysics see Chapter 2, page 15).

For Descartes it was a condition of consciousness that a thing be rational. Denying rationality to animals he also denied them consciousness and, therefore, the ability to feel pleasure or pain.[6]

Box 20.2 Case study: Animal emotions

When Dorothy, an elderly chimp, died staff of the Sanaga-Yong Chimpanzee Rescue Centre conducted her burial in full view of the other chimps. They rushed to the perimeter of their enclosure and stood silently in line with their hands on each others' shoulders (see Figure 20.1) to watch.

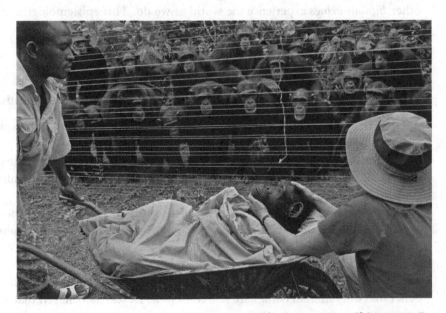

Figure 20.1 Dorothy and other chimpanzees at the Sanaga-Yong Chimpanzee Rescue Centre. © Monica Szczupider/*National Geographic* My Shot/National Geographic Stock.

You might think that Descartes' belief that animals don't suffer is abhorrent. But no belief can be abhorrent. Actions based on a belief might be abhorrent, but the belief itself is just that, *a belief*. You might more reasonably think that Descartes' belief is *false*. If, however, you are basing your claim on animal behaviour you might be accused of anthropomorphism: just because animals behave as we do does not necessarily mean they experience the world as we do.

Box 20.3 Activity: Web-research

Monkeys who lack a primary visual cortex, and who therefore experience *nothing* visually, nevertheless act *as if* they can see.

This phenomenon is called 'blindsight'. It demonstrates that the fact animals act *as if* they are conscious is not *conclusive* reason to believe they *are* conscious.

Put 'blindsight' into a search engine and find out more about it. You might start with this newspaper article:

http://www.timesonline.co.uk/tol/news/science/article5385633.ece.

When you have learned more discuss with a partner whether this supports Descartes' belief that animals are 'automata'.

Human beings 'experience' blindsight too: we can't even be certain therefore that other *human beings* experience the world as we do. This epistemological difficulty is known as the problem of 'other minds'.

Box 20.4 Philosophical background: The problem of other minds

Ask yourself: is it possible that only *I* experience the world, so others are merely automata who behave *as if* they experience the world?

You will almost certainly answer 'yes'. We never, after all, experience the minds of others, all we see are their behaviours. Even if their behaviour provides us with evidence that they have minds, this evidence is inconclusive.

The problem of other minds is predicated on the assumption that the mind is a private realm, its contents accessible only to introspection. These days philosophers question this.

But Descartes believed that unless there is an 'I', a *self*, aware of the contents of its own consciousness, there is no consciousness. On the basis of this, and the belief that only human beings are self-conscious, Descartes believed that animals are automata.[7]

But the problem of other minds is irrelevant in answering our question about how, morally, we should treat animals. Even if we cannot be certain that other human beings suffer, after all, we are morally obliged to assume they *do*. And as animals share our evolutionary history, behave in similar ways, and have a similar physiological make-up it seems reasonable also to assume they have similar experiences.

Animal preferences

We might still insist, however, that our only way of taking animals' experience into account is to put ourselves in their shoes. This is hopelessly unscientific.

But ethology, the science of animal behaviour, shows it is reasonable to claim we *can* 'ask' animals if they are suffering. Animals can be taught to put a 'price' on their preferences, for example, by pressing a lever, pecking a disc or swimming through a hoop to get food or avoid a shock. From the animal's willingness to work harder to achieve something we can determine how valuable this 'something' is to the animal.

For example, Marian Stamp Dawkins[8] presented to hens two different environments: a battery cage and an outside run. The hens could see both and were free to walk to either. Most hens chose the outside run. Those that didn't choose it first time chose it the second or third time (perhaps because the battery cage was the familiar environment). Dawkins argued this is an objective way of justifying the claim the hens preferred the outside run to the battery cage. Such work has generated an instrumental definition of suffering:

'Animal suffering: animals suffer if kept in conditions in which they are without something they will work hard to obtain, or in conditions they will work hard to escape, given the opportunity.'[9]

As it is reasonable to assume that animals *do* suffer, and as there are objective ways to determine what makes them suffer, we can now ask again whether causing them to suffer can be morally justified.

Deontology and animal rights

We shall start by considering what deontology might say about the moral acceptability of our treatment of animals. If you'd like to remind yourself what deontologists believes see Chapter 4, pages 37–42.

Direct and indirect duties

Kant says the mistreatment of animals is wrong.[10] This is not, however, because animals have the right not to be treated badly. Animals do not have rights, according to Kant, because only those who are ends in themselves have rights. It is a necessary condition of being an end in oneself that one be rational and animals, Kant says, are not rational.

Mistreating animals is wrong, says Kant, because a direct duty to ourselves generates an *indirect* duty to animals: we must not treat them badly because in doing so we brutalise *ourselves*. It is for *our own sake* that we must not mistreat animals.

Animal interests

The philosopher Joel Feinberg[11] argued that Kant's position wrongly assimilates our treatment of animals to our treatment of objects.[12]

For example, says Feinberg, we have a duty not to destroy the Taj Mahal, but no one would claim this is a duty *to* the Taj Mahal. Nothing *matters* to the Taj Mahal and so our duty to protect it is not a duty we have *for the sake of* the Taj Mahal itself: the Taj Mahal has no *sake*.

But, says Feinberg, things *do* matter to animals. Animals are sentient; they experience pleasure and pain. Animals, therefore, deserve protection *for their own sake*. Our duties to animals, according to Feinberg, are direct.

Feinberg strengthens his case by noting that whilst you cannot leave your money to the Taj Mahal, you can leave it to your cat. Your children might object but by the terms of your will the cat has a right to your money. If your children contest your will the court will appoint lawyers to represent your cat. In doing this, the court seems to be acting on a *direct* duty to your cat.

According to Feinberg, our duties to *objects* are nothing more than indirect duties to ourselves, but our duties to *animals*, because of their sentience, are more than this. Because of this, says Feinberg, animals can be said to have *interests* even if they can't be said to have rights.

> ## Box 20.5 Activity: Conceptual analysis
>
> Kant and Feinberg agree that animals do not have *rights* because they are not *rational*. Feinberg, however, believes they have *interests* because they are *sentient*.
>
> Can you express these ideas using the terminology of conditions 'necessary' and 'sufficient' for something?
>
> Answer: For Kant and Feinberg it is a necessary and a sufficient condition of having *rights* that one be rational. It is, for Feinberg, a necessary and a sufficient condition of having *interests* that one be sentient.

Animal rationality

Others agree that Kant is wrong. But they question his claim that animals aren't rational.

The idea that only humans are rational, we might think, contradicts our recognition that humans *are* animals. It makes us quite different from animals, sets us apart from them. Isn't it more realistic, we might ask, to think that rationality is a matter of *degree*? So humans are *more* rational than animals perhaps, or are rational in a different way, but this doesn't mean that animals are not rational *at all*. Even if we accept that the reasoning of humans is superior, or at least different, to the reasoning of animals, we needn't insist that animals are *incapable* of reasoning.

But the capacity for reason that interests us is the capacity, possession of which confers the status of being an end in oneself.

Rationality and personhood

The philosopher Roger Scruton[13] says that even if animals are rational they are not rational in the right way to be ends in themselves. For this it is necessary, says Scruton, to be a *person*, to have the potential for being a person or, at least to be the kind of thing capable of being a person.[14]

It is, Scruton allows, an empirical question whether there are or could be any non-human persons. But the evidence, he says, is against this. To be a person is to be the sort of thing that can negotiate, compromise and enter into agreement with other persons. In doing this persons create 'moral communities' in which each individual, despite his dependence on others, can live a life of his own choosing. Only human beings can create communities of this kind because the basis of these communities, says Scruton, is rational dialogue.

Rational dialogue depends on all parties being able to recognise good and bad reasons for a position, being prepared to make concessions, being free to take on duties to live up to agreements, and being able to act with the intention of honouring an obligation.

To suggest, says Scruton, that a dog should be accorded rights is to suggest that dogs are or could be equal partners with human beings in deciding how to live or that we could make an agreement with a dog and hold it to that agreement if it reneges. It is to suggest that it makes sense to impose duties on dogs, and to punish them, not simply in order to change their desires, but because they have failed in their duties.

But such things do not make sense. Dogs lack the mental capacities to be anything more than honorary members of a moral community. It is morally unacceptable, says Scruton, to impose on dogs, or on any other animals, duties they do not, and cannot, understand.

Like Kant, therefore, Scruton denies rights to animals. But like Feinberg he believes that in virtue of their sentience they have interests that confer on us direct duties towards them.

Box 20.6 Activity: Group Discussion

This house believes that even if animals are rational they are not rational in the right way to be accorded rights.

Participants might choose their own side, or they might be allocated a side.

They will need to have familiarised themselves with Scruton's argument before the discussion starts and they should be reminded that even if animals do not have rights, their interests might confer on us a duty not to mistreat them.

Deontological rights

The deontologist Tom Regan[15] believes, *pace* Kant, Feinberg and Scruton, that the sentience that suffices for possession of interests *also* suffices to ensure that animals are ends in themselves and that, therefore, they have rights. To Regan the fact animals are sentient gives them the same moral status as humans (see our brief discussion on moral status in Box 7.2).[16]

Box 20.7 **Activity: Evaluating arguments**

Regan's argument for the claim that animals have rights, set out logic-book style is:

Premise one: Anything capable of feeling pleasure or pain has interests.

Premise two: Anything that has interests is intrinsically valuable.

Premise three: Anything that is intrinsically valuable has inviolable rights.

Premise four: Animals are capable of feeling pleasure or pain.

Conclusion: Animals have inviolable rights.

Is this a sound argument (see Chapter 5, p. 57 for the definition of 'soundness')? If not identify what is wrong with it.

Notes: Something has an 'interest' if it has a stake in something, if it *matters* to that thing. You have an interest in your teacher being a good teacher and your dog has an interest in your being kind.

Something is 'intrinsically' valuable if it is valuable in and of itself, i.e. not as a means to achieving something else. Love is intrinsically valuable, money is only instrumentally valuable.

An 'inviolable' right can't be overruled (even by the benefits to be gained by overruling it).

Answer: The argument is valid, but it is not obvious that all its premises are true, so it is not obviously sound.

Regan, therefore, rejects the usual deontologist claim that ends in themselves must be rational and that rationality is required for rights. That he is a deontologist, however, is manifested in his belief that rights are *absolute* or *inviolable*. To treat animals solely as means to our own ends is morally abhorrent.

Box 20.8 **Activity: Analysing arguments**

Descartes, Singer, Feinberg and Scruton all reject Regan's argument as outlined in Box 20.7. Identify the grounds on which they would reject it.

Answer: Descartes would reject premise 4, Singer would reject premise 2 (utilitarians believe the only thing with intrinsic value is happiness), Feinberg might reject either premise 2 or premise 3 or both of them, Scruton would reject premise 3.

Animals' possession of rights does not entail they have the same rights we have. It is meaningless, Regan notes, to give males the legal right to abortion and just as meaningless to give dogs the right to vote. But animals do have the right not to be used as nothing more than means to our ends.

For society to adopt Regan's view of animals would arguably lead to a *huge* shift in our attitudes to animals. It would no longer be possible to use animals for scientific purposes, for example, unless we would use humans in the same way. Nor, would it be possible (without their consent) to eat them, use them for sport or recreation or keep them as pets.

There would be huge inconveniences attending this change in attitude. But a moral imperative is a moral imperative: it is not cancelled because it is inconvenient to respect it.

> ### Box 20.9 **Activity: Brainstorming**
> As a group participants should brainstorm on what we wouldn't be able to do to or with animals if they are ends in themselves and in possession of inviolable rights.

Utilitarianism and animal rights

Regan is unusual for a deontologist in believing that sentience is sufficient for rights. We might think that a utilitarian – who thinks of sentience rather than rationality as the fulcrum on which morality turns – would be more likely to think sentience sufficient for rights. It was a utilitarian, Peter Sïnger,[17] who started the 'animal liberation' movement in the 1970s.[18] Before we read about this you might like to remind yourself about utilitarianism by reading pages 42–45 in Chapter 4.

According to Singer to accept that animals experience pleasure and pain, is to be morally required to count animals when we decide which action produces the greatest happiness of the greatest number (GHGN).[19]

The right to be counted is not the same as the right deriving from being a deontological 'end'. Utilitarians do not recognise inviolable rights as deontologists do (Chapter 7, p. 102 to remind yourself of this). Adopting animal rights on utilitarian grounds would leave us morally free to use animals in any way at all so long as we were convinced that – counting animals – such uses would result in the GHGN.

But surely, we might ask, even if animals count, they don't count as much as human beings. Animals don't have the hopes and fears we have, they don't consider the future at all, their life-plans cannot be thwarted as ours can. They don't even *have* life-plans. There is no reason, therefore, to weigh animal interests as heavily as human interests.

Singer rejects this. The fact that animals' pains and pleasures differ, he says, is no reason to count their pains and pleasures for less. If the fact animals do not have life-plans means they can be killed with impunity, after all, then infants can also be killed with impunity. Black and female suffering counts as much as the suffering of white males, says Singer, and animal suffering counts as much as human suffering. To think anything else is speciesism[20] and as morally unacceptable as racism and sexism.

Box 20.10 Activity: Role play

For the purposes of this exercise participants should assume they are utilitarians and, in pairs, discuss whether or not they can justify eating meat.

After the discussion, which should take 10–20 minutes, participants should be invited to offer their views and in particular to say whether their views have changed.

Moral philosophy and the treatment of animals

Moral philosophers are therefore agreed, though for different reasons, in believing that there are moral constraints on our treatment of animals:

Kant: we have a direct duty not to brutalise ourselves which generates an indirect duty not to treat animals badly.

Feinberg and Scruton: animals, being sentient, have interests and this generates direct duties towards them.

Regan: animals, being sentient, have the inviolable rights of ends in themselves.

Singer: animals, being sentient, have the right to be counted in the utilitarian calculus.

If we ask how a virtuous person would treat animals it seems likely that he too would consider that the sentience of animals would generate moral constraints on our treatment of them.

Box 20.11 Activity: Discussion point

Christiaan Barnard, the South African heart transplant pioneer, once wrote:

'I had two male chimps who lived next door to each other in separate cages before I used one as a [heart] donor. When we put him to sleep in his cage in preparation for the operation, the other chattered and cried incessantly. When we removed the body to the operating room, the other chimp wept bitterly and was inconsolable for days. The incident made a deep impression on me. I vowed never again to experiment with such sensitive creatures.'[21]

Roger Scruton writes:

'certain actions are so distressing that a certain measure of callousness is required if they are to be performed. That which can be done only by a callous person should not be done.'[22]

Do you think the 'deep impression' described by Barnard is an indication of the fact that what he did could be done only by a callous person? A virtue ethicist would say that this makes it morally impermissible. Do you agree?

Unless we agree with Regan and accord the status of ends in themselves to animals (or at least to some animals), these moral constraints do not, however, forbid our use of animals. They require only that we mustn't brutalise ourselves, that we mustn't act against the interests of animals and/or that we must take the pains and pleasures of animals into account in the utilitarian calculus. What implications do these constraints have on our interactions with animals?

> ### Box 20.12 Activity: Great Ape Project and a committee of the great and the good
>
> In 1993 Peter Singer and Paola Cavalieri, an Italian philosopher, founded the Great Ape Project to secure, on behalf of the great apes, the right to 'life, liberty, and the prohibition of torture'.[23] The great apes, they argue, have such rights because they are intelligent beings with strong emotions like our own'.[24]
>
> This activity involves asking participants to form a committee with the following terms of reference:
>
> - to assess the arguments for and against according rights to the great apes.
>
> The following officers should be appointed:
>
> - a chairperson;
> - a scribe.
>
> Participants should be allowed time before the discussion to conduct some research. Boxes 20.3, 20.4 and 20.7 in this chapter may help.

The morality of using animals for research purposes

An interesting question for our purposes is whether these constraints are consistent with our using animals for research purposes.

Much research, of course, has no adverse impact on animals. The success of research involving the observation of animals behaving normally in their natural habitats, for example, depends on the animals' experience being the same as usual. Genetically modifying sheep or goats so their milk carries a human protein also seems benign: they would be producing the milk anyway. Unless using animals as 'bioreactors' is demeaning such procedures can't be objected to on the grounds of animal suffering.[25]

But most research is not benign. Sometimes we can't be sure the animals will suffer (for example, when animals are subjected to known mutagens to produce random mutations). At other times we can be certain animals will suffer anything from mild to severe pain and distress. We know that nearly all animals used will eventually be killed. How can we justify permitting such suffering?

We could argue that this will not brutalise us, so long as we are not callous. We might also say this is in their interests, assuming we feed and house the animals well, do not frighten or mishandle them, make sure their preferences are generally met and that our experiments contribute to veterinary science as well as human medicine.

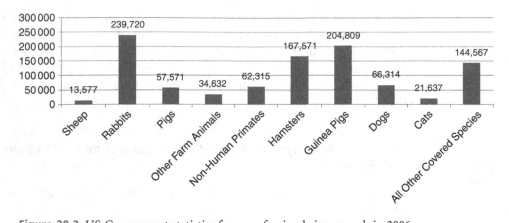

Figure 20.2 US Government statistics for use of animals in research in 2006 (http://speakingofresearch.com/facts/statistics/).

When it comes to calculating the greatest happiness of the greatest number, furthermore, the case seems made: in their 1988 White Paper on research using animals the American Medical Association claimed that:

'Virtually every advance in medical science in the twentieth century, from antibiotics and vaccines to anti-depressant drugs and organ transplants, has been achieved either directly or indirectly through the use of animals in laboratory experiments.'[26]

A huge amount of human suffering has been alleviated by the use of animals. Even taking into account the suffering of the animals used it seems reasonable to think in using them we promote the GHGN.

Box 20.13 **Factual information: Xenotransplantation**

The organ shortage described in Chapter 19, pages 385–387 may be alleviated by using pigs as organ sources.[27] Currently, though, humans suffer 'hyperacute' rejection when given pig organs. Another worry is the possibility of pig viruses infecting humans. To avoid this we would have to purpose-breed pathogen-free pigs.[28]

This would have welfare implications. The pigs may have to be delivered by Caesarean section, for example, and reared in isolation, a particularly stressful situation for pigs which are highly sociable.

The number of animals currently being used for research will be dwarfed by the number that *might* be used if xenotransplantation becomes possible.

For example approximately 9,200 kidneys would have been needed in 1994 alone (1,744 kidney transplants performed, 4,970 on the waiting list, and a conservatively estimated 2,485 who failed to meet the stringent conditions for getting on the list). It is not only kidneys, of course, that would be needed. Nor is it only organs: we also need cells and tissue.

To decide whether this is acceptable the happiness of millions of pigs must be included in the utilitarian calculus along with the undoubted happiness of the humans whose lives will be saved or transformed.

Before we take it that the case *has* been made, however, let's consider a claim to the effect that the use of animals for scientific research *doesn't* have the beneficial results claimed for it.

The scientific validity of animal research

We tend to think that animal research is scientifically useful and consistent with our moral duties to animals because:

(i) animals are similar enough to us to make it reasonable that they can act as experimental models for us;
(ii) the history of science demonstrates that animals *are* scientifically useful experimental models for human beings.

Hugh LaFollette and Niall Shanks[29] argue that both these claims are false.

(i) Animal–human similarity

Two false beliefs, say LaFollette and Shanks, mislead people into thinking that animals are good experimental models for humans:

(i) the belief that functional similarity guarantees causal similarity;
(ii) the belief that phylogenetic continuity implies causal similarity.[30]

The first belief misleads us, say LaFollette and Shanks, into assuming that because most animals have evolved some mechanism for, say, oxygenating the blood the causal mechanisms they use to perform this function will be similar. But as LaFollette and Shanks point out the peribronchial lungs of birds are very different from the alveolar lungs of mammals. Sameness of function does not entail sameness of causal mechanism underlying the function.

The second belief misleads us into assuming that phylogenetic continuity entails similarity of the causal mechanisms underpinning similar functions. Human beings are phylogenetically closer to pigs than rats, LaFollette and Shanks point out, but the way we metabolise phenol (80% by sulfation reactions and 12% glucoronidation conjugation reactions) is more like rats (45% through sulfation conjugation reactions) than pigs (95% through glucoronidation conjugation reactions).

The only way to be sure that animals *are* good models for human beings when it comes to the causal mechanisms underlying function, as opposed to the function itself, says LaFollette and Shanks, is to conduct experiments on humans. Animal testing is supposed to eliminate the need for this.

According to LaFolette and Shanks the undisputed functional similarities between animals predict that animals *will* be useful as *hypothetical analogical models* (HAMs) similar to the planetary model of the atom, for example, or the spiral staircase that helped Watson form his idea about the structure of DNA. Such models help to generate hypotheses that can then be tested (on humans). Much of the success of animal experimentation can, they say, be traced to the use of animals as HAMs.

But given the complexity of organisms, the way their systems and sub-systems have evolved separately and the fact that they interact with each other, say LaFollette and Shanks, animals are unlikely to be good *causal analogue models* (CAMs), good models for investigating the causal mechanisms that produce and direct the course of a disease or a condition. Many of the failures of animal experimentation – which according to LaFollette and Shanks often go unreported – can be traced to their misuse as CAMs.

In support of their contention LaFollette and Shanks cite numerous studies that have foundered because they were grounded on false assumptions of causal similarity. Such evidence demonstrates, they say, that inferences from animals to humans are not as well grounded as researchers might think.

But surely, we might think, animal research couldn't have been as successful as it has been if it is based on these false beliefs?

(ii) The history of research on animals

'There is considerable evidence,' say LaFollette and Shanks, 'that interventionist medicine has played only a relatively small role in lengthening life and improving health.' To support their contention they quote the *Lancet*:

'Public Health legislation and related measures have probably done more than all the advances of scientific medicine to promote the well-being of the community in Britain and other countries.'[31]

They also provide some figures:

'Life expectancy in the US increased 43% from 1900 to 1950 – before the advent of many medical treatment and vaccines. Since 1950 lifespan has increased 7.4%. Since the rate of mortality from motor vehicle accidents has decreased by more than 20% since 1950, that accounts for most of the increase in life expectancy.'[32]

But even if we accept this, we surely can't deny that 'interventionist medicine' has also had huge success?

Well, say LaFollette and Shanks, it depends how we measure success. This cannot be done, they warn, by 'tallying successes' as reported in literature surveys and histories. Such sources tend to draw on published data which represent a very small sample of experiments, and tend to be chosen by editors to cater for the tastes of readers.

Experimental failures, furthermore, are grossly under-reported. If a researcher spends time and effort trying to discover the nature of AIDS by examining rats and then discovers that rats don't develop AIDS, they point out, this is unlikely to get a mention. Finally, they argue:

'Many biomedical historians are members of the disciplines about which they are reporting. Since vivisection is integral to these disciplines we should not be surprised that these histories often emphasise its successes.'[33]

LaFollette and Shanks believe that animal research is nowhere near as scientifically useful as people believe and that we often, therefore, cause scientifically unnecessary animal suffering. If LaFollette and Shanks are right then even allowing that use of animals for research can be consistent with our duties to animals, this does not mean that our current uses of animals *are* morally acceptable.

Alternatives to the use of animals for scientific research

Those who are unhappy about the use of animals in research, or who believe that many uses of animals are morally unacceptable, usually suggest that scientists do not pay enough attention to alternatives to the use of animals.[34] Alternatives currently available include:[35]

- Experimenting on cell cultures instead of whole animals;
- Using computer models;
- Studying human volunteers;
- Using epidemiological studies.

Few would accept that such alternatives could, at the moment, replace the use of animals in research. But it seems clear that our duties to animals require us to search diligently for more and better alternatives.

Box 20.14 Activity: Research and discussion

Divide participants into two groups.

Group One: should conduct research into the arguments of those who believe that the use of animals in medical science is less useful than we might think.

Group Two: should conduct research into the successful use of animals in medical science.

Both groups should prepare to present those arguments in the following debate:

This house believes that the use of animals in medical science does not promote the GHGN.

The moral acceptability of using animals

It seems clear that justifying the claim that a given use of animals is morally acceptable depends on our asking many questions about that particular use of animals. We need to know, broadly, that *it* will not brutalise those performing it, that *it* is consistent with the interests of the animals used, and that *it* will promote the GHGN. Acquiring such knowledge will depend on our asking, and answering satisfactorily, the right questions. In Box 20.15, you will find a description of the regulatory regime current in the UK, a regime that relies on this process.

Box 20.15 Factual information: Animal protection in the UK

The approach taken in the UK to animal welfare, especially in scientific research, is grounded on the 'three Rs'.[36] This requires that before a 'procedure' (experiment on animals) will be licensed (and every procedure must be licensed) three questions must have been answered:

- **Refinement:** can we refine the procedure to reduce animal suffering?
- **Reduction:** can we use fewer animals, of types less likely to suffer?
- **Replacement:** can we achieve our aim without using animals?[37]

The answer to each of these questions must be 'no' before the procedure will be licensed.

Each procedure furthermore can be conducted only:

- by an individual licensed to conduct that procedure on those animals (no one can remove the toe of a frog for identification purposes unless they have been trained to remove the toes of frogs for identification purposes);
- in an institution licensed to keep and use animals for research and to satisfy all the animal welfare regulations imposed (no institution will be licensed unless they demonstrate that trained individuals feed, house, entertain and care for the animals in accordance with their needs and preferences).

Licences are issued by the Home Office only when it is satisfied that individuals are properly trained, institutions properly run, and the three Rs properly considered.[38]

The questions we must ask about any given use of animals must cover not only the procedure, but also the care animals receive before and after the procedure. If the way we capture, transport and train them distresses them this counts. If they are social animals but housed individually this counts. If they are playful animals who aren't given toys, this counts. If they are killed clumsily this counts. From the moment an animal comes into our hands, to the moment it is released, or killed, its care must be scrutinised to ensure it is consistent with our duty not to cause unnecessary suffering.

Whether suffering counts as necessary will not always be obvious. It is not possible, for example, to say what suffering will be caused by subjecting animals to known mutagens to produce random mutations, or by using them to test a drug for side effects. Failure to achieve our experimental aims will not automatically lead to unnecessary suffering because we can learn a lot from failures, but we wouldn't want to have too many, so the chances of success must be considered. Sometimes the hoped-for benefit of a procedure might be large enough to justify a high risk of failure.

Even if answering our questions is not always easy, however, the important point is that the questions are asked. It is only by asking them of every procedure, and by making sure they are answered satisfactorily, that we can be sure our uses of animals for scientific research are justified.

Box 20.16 Activity: Identifying the right questions

Participants should read this case study, adapted from one provided by the National Council of Bioethics, then decide which questions would need to be answered to decide whether this use of animals is morally acceptable.

This particular procedure uses 18-month-old macaque monkeys. Its aim is to understand how activity in groups of brain cells in the motor cortex controls specific hand and finger movements.

Before the research starts the monkeys are trained, and 3D scans of their skulls and brains are taken. This permits accurate targeting of the brain areas from which recordings will be made.

Once a monkey is trained a head restraint device and recording chamber are attached to it by means of four bone screws of 3 mm diameter, threaded through holes in its skull and secured from within. These weigh 150 g and consist of a metal ring 10 cm diameter and 1 mm thick. Electrodes are also implanted to record the activity of nerve cells and muscles.

During the procedure itself the monkey is restrained by connecting the ring screwed to its skull to a metal disc attached to a steel chair. It can move its jaw and body but its head is immobilised to allow for stable recording of the activity of single neurones.

Multiple micro-electrodes are inserted through the implanted recording chamber into the monkey's brain. The electrodes are attached to a computer and to devices recording the muscle activity in the monkey's arm and hand.

The monkey is then required to use its thumb and index fingers to squeeze two levers. Once sufficient data are obtained on the link between one neural area and the hand movements, the electrodes are inserted into a new area of the brain.

Each week there are 3–5 sessions lasting 3 hours each. Over 18 months each monkey provides 100–200 fully analysed neurones.

At the end of the procedure the monkey is given a deep anaesthetic from which it does not recover. This permits researchers to verify the position of the electrodes.[39]

Answer: These are very broad questions that should be asked. Under each broad question are many more specific questions that might be brought out in discussion. The answers to many of the questions that will be asked will be found in the original case study.[40]

(i)   Do we have to use primates in this experiment or might we use other, less sensitive, animals?
(ii) Could the number of monkeys used be reduced? Might we achieve our aims by other means?
(iii) Might the experiment, or activities surrounding it, be refined to reduce the monkeys' suffering?
(iv) What benefits will be derived from this experiment?
(v)   Are the benefits accompanied by any risks?

(vi)   What is the likelihood of successfully achieving the aim of this experiment?
(vii)   Does this experiment duplicate existing work?
(viii) Are the monkeys' preferences catered for before, after and where possible during the experiment?
(ix)   Are safeguards in place to protect 'whistleblowers'?
(x)   Are staff emotionally 'alive' to the monkeys' suffering?
(xi)   Are we overriding strong intuitions against this use of monkeys?

The public perception of the use of animals for research

One unfortunate result of the activities of the less law-abiding parts of the animal liberation movement since the 1970s[41] has been to encourage researchers using animals to go 'underground' (sometimes literally[42]). In fear of their livelihoods, or even their lives, researchers have been reluctant to subject their activities to public scrutiny.[43]

Arguably the effect of this has not been conducive to public acceptance of animal research; many suspect this lack of transparency is prompted by arrogance and rejection of the idea that such research needs justification. Such suspicions are exploited by animal rights' extremists.

The case for animal research has not been helped by the results of various undercover operations by animal rights' activists. Some of these have led to public outrage, prosecutions and the revoking of licences.

Box 20.17 Case studies: Undercover investigations of animal abuse

In 1996 Huntingdon Life Sciences was infiltrated by a journalist who filmed a member of staff punching a beagle held by another member of staff.[44] Two employees, admitting to charges of 'cruelly terrifying' dogs, were prosecuted under the Protection of Animals Act 1911 and dismissed.

The National Anti-Vivisection Society undertook an undercover investigation into the Charing Cross and Westminster Medical School in 1994–95.[45] They presented their report to the Home Office. The resulting investigation found 'irregularities in the application of approved methods for the humane killing of animals and deficiencies in middle management'. The school's licence for keeping animals for research purposes was revoked until it had retrained staff and made changes to its arrangements for animal care.[46]

A few institutions[47] are starting, as a result of this, to increase transparency. Huntingdon Life Sciences, for example, has instituted a programme of visits by schools, colleges and the local community as well as MPs. They have also helped to make several television documentaries on animal use in research. The Nuffield Council on Bioethics has welcomed such initiatives, arguing that freedom of information is essential to debate:

'It would be desirable for the public to have, as far as possible and subject to appropriate levels of safety for those involved in research, access to detailed information about the kinds of animal research, the numbers and species of animals used in specific research projects, the full implications in terms of pain, suffering and distress for the animals involved, and the intended benefits of the work.'[48]

Another move that would help would be to take steps to facilitate and reward whistle-blowing. If those employed in institutions which use animals are encouraged to report abuses – intentional or otherwise – of animals, and rewarded for doing so, this would send the important message that such abuse is unacceptable.

> ### Box 20.18 **Activity: Brainstorm**
>
> Participants should brainstorm on ways scientists might help to change the public perception of research using animals.
>
> Participants might prepare by reading about Pro-Test. This is a group that was started by 16-year-old Laurie Pycroft who was frustrated by the way animal rights activists were dominating the public debate:
>
> http://www.pro-test.org.uk/.

We have considered the importance of the public perception of science elsewhere (see Chapter 17, page 338ff.). The public perception of the use, by science, of animals is a particularly important area: the only way science can be sure of avoiding adverse publicity in respect of its treatment of animals is to live up to its duties to animals, and to be seen to do so.

Summary

In this chapter we have considered the moral acceptability of using animals for our own ends. In particular we have:

- considered Descartes' claim that animals are not conscious;
- noted that we can reasonably claim to have objective means of determining animal preferences;
- reflected on deontological positions regarding the use of animals especially:
  - Kant's claim that we brutalise ourselves in mistreating animals;
  - Feinberg's claim that animals have interests because they are sentient;

- Scruton's claim that animals are not persons, but their interests constrain our treatment of them;
- Regan's claim that animals are ends in themselves.

- learned about Singer's utilitarian position and his development of the 'animal liberation movement';

- reflected on the difference between the rights ascribed to animals by Regan and Singer;

- examined the claim that animal experimentation is not as scientifically valid as people think;

- asked whether killing animals could be consistent with their interests;

- looked at the alternatives to using animals in research;

- learned about the Great Ape Project;

- reflected on animal rights activism and the public perception of using animals for research.

Questions to stimulate reflection

Why should anyone think that animals are capable of experiencing pleasure and pain? Are there any considerations that tell against this?

Should we agree that anything capable of experiencing pleasure and pain is intrinsically valuable? If so should we accord it absolute rights?

Is there reason for or against thinking the interests of animals should count for less in the utilitarian calculus than the interests of human beings?

Is speciesism really as morally unacceptable as racism or sexism?

Are our duties to animals indirect duties to human beings or direct duties to the animals themselves? Does this matter?

What would a virtue ethicist have to say about the use of animals for scientific research?

Can you describe three different deontological views on the proper use of animals?

What are the conditions under which a utilitarian would refuse to use an animal for a given procedure?

Additional activities

If you are in, near or can travel to an institution that conducts experiments on animals, see if you can take a guided tour of their facilities or conduct an interview with one of the researchers about the welfare of their animals.

Conduct an opinion poll among family and friends on the use of animals in research.

Write to the government department with responsibility for implementing regulation on animal research in your country. Ask them whether the regulations they implement rule out unnecessary animal suffering.

Write to an animal rights organisation in your country asking them why the regulations governing research on animals in your country do not, in their opinion, prevent unacceptable uses of animals.

Try not to eat meat for a week. Look into the economic case for vegetarianism and consider the ethical case. At the end of the week write 500 words on why you have decided (on not) to become a vegetarian.

Notes

1 Abbot, A. in *Nature*, **432**, 541
2 http://www.understandinganimalresearch.org.uk/resources/videos_library/details/265/mice_in_medical_research/.
3 http://iowa.sierraclub.org/icag/2004/1104quotes.pdf.
4 Dawkins, R. (1993) Gaps in the mind. In P. Cavalieri and P. Singer (eds), *The Great Ape Project*. New York: St. Martin's Griffin, pp. 81–87.
5 http://renedescartes.com/.
6 http://www.iep.utm.edu/anim-eth/#SH1c. Descartes' views on animals from the *Internet Encyclopedia of Philosophy*.
7 http://plato.stanford.edu/entries/other-minds/. The *Stanford Encyclopedia of Philosophy* on other minds.
8 http://users.ox.ac.uk/~snikwad/. Marian Stamp Dawkins' webpages.
9 Stamp Dawkins, M. (2006) Scientific basis for assessing suffering in animals. In P. Singer (ed.), *In Defence of Animals*. Oxford: Blackwell, p. 28.
10 http://www.people.fas.harvard.edu/~korsgaar/CMK.FellowCreatures.pdf. A philosophical essay on Kant's view of animals. Accessible to non-philosophers.
11 http://www.nytimes.com/2004/04/05/us/joel-feinberg-77-influential-philosopher.html. An obituary of Joel Feinberg in the New York Times.
12 Feinberg, J. (1980) The rights of animals and unborn generations. In J. Feinberg (ed.), *Rights, Justice, and the Bounds of Liberty: Essays in Social Philosophy*. Princeton, NJ: Princeton University Press, pp. 159–84, at 166–7 [essay first published in 1974].
13 http://www.roger-scruton.com/. Roger Scruton's website.
14 Scruton, R. (2000) *Animal Rights and Wrongs*. London: Claridge Press.
15 http://www.animalsvoice.com/TomRegan//regan.html.
16 Regan, T. (2004) *The Case for Animal Rights*. Berkeley, CA: University of California Press. Also Regan, T. (2007) *Defending Animal Rights*. Champaign, IL: University of Illinois Press.
17 http://www.princeton.edu/~psinger/. Peter Singer's webpages.
18 http://www.utilitarian.org/texts/alm.html. The Animal Liberation Movement. Singer, P. (1995) *Animal Liberation*. London: Pimlico.
19 http://www.philosophybites.libsyn.com/category/Peter%20Singer. Peter Singer on human uses of animals for Philosophy Bites.

20 http://www.bbc.co.uk/ethics/animals/rights/speciesism.shtml. The BBC on speciesism.

21 http://ruralgrocery.com/womenscenter/W.A.R/Animal%20Quotes.pdf.

22 http://ruralgrocery.com/womenscenter/W.A.R/Animal%20Quotes.pdf, p. 76.

23 http://www.youtube.com/watch?v=30DOJZHg4qA. A video on the Great Ape Project.

24 http://www.utilitarian.net/singer/by/200605–.htm.

25 http://cfhs.ca/info/genetic_modification_of_livestock/.

26 AMA (1988) The use of animals in biomedical research: the challenge and response. AMA White Paper, p.16.

27 http://news.bbc.co.uk/1/hi/sci/tech/425120.stm. The BBC on xenotransplantation.

28 http://www.pbs.org/wgbh/pages/frontline/shows/organfarm/etc/faqs.html.

29 Lafollette, H. and Shanks, N. (1995) Two models of models in biomedical research. *The Philosophical Quarterly,* **45**(179), 141–160. http://www.hughlafollette.com/papers/two.models.of.models.pdf.

30 Lafollette, H. and Shanks, N. (1997) *Brute Science: Dilemmas of Animal Experimentation.* London: Routledge.

31 *The Lancet,* August 1978, p. 354.

32 Lafollette, H. and Shanks, N. (1995) Utilising animals. *Journal of Applied Philosophy,* **12**(1), 13–25.

33 Lafollette and Shanks (1995) Utilising animals.

34 http://www.nc3rs.org.uk/downloaddoc.asp?id=1013.

35 http://www.aboutanimaltesting.co.uk/new-technologies-alternatives-animal-testing.html.

36 http://www.nc3rs.org.uk/landing.asp?id=2. The National Association for the 3Rs (NA3Rs).

37 http://www.nc3rs.org.uk/page.asp?id=7. An explanation of the three Rs.

38 Animals (Scientific Procedures) Act 1986.

39 Adapted from Box 5.4 of *The Ethics of Research Involving Animals,* the Nuffield Council of Bioethics, 1996.

40 Case study adapted from Box 5.4 of *The Ethics of Research Involving Animals,* the Nuffield Council for Bioethics, 1996.

41 http://news.bbc.co.uk/1/hi/england/7795558.stm.

42 http://www.the-scientist.com/blog/display/55764/.

43 http://news.bbc.co.uk/1/hi/uk/6610429.stm.

44 http://www.independent.co.uk/news/uk/politics/the-laboratory-huntingdon-life-sciences-702932.html.

45 http://www.navs.org.uk/about_vivisection/27/42/336/.

46 Adapted from Box 2.5 of *The Ethics of Research Involving Animals,* the Nuffield Council of Bioethics, 1996.

47 http://news.bbc.co.uk/1/hi/health/7721919.stm. A BBC report on Oxford University's animal labs.

48 *The Ethics of Research Involving Animals,* the Nuffield Council of Bioethics 1996, p. 29.

Further reading and useful websites

DeGrazia, D. (2002) *A Very Short Introduction to Animal Rights.* Oxford: Oxford Paperbacks.

Gluck, J., DiPasquale, P. and Orlans, F. B. (eds) (2000) *Applied Ethics in Animal Research: Philosophy, Regulation and Laboratory Applications.* West Lafayette, IN: Purdue University Press.

Orlans, F. B., Beauchamp, T. L., Dresser, R., Morton, D. B. and Gluck, J. P. (2008) *The Human Use of Animals: Case Studies in Ethical Choice.* New York: Oxford University Press USA.

Singer, P. (2005) *In Defense of Animals: The Second Wave.* Oxford: Wiley Blackwell.

http://www.debatingmatters.com/topicguides/topicguide/animal_experimentation/. A topic guide with resources from Debating Matters.

http://www.nuffieldbioethics.org/go/ourwork/animalresearch/introduction. The ethics of research involving animals, the Nuffield Council of Bioethics 1996 (also see: http://www.nuffieldbioethics.org/education/education-teaching-resource-use-animals-research).

http://www.philosophybites.libsyn.com/jeff_mc_mahan_on_vegetarianism. A discussion of vegetarianism by philosopher Jeff McMahon.

21 The living and non-living environment: Spaceship Earth

Objectives

In reading this chapter you will:

- consider why we might believe we have duties to the environment;
- reflect on the source of these duties;
- consider how the different moral theories would view duties to the environment;
- examine the nature of these duties;
- examine the threat of climate change and the duties it imposes;
- reflect on climate-change scepticism;
- reflect on the threat of mass species extinction.

There are broadly three positions we might take on our duties to the environment:[1]

Anthropocentrism: we have direct[2] duties to ourselves; everything else is only of instrumental value;

Biocentrism: we have direct duties to ourselves and to (certain) other living things; the non-living environment is only of instrumental value;

Ecocentrism: we have direct duties to ourselves, other living things *and* the non-living environment.

Plenty of people would add to or cross-cut these distinctions. But let's consider each in turn.

Anthropocentrism

Human beings, like other living things, have always used nature as a resource. Some think that until the Industrial Revolution we acted in harmony with nature, but that since then our activities have thrown nature comprehensively out of balance. The latter part of this claim, at least, seems justified if we believe those who say our activities are implicated in climate change and in the sixth great extinction of planetary history. We shall discuss both below.

Our belated recognition of the possible consequences of our disregard for nature means that anthropocentrism, understood as grounding our right to use nature unthinkingly, has become untenable. There are few anthropocentrists who would these days make such a claim. Enlightened anthropocentrism[3] argues that the only *direct* duties we have are to other human beings, but that we should recognise many *indirect* duties to other parts of nature. These duties require us to use nature only in such a way that as much and as good is left for future generations.

> ### Box 21.1 Activity: Web-wandering
>
> Put 'stewardship' and 'environment' into an online search engine together with the name of the religion of your family or culture.
>
> Identify, read about and reflect on how members of this religion would justify an enlightened anthropocentrism.

Perhaps counterintuitively it has been suggested, by the philosopher William Grey,[4] that adopting an enlightened anthropocentric viewpoint is a necessary condition of being an environmentalist. It is only from this viewpoint, says Grey, that our activities can properly be seen as 'damaging' to the planet. The disaster that led to the death of the dinosaurs, for example, wiped out 85% of all species.[5] But for the planet this was just another incident. The extinction of all those species merely paved the way for other species to flourish.

What worries us, says Grey, and rightly so, is that our activities might render the planet uninhabitable *for us* and for the species we rely upon and care about. If we take ourselves out of the equation, says Grey, then there is no *right* and *wrong* way for the planet to continue, no way of saying that it is *good or bad* that certain species evolve and others do not, or that the climate is *too* hot or *too* cold.

> ### Box 21.2 Activity: Discussion topic
>
> *Adopting an anthropocentric position is a necessary condition of claiming that we are damaging our planet.*
>
> Participants should discuss this in pairs or as a group.

Biocentrism

There are three biocentric positions:

Mild biocentrism: rational living things matter morally.
Moderate biocentrism: sentient living things matter morally.
Radical biocentrism: all living things matter morally.

The first two positions were discussed in the last chapter (although in connection with animals, and not under the title 'biocentrism'). In this chapter, therefore, we shall discuss only the final position.

Radical biocentrism

The radical biocentrist argues that *all* living things matter morally. If this is true we owe direct duties not just to human beings and to rational and sentient animals, but also to centipedes, ants and spiders, to mussels, nematodes and sea slugs, to maize, cauliflowers and roses, woodworm, Japanese knotweed and the HIV virus (if viruses are living things). Why, though, should we accept that such things matter morally?

Paul Taylor[6] argues that each individual living thing is a 'teleological-centre-of-life' because it has 'a good of its own'. Having goods of their own, says Taylor, living things have *interests* and are therefore ends in themselves.[7] Like Tom Regan, therefore (see Chapter 20, pp. 401–403) Taylor thinks that having interests suffices for being an end, but he rejects the idea that sentience (never mind rationality) is necessary: it is a sufficient condition, he thinks, for having interests, that a thing be *alive*.

One way to make sense of this is to see that if we feed and water roses well they flourish. If we do neither, they sicken and die. There are conditions we might say, in which they 'choose' to live, and other conditions in which they 'choose' to die. For Taylor this amounts to an interest in being fed and watered well. This is not a *subjective* interest, i.e. roses don't literally *care* about being fed and watered, but it is still an interest.

> ### Box 21.3 Activity: Personal reflection
>
> If we allow that non-sentient, non-rational things have *interests* might this impact on other moral problems such as abortion and therapeutic cloning?

We might want to object that radical biocentrism extends moral status to too many things. To embrace it, for example, is to think that not only embryos, but also eggs and sperm, and possibly viruses, like the HIV virus, are ends in themselves. We might also think that it would leave us very hungry: how after all can we justify *eating* something that is an end in itself?

But just as the utilitarian can justify causing unhappiness in pursuit of greater happiness a radical biocentrist can justify taking life to promote life. Radical biocentrism locates intrinsic value in the consequences of our actions for *life* rather than happiness. On page 43 we considered various types of consequentialists. The radical biocentrist is a consequentialist. This has radical implications for our behaviour. It is impossible to argue, for example, that we need to eat meat to stay *alive*. Indeed eating meat probably *costs* lives given the detrimental effects of saturated fat. It would be difficult to be a radical biocentrist without being a vegetarian.

So the radical biocentrist would not starve to death. Nor would he be forced to preserve the HIV virus at the expense of human lives.

There is something compelling, furthermore, about the idea that life is *itself* intrinsically valuable. When we send probes to other planets one of the things we are most interested in finding is *life* of some – any – kind. If *all* life is intrinsically valuable, however, our conception of our place in nature would have to change dramatically. As with racism and sexism however these radical changes in attitude might be morally required.

> ### Box 21.4 Activity: Paired reflection
>
> If we go along with Singer (Chapter 13, pages 227–230) in thinking that it is the *quality of life* that matters does this mean we can't be radical biocentrists?

Ecocentrism

The ecocentrist is even more generous than the radical biocentrist in his account of moral status. He believes it is not just individual living things that matter but also whole ecosystems and species, and for some ecocentrists, even the built environment; cities, towns, opera houses and football stadia. To the ecocentrist a tropical rainforest, a mountain and a stream are as intrinsically valuable as human beings.

The main difficulty for the ecocentrist is motivating this claim. Even if we incline towards according intrinsic value to things that have cognition, are sentient or are alive, we might baulk at according *intrinsic* value to mountains, streams, deserts and forests, never mind buildings.

Many attempts have been made to motivate this claim. Goodin,[8] for example, following Rolston,[9] has argued that ecosystems are intrinsically valuable because of the naturalness of the historical processes that have produced them. Our arguments in Chapter 6, pages 22–76, undermine this argument: we saw there that being natural is neither necessary nor sufficient for something's being morally good. Earthquakes, after all, are natural, and hospitals are not.

Rodman argues that things that have a capacity for *autopoiesis*,[10] internal self-direction and self-regulation, are intrinsically valuable.[11] Fox suggests that 'responsive cohesion' is the key[12] believing this demonstrates that the built environment is also intrinsically valuable (so long as it is responsively cohesive, i.e. structured in such a way that its constituents are flexibly responsive to each other).[13]

These claims suggest that the planet itself, which is undeniably natural, self-regulating and responsively cohesive, is intrinsically valuable independently of whatever lives on it. But why we should accept that being natural, and/or self-regulating and/or responsively cohesive, is a sufficient condition for being *intrinsically* valuable? Arguably the HIV virus satisfies all these conditions but is it intrinsically valuable?

Another way of motivating the ecocentrists' claim is to argue that *everything* is constituted by its relations to everything else. This suggests that our intuitive desire to see the individual as primary is wrong. The individual is nothing more than a 'node' in a network of relationships. It is the relationships that are primary. One way of understanding this is to think of a spider's web, where the slightest impact on any part of the web affects every other part of the web.

Such claims are made by people like Arne Naess,[14] Aldo Leopold,[15] Richard Routley[16] (later Sylvan) and James Lovelock,[17] leaders of the 'deep ecology movement'.[18] Some deep ecologists (for example, Naess) believe that the planet is akin to a living system, others believe the whole planet *is* a living system (Lovelock). To deep ecologists the destruction of *anything* impacts on *everything*.

Deep ecology is set against 'shallow ecology', the fight against pollution and resource depletion. This distinction cross-cuts that between anthropocentrists, biocentrists and ecocentrists: Lovelock, for example, because he believes that the planet is a living system, might be counted as a biocentrist rather than an ecocentrist.

Box 21.5 Activity: Thought experiment: the last person

Imagine that a catastrophe has left only one living thing – a person – on earth. This person is dying.

As his last act this person destroys the planet.

The question to be answered is: did he do anything *wrong*?

If your intuition suggests he did do wrong does this demonstrate that the planet itself, independently of the living things it supports, has value? If not how would you explain this intuition?

This thought experiment, known as 'The Last Man Argument', is adapted from that used to stimulate discussion at a conference in 1973 by Richard Routley.

Environmental ethics

On *none* of the positions discussed is it acceptable for humankind to act as if the only thing that matters is the immediate needs of human beings. It is not necessary to be an ecocentrist, for example, to believe that we have duties – perhaps indirect ones – to the non-living environment, or a radical biocentrist to believe we have duties – again perhaps indirect – to all living things.

Identifying these duties, however, is not a simple matter. Even if we need only take into account the direct effect on *us* of our interactions with the environment we still need to know much more about how the environment works, about the resources we use and about the effects of our actions on the environment.

All of these questions, of course, are empirical questions. In environmental ethics (as elsewhere) science and philosophy must work together to identify how we should act.

In the rest of this chapter we shall consider two problems in environmental ethics – climate change and species extinction – to see how our duties to the environment might impact on our behaviour, and on how biotechnology can help (or hinder).

Climate change

The climate on Earth has changed many times in the past.[19] It will continue to do so too, thanks to the 'Milankovitch cycles',[20] variations in the way the earth's eccentricity, axial tilt, and precession affect the earth's circumnavigation of the sun. Once there was no ice even at the poles. Once there was ice over Europe, much of Asia and even parts of Africa. Climate change is nothing new.[21]

But the climate is currently undergoing a change that *is* new. A change for which, arguably, *we* are responsible. Since the Industrial Revolution our economies, at least in the developed world, have been driven by the burning of fossil fuels:[22] coal, gas and oil.[23] The emissions produced by burning such fuels, together with our destruction of the rain forests (which act like 'sinks' to soak up CO_2),[24] are thought to be producing an effect on the atmosphere of the earth that is producing global warming: a significant and worrying increase in the average temperature around the globe.

To see how this works we need to understand the so-called 'greenhouse effect'.

The greenhouse effect

The earth's atmosphere is surrounded by a layer of gases that let the sun's heat through to earth then, like a greenhouse, trap just enough of it inside the earth's atmosphere to keep the average global temperature comfortable. These gases include water vapour, methane, carbon dioxide (CO_2) and nitrous oxide.

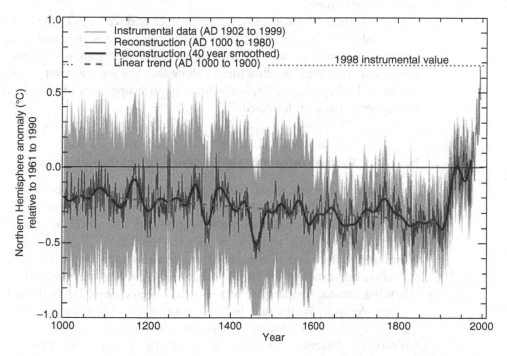

Figure 21.1 The so-called 'hockey stick' graph suggesting that climate change is the result of industrialisation. Source: *IPCC Third Assessment Report – Climate Change 2001.* UNEP/GRID-Arendal.

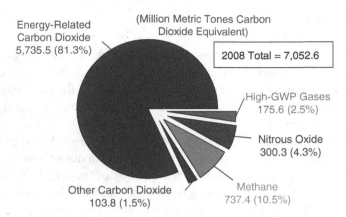

Figure 21.2 US greenhouse gas emissions by gas, 2008. Source: Emissions of Greenhouse Gases in the United States Report, US Energy Information Administration (2008).

Our activities, however, have greatly increased the concentration of some of these greenhouse gases, especially CO_2, thereby producing an *enhanced* greenhouse effect.[25]

Much more of the sun's heat is now trapped in our atmosphere, increasing temperatures around the globe. Studies show, for example, that the average global temperature has increased by 0.75% over the last 100 years. It won't be long, if we continue as we are, before the temperature becomes high enough to have effects that could be catastrophic.

Global warming[26] has already, for example, caused sea levels to rise by 10 cm.[27] This is not only because the glaciers, permafrost and ice caps are melting and releasing more water into the oceans,[28] it is also because water expands as it warms and absorbs more heat than land. Satellite images show that the sea-ice cover in the Arctic has decreased by 30% since 1978, and submarine measurements suggest the thickness of the ice cover has also decreased.[29]

Box 21.6 **Factual information: Evidence for global warming**

Temperature increase: global temperatures have increased by about 0.75°C over the past century and 2000–09 was the warmest decade on record.

Changes in rainfall patterns: wetter regions of the world are generally getting increasing rainfall, and drier regions less rainfall.

Humidity: surface and satellite observations show moisture in the atmosphere has increased over the last 20–30 years, meaning all the more water to fall in rain.

Warming oceans: temperature increases have been observed over the last 50 years in the Atlantic, Pacific and Indian Ocean basins. These cannot be attributed to changes in solar activity, volcanic eruptions or variations in ocean currents.

Salinity: the Atlantic Ocean is becoming saltier in sub-tropical latitudes thanks to an increase in ocean evaporation. In the long-term the melting of ice and increase in rainfall is expected to make ocean regions at higher latitude less salty.

Sea-ice: summer minimum of Arctic sea-ice is declining at a rate of 600,000 km^2 per decade, an area approximately the size of Madagascar.

Antarctic: sea-ice in the Antarctic has increased slightly since the satellite record began in 1978. This is consistent with the combined effects of greenhouse gas increases and reductions in the ozone layer because these cause increases in some regions, such as the Ross Sea, and decreases in others, such as the Amundsen-Bellingshausen Sea.[30]

Half of the world's population (1.5 billion people) live on the coast.[31] A dramatic rise in sea level will produce flooding on a grand scale and make large tracts of land uninhabitable.[32] Flooding on this scale will not just affect the fishing villages of East Asia, but cities like London, New York, Sydney and Tokyo. The British Government's Office for Science imagines people having to move from the south-east of England to new cities in Dumfries and Galloway, Northumberland and Powys.[33] Such mass migrations have happened before, but rarely from places like London.

A rise in sea temperature will also increase the frequency and intensity of hurricanes, tornados and other severe weather. It will also disrupt ocean currents, and make some places hotter and drier. Rivers and lakes will dry up leading to drought, forest fire,[34] and in some places, famine.

Recently it has been discovered that methane levels, over thousands of square miles of the Siberian continental shelf, are 100 times background levels.[35] This has prompted fears that the 100s of tonnes of methane trapped in the permafrost is being released as the permafrost melts. This would greatly accelerate global warming. Methane is a more powerful greenhouse gas than CO_2.

Climate change 'denial'

Not everyone accepts that global warming is happening, and many people deny that climate change is down to us.[36]

About 47% of Americans, 37% of Chinese and 26% of Britons believe it is a conspiracy on the part of the green lobby to halt or reduce global development, for example, Melanie Phillips of the *Daily Mail* says:

'Global warming is a massive scam based on flawed computer modelling, bad science and an anti-western ideology . . . The majority of well-meaning opinion in the western world believes a pack of lies and propaganda.'

For climate change and global warming to be a conspiracy, though, given the consensus on climate change, would be for the green lobby to have most of the world's scientists in its pocket. This seems unlikely.

Others, however, are worried by what they see as the evidence of their own eyes. The last two winters in the northern hemisphere, for example, have been extremely harsh. Many people believe this is inconsistent with global warming.

But this confuses the *weather* with the *climate*.[37] The weather consists in the temperature and precipitation (wind, rain, sleet, snow) at a time or over a relatively short period. The weather changes every day and every hour (and in the UK every minute). Changes in the weather are constant and a threat only to our barbecues and picnics.

The climate, on the other hand, is a function of the average temperature over the whole surface of the earth taken over time. And this in turn is a function not only of the heat of the sun but also of the way the ocean, which covers 71% of the earth's surface, takes water heated by the sun from the equator to the poles and around the globe.

Since 1992 the thermohaline circulation[38] in the Atlantic has slowed by one third. Computer models suggest this will continue. If it does the temperature in north-western Europe might fall by 3–4%.[39] Winters will become extremely harsh.[40] It is possible this is the result of global warming. It is also possible it is contributing to global warming. Either way, it is consistent with global warming, and the idea that global warming is causing climate change.

Some people allow that global warming is happening, but deny that *we* are responsible for it. Václav Klaus, for example, the President of Czech Republic, claims that climate change is caused 'not by human behaviour but by various exogenous and endogenous natural processes (such as fluctuating solar activity)'.[41]

A recent study by senior scientists from The Met Office Hadley Centre, the universities of Edinburgh and Melbourne and Victoria University in Canada, however, concluded that there is only a 5% chance that natural variations in the climate are responsible for the changes that justify claims about global warming.[42] In 2007 the Intergovernmental Panel on Climate Change (IPCC) assessed more than 100 recent peer-reviewed papers. The overwhelming majority, they found, demonstrated clear evidence of human influence on the climate.[43]

Given this, why do so many people believe, in the words of John Houghton, the former CEO of the Met Office, that 'they are being steam-rollered into believing something false or flakey that will make them poorer or stop them flying'?[44]

Is it that the science is difficult for non-scientists to understand? Is it because people are reluctant to accept that their comfortable way of life must change,[45] because scientists are not successfully explaining the science,[46] or because governments are failing to convince people of the need for change?[47] Or is it some combination of these things?[48]

Box 21.7 Activity: Research and discussion: climate-change scepticism

Recently climate-change scepticism has been on the increase. There are three reasons for this:

(i)   The leaking of emails between climate-change scientists, that seemed to suggest that 'tricks' were being used to suppress research suggesting a decline in global temperatures;

(ii) A UN report, based on an article in the *New Scientist*, which falsely claimed that the Himalayan glaciers would melt by 2035. The article was later discovered to rest on a telephone conversation with an Indian scientist, who admitted he had no evidence to support his claim.

(iii) When the Met Office in England published on its website all its land-based temperature records, bloggers immediately found many mistakes.

Participants should conduct research on climate-change scepticism, and in particular these three reasons for it, then discuss, or write essays on, the following questions:

1. What is the scientific evidence for the claim that the climate is changing and that we are responsible?
2. What, other than the activities of human beings, might have caused global warming?
3. How good is the evidence for the claim we are causing it (how many scientists have corroborated it, are the credentials of these scientists good, do the different forms of evidence support each other)?
4. Why do the three events described above undermine this evidence?
5. Are there comparisons to be made and lessons learned from comparing the debate about climate-change with the debate about GM food?
6. What might be done by scientists to combat the idea that the climate is not changing and/or the idea that we are not responsible?

If the climate is changing this threatens our way of life. If we can avert this, it seems reasonable to think we have a moral duty – to future generations, if not to the planet itself – to try to avert this.

Preventing, mitigating or adapting to climate change

There are three responses we might make to prevent, or reduce the impact of, climate change:

(i)   we might reduce the emissions that contribute to the greenhouse effect;[49]
(ii) we might engage in geo-engineering to mitigate the enhanced greenhouse effect;[50]
(iii) we might accept and adapt to the changes in our climate.[51]

Reducing our carbon footprint

If the enhanced greenhouse effect is causing global warming, then we will have to stop emitting the gases that produce it, or find a way of capturing such emissions before they do more damage. We will have to stop burning fossil fuels or find a way of doing it more cleanly.

We will have to change our behaviour: no more driving to the shops, flying to Paris[52] or buying Peruvian asparagus,[53] no more felling the rain forests for garden furniture.[54]

Changing behaviour

But such small adjustments won't be enough. We'll probably have to stop using cars altogether or at least cars that run on fossil fuel, either directly (petrol or diesel) or

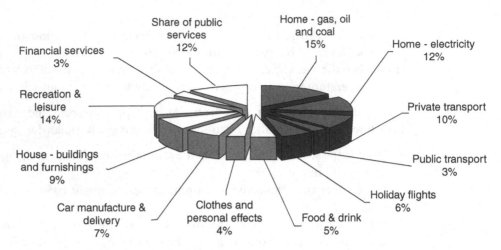

Figure 21.3 The main elements which make up the total of an typical person's carbon footprint in the developed world. Courtesy of www.carbonfootprint.com.

indirectly (fossil-fuel generated electricity or first generation biofuels).[55] Certainly we'll have to conduct our global business without the personal contact that is so costly in terms of aviation fuel.[56] We'll also almost certainly have to rethink our diet. At the very least we'll have to eat more seasonal and locally produced produce, more likely we'll all have to become vegetarians.

> **Box 21.8 Activity: Creative writing**
>
> Write 500–1,000 words on life without fossil fuel.

The difficulty, of course, is that no one likes change. Especially not changes that we perceive as making us less comfortable. It is all too easy to persuade ourselves that *this* drive to the shops, *this* holiday abroad, *this* roast lamb, couldn't possibly make much difference. And of course we are right, taken individually these acts won't make much difference. If everyone thinks like this, of course, then this approach to climate change is hopeless.

> **Box 21.9 Activity: Personal reflection**
>
> How many other activities can you think of that are not harmful if done by one person, but very harmful if done by many?
>
> How might we persuade people that *they* should not do something if *their* doing that thing will not be harmful?
>
> Do you think any of the theories discussed in Chapter 4 might have an answer to this?

The job of persuading significant numbers of people these changes are really necessary is likely to be achievable only by using the sort of levers – for example, education and taxation – available to the state. The media also have a major role to play. Some recent documentaries (for example *The End of the Line*[57] premiered at the Sundance Film Festival) have had serious awareness-raising success, as have 'edutainment' programmes[58] that seriously examine the cases for and against climate change, board games[59] and mobile phone 'apps'.[60]

Box 21.10 Factual information: The 'cap and trade' route to reducing emissions

Governments can encourage industry to reduce emissions by (i) setting a legal limit on the volume of greenhouse gases (GHG) that they will allow to be produced on their territory over a set duration, and then (ii) selling or giving permits to various companies allowing them to emit a negotiated share of this total.

If the company's emissions are higher then expected it will run out of permits. It must then do one of three things:

(i)   reduce its emissions;
(ii) buy permits from a company with emissions lower than expected;
(iii) earn credits by funding development in a poorer country (for example, by paying to plant a forest, or introduce green technology).

Permits and credits are traded like stocks and shares. If prices rise, they are more expensive, giving companies the incentive to be cleaner.

But if prices drop it can become cheaper to buy credits and continue burning coal than to invest in renewable energy. In Europe a tonne of carbon can currently be emitted for 13 Euros.

There are also other counterintuitive side effects of this market. Corus, the British steelmaker, recently decommissioned one of its steel plants. This meant it no longer needed its permits, and was able to sell them for a huge profit.

A recent evaluation of the European carbon credit scheme,[61] however, demonstrates it has been a huge success: cutting GHG emissions by 300 million tonnes over a 3-year period. This is equivalent to half the UK's annual emissions.

Could this scheme work globally to reduce emissions whilst supporting development?

Alternative sources of energy

One of the ways governments can help is by funding scientific research into alternative sources of energy.[62] As fossil fuel is running out even the so-called 'climate change deniers' have reason to support these initiatives.

Scientists are working on getting power from the waves,[63] the wind[64] and the sun.[65] As we saw in Chapter 17 our first attempts to get fuel from crops have not been an unmitigated success, but we are working on turning waste or algae into fuel and on producing cars that will run on electricity that is itself produced from sustainable sources.

Unfortunately, the alternative sources of energy we are currently considering are unlikely to fulfil our needs. The Institute for Energy Research in Germany recently found, for example, that Germany's renewable energy policy resulted in 'massive expenditures that show little long-term promise for stimulating the economy, protecting the environment or increasing energy security'.[66]

Box 21.11 Factual information: Wind power

Many wind farms, often found in the most beautiful parts of the UK, were given planning permission on the basis of an estimated maximum power output.

Unfortunately, according to Ofgem, the UK's energy regulator, no wind farm produces 100% of its maximum power output. The most realistic estimate of operating maximum power is 50%. But many wind farms fall below even this, producing 25–30% on average, and sometimes less than 10%. These low outputs add significantly to the costs of wind power, the generation of which is already extremely costly.

Nuclear power could help enormously.[67] Unfortunately, people are frightened by it. This is partly because the processes used to create nuclear energy (notably enrichment and reprocessing of used fuel) could also be used to produce weapons, but also because of the environmental disasters produced by the accidents at Three Mile Island[68] and Chernobyl[69] and by the earthquake and tsunami that hit Fukushima in Japan.[70]

The combination of Hiroshima[71] and Chernobyl, especially in these days of terrorism, is a potent mix. The catastrophic environmental impact of the explosion on the Deepwater drilling rig in the Gulf of Mexico[72] demonstrates, however, that it is not only nuclear energy that can result in environmental disaster. If nuclear energy is to help in the fight against climate-change, however, it must first undergo a public relations make-over.

Interestingly the potential disaster triggered by the huge earthquake and tsunami in Japan in 2011, and their impact on the nuclear reactors at Fukushima, prompted one green activist, George Monbiot, to change his stance on nuclear energy. He is now . . . supportive. Acknowledging the potential for disaster represented by the damage to the reactors, he says:

'Yet as far as we know no one has yet received a lethal dose of radiation . . . Atomic energy has just been subjected to one of the harshest of possible tests and the impact on the people and the planet has been small.'[73]

Nuclear fission vs. fusion

It is only nuclear *fission* that is such a threat to the environment. There are scientists who hope that nuclear *fusion* will solve all our problems. Nuclear fusion, should we succeed in finding a way to get out more energy than we put in, will provide a cheap, clean, green source of energy that will fuel the world on little more than sea water (and the industrial plants which will turn the sea water to usable energy). To this end 34 nations have worked together to fund and stuff the International Thermonuclear Reactor (ITER) at Cardarache, in France. It is estimated the project's ten-year construction phase alone will cost 13 billion euros. There are scientists, however, who believe this money will be based because in worlds often quoted (the source of which is unclear): 'nuclear fusion has been the energy of the future for decades and it always will be!'[74]

Box 21.12 Activity: Presentations

Participants should be divided into small teams. Their task is to pretend to be a PR company charged by the government to develop a strategy to rehabilitate nuclear fuel as a potential solution to global warming. It is vital that such strategies take seriously:

(i) people's worries about nuclear power (as a weapon and in accidents);
(ii) the world's need for clean energy.

Each team should be given a week to come up with a 10-minute presentation of their strategy.

Justice for the developing world

Another major problem with trying to deal with climate change by controlling emissions is that it is perceived by many developing countries to be unfair. It must seem to countries in the Indian sub-continent,[75] China[76] and Brazil[77] that just as they are beginning to get somewhere, the developed world is pulling up the ladder behind it. We used fossil fuels as if the supply was infinite. We are now telling them drastically to reduce their carbon emissions in pursuit of 'sustainable' development. Is it any wonder that they are insisting that the wealthiest industrialised nations radically reduce *their* carbon emissions first?[78]

Is it acceptable for us to ask the developing world to reduce its emissions, thereby threatening its development, when it was our profligate use of fossil fuel that caused this crisis?

Box 21.13 Activity: Group discussion

Participants should be asked to consider the barriers to reducing carbon emissions, and how, if at all, these barriers might be removed.

Geo-engineering

An entirely different approach to climate change, geo-engineering, involves deliberate, large-scale manipulation of the environment.[79] Here are some of the ideas that have been suggested:

- erecting giant umbrellas between the planet and the sun;
- injecting sulphur particles into the stratosphere, mimicking a major volcanic eruption;
- painting all the planet's roofs white and covering the deserts with aluminium foil;
- installing mirrors in space to reflect the sun;
- seeding clouds to make them whiter and more reflective;
- fertilising plankton so it consumes more CO_2.

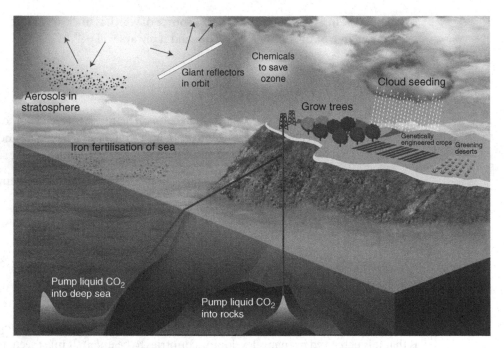

Figure 21.4 A schematic representation of various geoengineering and carbon storage proposals. Courtesy of Lawrence Livermore National Laboratory, USA.

Bill Gates has recently contributed $300,000 to fund a trial of 'cloud seeding'. The trial, run by 'Silver Lining', a research body in San Francisco, involves ten ships and 10,000 km^2 of ocean. Machines will be developed to convert seawater into microparticles that will be blown from tall funnels into the clouds increasing the number of nuclei and so whitening them and making them reflect more sunlight.

Some believe that given the difficulties of changing human behaviour, huge projects like this might have a better chance of success than the attempt to reduce gas emissions.

The potential for environmental disaster

Others, however, have suggested that geo-engineering could have catastrophic consequences.[80] What, for example, might be the effect on marine life of spraying iron sulphate over the ocean to multiply the phytoplankton that absorb CO_2 as they grow (which could remove a billion tonnes of carbon a year from the atmosphere)? This would reduce the oxygen in deep water and make the ocean more acidic thereby destroying many habitats. It might even result in an increase in the emissions of nitrous oxide, a greenhouse gas even more powerful than CO_2.[81]

Governance

Another difficulty is the fear that one of the richer nations might decide unilaterally to employ such a technology to choose a temperature to suit it.[82] Are we prepared for the hand of China or Russia to be on the planet's thermostat? Would they be happy for America to control it? The similarities with the unilateral use of nuclear weapons are inescapable. The world has so far successfully negotiated this concern. Will it be as successful in the case of geo-engineering?[83]

> **Box 21.14 Activity: Group discussion**
>
> Participants should be asked to conduct some basic research into the different methods of geo-engineering. They should then be asked to discuss whether geo-engineering is a better solution to climate change than the attempt to reduce emissions of greenhouse gases.

Adapting to climate change

Some believe that human beings are infinitely adaptable and whatever happens we'll deal with it. If this means we can just be complacent and sit back, it is undoubtedly wrong. If, however, it means nothing more than that we shouldn't worry because the chances of our dealing successfully with climate change are good it might well be correct.

Matt Ridley believes that 'rational optimism' is the best attitude to take to the threat of climate change.[84] He argues that the peculiarly human capacity to exchange ideas, goods and services, permits specialisation and so drives an ability to adapt that has disarmed every threat with which we have been faced for the last 10,000 years. Acknowledging we cannot continue as we are, Ridley believes we will soon find ways of living with the new realities posed by climate change. The oil might run out, but we will find other ways of keeping warm and getting around.

Ridley's optimism is attractive. But to what extent is it likely that we will eventually deal with climate change *because* we are frightened of it?

> **Box 21.15 Activity: A thought experiment**
>
> The philosopher Derek Parfit says that just as we wouldn't be here if our mums and dads hadn't got together when they did, the people who will exist 200 years from now will be the people they are only because of what we do now.
>
> This suggests that as those people who exist in 200 years wouldn't exist except for *whatever* we do now, there is no reason to think they won't be grateful to us whatever the world we bequeath to them.
>
> Question: is this a reason not to change our behaviour?

Species extinction

Climate change is one contributing factor to such a loss of biodiversity that some think we are undergoing the sixth mass extinction in the planet's history.[85] This, however, will be the first mass extinction for which *we* are responsible.

Despite huge disagreement about how to measure biodiversity most estimate there are between 5 and 15 million different species,[86] fewer then 2 million of which have been described.[87] Even within a species the genetic diversity is immense. Think of all the human beings you know and how they differ, physically, psychologically, emotionally and behaviourally. This living diversity is supported by an equally astonishing array of ecological diversity from biomes to habitats, bioregions, landscapes and ecosystems, populations and communities. 'Biodiversity' consists in the totality of these three elements:[88]

- species diversity;
- genetic diversity;
- ecosystem diversity.

From micro-organisms to elephants, from coral reefs to the snowfields, from the Inuit in Alaska to the San Bushmen of Sub-Saharan Africa, this biodiversity is the engine of evolution. It is also the earth's support system; without it our air would not be pure, our water fresh, our soil fertile, our crops pollinated and our waste recycled.

But biodiversity is under serious threat. Measuring the rate at which we are losing species is as difficult as measuring species in the first place. But we seem to be losing species 1000 times faster than we should be,[89] at the rate of one per hour.[90]

Soon there may be no Siberian tigers.[91] The polar bear is dying out.[92] So is the jaguar.[93] But it is not just the big and impressive creatures that are under threat. Nor is it just the mammals, though over the last 500 years we have lost 83 species of mammal from Britain alone.[94] The sea creatures are also losing the battle for life: the cod, the squid, the bluefin tuna and the marlin.[95] Insects and other invertebrates are also under threat:[96] butterflies, spiders, beetles and the honey bee.[97] A total of 113 species of British birds have become extinct since 1880. 'One by one,' said Lord Robert May in his 2001 lecture to the Natural History Museum, 'the lights are winking out'.

The unenlightened anthropocentrist might ask why this should matter so long as the species dying out are not ones we care about or rely upon.

But this is short-sighted. Even if the species we care about were not directly threatened, they would be threatened indirectly from the extinction of species on which *they* depend. The bees, for example, are dying. If the bees do not pollinate plants, the plants will die out, as will everything that depends on these plants for food. The ecosystem is one vast web of dependence: one is reminded of the old nursery rhyme: for want of a nail the shoe was lost. . .

Then there are the species we may not care about or rely upon at the moment, but only because we haven't yet discovered them or their value to us. It has recently been discovered, for example, that the tropical cone snail contains toxins a thousand times more potent than morphine for pain relief.[98] Currently, however, millions of cone snails are killed annually for their shells. How many more opportunities are we losing as species die out before we have even described them?

Anyway, we *are* losing species that are important to us. We have fished the North Sea cod virtually to extinction. Our grandchildren may never taste it. Nor are they likely to taste Ilex squid or bluefin tuna. Our modern fishing boats carry radar so there is nowhere for fish to hide. Their largest nets are large enough to take three jumbo jets. These are often trawled along the seabed to catch whatever is going. Annually 700 million tonnes of 'waste' – jellyfish, sponges, coral, turtles, dolphins – are thrown over the side.[99]

The result is not merely an inconvenience necessitating a change of diet. For some it is the loss of a livelihood. In the seas around the Falkland Islands it used to be possible to catch 200,000 tonnes of squid. In 2009 only 45 tonnes were found.[100] The Southern blue whiting, worth about £650 a tonne, is also dying out. The loss of revenue to the Islands is profound. Thousands of fishermen in Canada, the UK and Iceland are out of work as a result of the demise of the cod.

The causes of species extinction

It is thought that at least some of the earth's previous mass extinctions were caused by the earth's colliding with a massive meteor. But that is not the cause of this extinction. It seems likely that just as this change in our climate is down to us, so is this mass extinction. Ironically, this is because *we* are the most successful species ever to have lived; there is no sign that *we* are on the verge of extinction.

The earth's human population hit 1 billion in 1880. In 50 years it doubled. It doubled again in the next 40 years, hitting 4 billion in 1970. During the 70s it grew at a rate of 2% a year. Now it is about 1.4% per year. There are now approximately 6 billion people on earth. These people have to have somewhere to live and they need food and water, energy, employment and manufactured goods. The resources needed to provide all this are huge.

In addition to climate change, all the following factors are implicated in species extinction, mainly (though not always) because such activities destroy habitats:[101]

(i)   **Urbanisation:** By 2015 the six largest cities in the world are expected to have approximately 20 million inhabitants each. Our towns and villages are growing too. To facilitate this land is cleared, destroying the habitats of every creature unable to adapt quickly enough to survive.

(ii) **Industrialisation:** The demand for energy, employment and manufactured goods generates water, air and soil pollution. For example, waste might leak into the water table and kill many aquatic creatures, or pour from factory chimneys as the acid rain which kills the forests.

(iii) **Deforestation:** We also kill the forests, including the rain forests, directly in our greed for timber for building, fuel and paper. But trees, especially in the tropical rain forests, capture CO_2 and help to prevent the toxic 'run-off' of pollutants into our soil. A single oak tree, furthermore, may be home to 400 different species of insect.

(iv) **Afforestation:** We do plant trees but for commercial purposes. Instead of creating forests with many varieties of trees, our forests consist in just a few species, all quickly harvested for timber and paper, and planted so closely together that only shade-loving species can thrive.

(v)   **Agriculture:** Modern farming techniques are intensive, tend to monoculture, and over-use of pesticides and fertilisers which contribute to soil, air and water pollution (see Chapter 17).

(vi) **Alien species**: many non-native species introduced by us are flourishing and threatening to kill off native species by competing successfully with them for prey.[102]

(vii) **Hunting:** we use animals for their skins, teeth, hair, bones, flesh, shells and just about everything else. We also use them as pets and for scientific research. Unless we hunt and trade animals and their parts with regeneration in mind we risk hunting to extinction.[103]

Box 21.16 Case study: Swamp stonecrop

Swamp stonecrop[104] was brought into Britain as an aquarium plant. It wasn't long before it appeared in the wild. It forms carpets, with 100% coverage, over ponds and waterways and kills off all competing wildlife. It is a major threat to British aquatic life.

The herbicides that would deal with swamp stonecrop have been banned for use except under (rather expensive) licence. Removing this weed by mechanical means does not work. In the meantime the birds are spreading it exponentially...

If we are responsible for the sixth mass extinction, and if we have a duty to do something about it, what *can* we do about it? And are there any moral problems associated with the behaviours that are needed?

Population control

We could have fewer children. In the developed countries we are already restricting family size. In many developing countries, however, having children is still the only way to secure one's own future.

Zoos, game and nature reserves and sanctuaries

We can intentionally conserve species in land set aside for this purpose. Such 'institutions' see the education and pleasure of humans as secondary to their conservation aims. Not everyone, however, thinks that keeping animals in zoos or reserves can be justified even in terms of conservation.[105]

Box 21.17 Case study: Madikwe Game Reserve

Near the border with Botswana, in the shadow of the Dwarsberg Mountains, is the fourth largest game reserve (75,000 hectares) in South Africa. There are 16,000 mammals with 95 different species in Madikwe, thanks to Operation Phoenix, the largest reintroduction of game ever undertaken in Africa.

This involved the relocation of entire breeding herds of elephant, buffalo, rhino, hyena, wild dog and various species of antelope.

At least 340 bird species, 54 reptile species, 20 frog species and many spiders and insects have been recorded in the park since 1992. All the 'big five' (elephants, lions, buffalo, rhino and leopard) can be found, together with the cheetah, and the wild dog (a huge success story for Madikwe).

The reserve constantly monitors all the components of its ecological systems (flora, fauna, fire, hydrological processes, erosion, etc.) to ensure it is successfully managing the reserve in accordance with its aim to ensure the continuation of the biodiversity in the area.

An important part of this is its wild-life based tourism, which is believed to be the most cost-beneficial option for achieving the aims of the reserve.[106]

Seed banks

By collecting and storing examples of seeds we should be able, even if species become extinct, to regenerate them and return them to the wild.[107]

Organic farming

Organic farmers eschew the use of pesticides, synthetic fertilisers, feed additives and anything else that might be harmful to humans or the environment. But, for this reason, organic food is expensive. Is it reasonable to ask the poor to pay higher prices to protect the environment?

Legislation

Many governments are introducing legislation in the hope of preserving habitats, preventing illegal trade in endangered species and funding initiatives such as seed banks and nature reserves.

Biotechnology and species extinction

Maybe, though, biotechnology will come to the rescue? Here are some ways it might help to avert the loss of biodiversity, and even perhaps increase it:

Genetic engineering (see Chapter 17): could help increase agricultural yields whilst decreasing the land required for farming and minimising the use of pesticides and fertilisers. It might also enable us to modify plants and animals the better to adapt to new habitats.

Cloning (see Chapters 7 and 8): would enable us to increase stocks of existing species (albeit without increasing the genetic diversity within the species) and even perhaps to bring back species that have already lost the battle.

Synthetic biology (see Chapter 16): could be used to create entirely new species and perhaps to mitigate the threat to existing species by means of bioremediation.

Box 21.18 **Case study and activity: Group discussion**

In 2010 Dr Craig Venter was the first to create artificial life by means of synthetic biology. 'Synthia' was created after Venter produced a 'minimal organism', one from

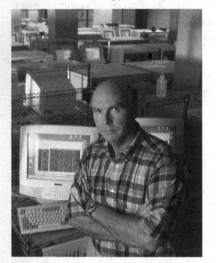

Figure 21.5 Dr Craig Venter. ©
Volker Steger/Science Photo Library.

which all unnecessary genes had been removed to produce a 'chassis' on which to build a new genome. Venter then introduced the synthetic chromosome into a cell from which the existing one had been removed.[108]

Dr Venter hopes that Synthia will eventually help us turn algae into clean energy, be instrumental in developing vaccines, or help remove pollution from the oceans.

In response to those who fear that Synthia might replicate and run amok, he has inserted a 'watermark' so all such organisms can be traced to their source. It should eventually be possible to insert a 'destruct' code into Synthia and her progeny so they would not survive outside a given habitat.

Participants should familiarise themselves with the arguments for and against the creation of Synthia and then discuss the following questions:

This house believes that only God should create life.

Could it be that it is only by using technologies that many have rejected as 'unnatural' that we will be able to alleviate the damage we have done to our planet?

Summary

In this chapter we have considered our duties to the non-living environment and how biotechnology can help. In particular we have:

- reflected on different environmentalist positions;

- distinguished 'dominion' from 'stewardship' and related them to unenlightened and enlightened anthropocentrism;

- noted how radical biocentrism differs from mild and moderate biocentrism, and considered the arguments for it;

- considered ecocentrism and the motivation of its claim that the non-living environment has intrinsic value;

- learned about climate change, considering the views of the denialists, and looked at how scientists might inadvertently have furthered their case;

- asked how we might respond to climate change, and in particular how biotechnology might help;

- learned about biodiversity, its importance, and the threat to it from species extinction;

- reflected on the causes of species extinction and the possible remedies;

- noted how biotechnology could be of help in our response to species extinction;

- considered whether science is in danger of playing God and if so whether this is morally unacceptable.

Questions to stimulate reflection

Do you think anthropocentrism can ever be 'enlightened'? What do you think of the claim that environmentalism *depends* on anthropocentrism?

Do *all* living things have intrinsic value? Even cockroaches? How might this claim be justified?

Does the non-living environment have intrinsic value? How can this be the case?

What would you say to someone who argued that environmental ethics is new-fangled nonsense?

Is it acceptable for human beings to create totally new life forms?

Is global warming the work of humans? If so should we try to reverse it, mitigate it or learn to live with it?

Do you think it matters that so many species are dying out despite its having happened before without causing (us) too many problems?

Do you think the use of genetic engineering, cloning or synthetic biology to preserve biodiversity is morally permissible?

Do you think it is morally unacceptable for human beings to 'play God'?

Additional activities

Find out whether there are any car pools or car-sharing clubs in your area. If not might you start one? Conduct some research into how it might work.

Find out if your energy supplier provides free energy meters. If so get one, monitor your energy use and see where you might reduce it.

Start a compost heap or a wormery in your (parents') garden. And/or build a pond. See how many different forms of wildlife you can attract.

See how many different uses you can find for plastic bags from the supermarket.

Keep a log of the birds that visit your garden. Set up bird tables, bird feeders and nesting boxes. Do the same for insects.

Consider taking a course in bee-keeping, starting a hive and producing your own honey.

Learn whether any invasive species has appeared in your neighbourhood and keep an eye out for it in your garden.

Visit a national park, wildlife sanctuary or zoo and find out about their conservation efforts.

Notes

1 http://www.iep.utm.edu/envi-eth/. *The Internet Encyclopedia of Philosophy* on environmental ethics.

2 For a reminder about direct versus indirect duties see Chapter 20.

3 See Norton, B. (1991) *Towards Unity With Environmentalists*. New York: Oxford University Press.

4 Grey, W. (1993) Anthropocentrism and deep ecology. *The Australasian Journal of Philosophy*, **71**(4), 463–475.

5 http://www.firstscience.com/home/articles/origins/death-of-the-dinosaurs_27907.html. On the death of the dinosaurs from First Science.com.

6 http://www.sunypress.edu/p-4109-with-respect-for-nature.aspx. The webpage for Paul Taylor's book *Respect for Nature*.

7 Taylor, P. (1986) *Respect for Nature*. Princeton, NJ: Princeton University Press.

8 Goodin, R. (1991) A Green Theory of Value. In D. J. Mulvaney (ed.), *The Humanities and the Australian Environment*. Canberra: Canberra Australian Academy of the Humanities.

9 Rolston, H. (1975) Is there an ecological ethic? *Ethics*, **85**, 93–109.

10 http://supergoodtech.com/tomquick/phd/autopoiesis.html. A definition and account of autopoiesis.

11 Rodman, J. (1983) Four forms of ecological consciousness reconsidered. In T. Attig and D. Scherer (eds), *Environmental Ethics*. Buffalo, NY: Prometheus.

12 Fox, W. (2007) *A General Theory of Ethics: Human Relationships, Nature and the Built Environment*. Cambridge, MA: MIT Press.

13 http://ndpr.nd.edu/review.cfm?id=11543. A review of Fox's book by Andrew Brennen of LaTrobe University.

14 Naess, A. (1973) The shallow and the deep, long range ecology movement. Inquiry, **16**. Reprinted in *Sessions* 1995.

15 Leopold, A. (1949) A land ethic. In *A Sand County Almanac*. Oxford: Oxford University Press.

16 Routley, R. (1973) Is there a need for a new environmental ethic? *Proceedings of the 15th World Congress of Philosophy*, **1**: 205–210.

17 Lovelock, J. (1979) *Gaia: A New Look at Life on Earth*. Oxford: Oxford University Press.

18 http://www.deepecology.org/. The website of the Deep Ecology Movement.

19 http://www.bbc.co.uk/news/10342318. A BBC report on the view that even ancient climate change was linked to CO_2.

20 http://geography.about.com/od/learnabouttheearth/a/milankovitch.htm. An account of the Milankovitch cycles.

21 http://news.bbc.co.uk/1/hi/in_depth/sci_tech/2009/copenhagen/8386319.stm. The BBC on the history of the climate on earth.

22 http://www.discoveringfossils.co.uk/fossilfuels.htm. All about fossil fuels.

23 http://news.bbc.co.uk/1/hi/sci/tech/8285247.stm. A BBC history of climate change.

24 http://news.bbc.co.uk/1/hi/world/americas/3499500.stm. The BBC on the rainforests acting as carbon sinks.

25 http://www.bbc.co.uk/climate/evidence/greenhouse_effect.shtml. The BBC on the evidence for the greenhouse effect.

26 http://www.bbc.co.uk/weather/features/global_warming1.shtml. The BBC on global warming.

27 http://www.sciencedaily.com/releases/2009/01/090108101629.htm. *Science Daily* on the rising sea levels.

28 http://news.sky.com/skynews/Home/World-News/British-Rsearch-Team-Discovers-Greenland-Ice-Caps-Are-Melting-At-An-Accelerated-Rate/Article/201007415674119. A Sky News report on the melting of the ice caps.

29 http://www.nasa.gov/topics/earth/features/arctic_thinice.html. NASA report on the thinning of Arctic ice.

30 http://www3.interscience.wiley.com/journal/123310513/abstract. Stott, P. A., Gillett, N. P., Hegerl, G. C. *et al.* (2010) Detection and attribution of climate change: a regional perspective. *Wiley Interdisciplinary Reviews: Climate Change*, 1, 192–211.

31 http://www.theglobaleducationproject.org/earth/human-conditions.php. Interesting facts about human beings on our planet from the Global Education Project.

32 http://www.bbc.co.uk/news/science-environment-10958760. A BBC discussion of the extent to which climate change is implicated in the disastrous floods in Pakistan in 2010.

33 The Office for Science (2010) Land use futures: making the most of land in the 21st century. Report.

34 http://www.bbc.co.uk/news/science-environment-10919460. The BBC reporting a claim that climate change is implicated in the Russian forest fires of 2010. http://www.livescience. com/6875-russia-wildfires-due-climate-change-scientists.html. A report to the effect that climate change is *not* implicated in Russia's forest fires.

35 http://www.independent.co.uk/environment/climate-change/exclusive-the-methane-time-bomb-938932.html. An *Independent* newspaper report on the release of methane gas from the permafrost.

36 http://www.guardian.co.uk/environment/georgemonbiot/2009/mar/06/climate-change-deniers-top-10. A list of 10 'climate change deniers' from George Monbiot.

37 http://www.metoffice.gov.uk/climatechange/guide/. UK Met Office guide to climate change including a distinction between the weather and the climate.

38 http://www.cru.uea.ac.uk/cru/info/thc/. About thermohaline circulation from the Climate Research Unit at the University of East Anglia.

39 http://www.bbc.co.uk/weather/features/science_nature/the_day_after_tomorrow.shtml.

40 http://news.bbc.co.uk/1/hi/sci/tech/4485840.stm. The BBC on the possibility of abrupt climate change.

41 http://www.guardian.co.uk/environment/2009/mar/09/climate-change-deniers. The *Guardian* on Vaclav Klaus' claims.

42 Stott, P. A., Gillett, N.P., Hegerl, G.C. *et al.* (2010), Detection and attribution of climate change: a regional perspective. *Wiley Interdisciplinary Reviews: Climate Change*, 1, 192–211.

43 http://www.scientificamerican.com/article.cfm?id=seven-answers-to-climate-contrarian-nonsense. *Scientific American* responds to climate change denial.

44 http://www.timesonline.co.uk/tol/comment/columnists/guest_contributors/article7061646.ece. A *Times* article on climate change denial.

45 http://www.guardian.co.uk/science/2010/mar/29/james-lovelock-climate-change. James Lovelock claiming humans are too stupid to deal with climate change.

46 http://news.bbc.co.uk/1/hi/sci/tech/8451756.stm. The BBC on the need to end 'climate confusion'.

47 http://www.guardian.co.uk/environment/2009/may/22/hay-climate-change-giddens. Criticism of the government for failing to convince people of the need for change.

48 http://www.beep.ac.uk/content/215.0.html. The Bioethics Education Project on Climate Change including a video from David King, the Chief Science Advisor to the UK.

49 http://www.carbonfootprint.com/. How to reduce one's carbon footprint.

50 http://www.oxfordgeoengineering.org/. A site on geo-engineering from the University of Oxford.

51 http://www.scidev.net/en/features/climate-change-adapting-is-crucial-too.html. An article on adapting to climate change.

52 http://www.seat61.com/CO2flights.htm. Calculating the carbon costs of flying.

53 http://www.dailymail.co.uk/news/article-1277180/Tesco-selling-asparagus-Peru-town-famous-producing-vegetable.html. The *Daily Mail* on the carbon cost of flying in asparagus from Peru.

54 http://www.bbc.co.uk/gardening/today_in_your_garden/ethical_wood.shtml. Rainforest friendly garden furniture.

55 http://www.greencarsite.co.uk/. A comparison of 'green' cars.

56 http://www.accaglobal.com/page/3274981. The global body of professional accountants asking whether the corporate world is doing enough to reduce carbon emissions.

57 http://endoftheline.com/. The End of the Line.

58 http://www.bbc.co.uk/pressoffice/proginfo/tv/wk38/feature_earth.shtml. A discussion of the BBC's programme *The Climate Wars*.

59 http://www.guardian.co.uk/technology/gamesblog/2010/feb/16/pc-games. A Guardian report on a new board game on climate change.

60 http://www.guardian.co.uk/environment/blog/2010/feb/17/iphone-app-climate-change. A *Guardian* report on a new mobile 'app'.

61 Ellerman, A. D., Convery, F. J., de Perthuis, C. *et al.* (2010) *Pricing Carbon.* Cambridge: Cambridge University Press.

62 http://www.youtube.com/watch?v=r94xoS80ykk . An introduction to renewable energy by podcast from UC Berkeley.

63 http://www.bbc.co.uk/learningzone/clips/wave-power-hydroelectricity-and-wind-farms/475.html. BBC learning zone on wave power.

64 http://www.bbc.co.uk/climate/adaptation/wind_power.shtml. BBC on wind power.

65 http://www.uk-energy-saving.com/advantages-disadvantages-solar-energy.html. A site considering the advantages and disadvantages of solar power.

66 Frondel, M., Ritter, N., Schmidt, C. M. and Vance, C. (2010) Economic impacts from the promotion of renewable energy technologies: the German experience. http://ideas.repec.org/p/rwi/repape/0156.html.

67 http://news.bbc.co.uk/1/hi/sci/tech/4216302.stm. The BBC on nuclear power.

68 http://news.bbc.co.uk/onthisday/hi/dates/stories/march/28/newsid_2734000/2734499.stm. The BBC on Three Mile Island.

69 http://news.bbc.co.uk/1/shared/spl/hi/guides/456900/456957/html/nn1page1.stm. The BBC on Chernobyl.

70 http://www.bbc.co.uk/news/world-asia-pacific-12720219.

71 http://news.bbc.co.uk/onthisday/hi/dates/stories/august/6/newsid_3602000/3602189.stm. The BBC on the dropping of the bomb on Hiroshima.

72 http://www.bbc.co.uk/news/10177716. The BBC on deepwater drilling after the Deepwater Horizon disaster.

73 http://www.guardian.co.uk/commentisfree/2011/mar/21/pro-nuclear-japan-fukushima.

74 http://www.iter.org/
http://www.bbc.co.uk/schools/gcsebitesize/science/add_aqa_pre_2011/radiation/nuclear-fissionrev1.shtml

75 http://www.guardian.co.uk/environment/interactive/2009/nov/06/oxfam-bangladesh-cyclone-aila.

76 http://www.bbc.co.uk/worldservice/documentaries/2009/12/091201_wednesdaydoc_chinagreen.shtml.

77 http://www.scidev.net/en/policy-briefs/brazil-climate-change-a-country-profile.html.

78 http://www.opendemocracy.net/globalization-climatechange/article_252.jsp.

79 http://news.bbc.co.uk/1/hi/sci/tech/8231387.stm.

80 http://www.timesonline.co.uk/tol/news/environment/article6817280.ece.

81 http://news.bbc.co.uk/1/hi/sci/tech/7133619.stm.

82 http://www.oxfordgeoengineering.org/pdfs/geoengineering_quarterly_first_edition.pdf.

83 http://royalsociety.org/Royal-Society-launches-major-study-on-the-governance-of-geoengineering/.

84 Ridley, M. (2010) *The Rational Optimist: How Prosperity Evolves.* London: Fourth Estate.

85 http://www.telegraph.co.uk/science/dinosaurs/7885635/Earth-hit-by-mass-extinctions-every-27m-years.html.

86 http://environment.uk.msn.com/climate-change/gallery.aspx?cp-documentid=10223754&imageindex=7.

87 http://www.guardian.co.uk/environment/2009/sep/29/number-of-living-species.

88 http://www.ukbap.org.uk/.

89 http://www.telegraph.co.uk/earth/earthnews/7397420/Worlds-nature-becoming-extinct-at-fastest-rate-on-record-conservationists-warn.html.

90 http://www.timesonline.co.uk/tol/comment/columnists/simon_barnes/article7106699.ece.

91 http://www.bbc.co.uk/nature/species/Tiger.

92 http://www.bbc.co.uk/nature/species/Polar_bear.

93 http://www.bbc.co.uk/nature/species/Jaguar.

94 http://www.guardian.co.uk/environment/2010/mar/11/extinct-species-england.

95 http://www.guardian.co.uk/environment/2010/aug/02/census-marine-life-sea.

96 http://news.sky.com/skynews/Home/UK-News/Butterflies-New-Threat-To-Endangered-Insects-In-UK-Countryside/Article/200807315039444.

97 http://www.guardian.co.uk/environment/2010/may/24/honeybees-winter-decline.

98 http://news.bbc.co.uk/1/hi/sci/tech/3207632.stm.

99 http://www.animalaid.org.uk/h/n/CAMPAIGNS/vegetarianism/ALL/652/.

100 http://www.antarctica.ac.uk/press/press_releases/press_release.php?id=3.

101 http://library.thinkquest.org/5736/causes.htm.

102 http://news.bbc.co.uk/1/hi/sci/tech/2730693.stm.

103 http://notes.utk.edu/bio/unistudy.nsf/0/2c2ce274f56bea1185256f8e005f6a31?Open Document.

104 http://www.chiltern.gov.uk/site/scripts/documents_info.php?documentID=621&page Number=3.

105 http://www.zsl.org/conservation/carnivores-and-people/conservation-support-from-zoos, 40,AR.html.
http://www.game-reserve.com/.
http://news.bbc.co.uk/1/hi/uk/8658664.stm.
106 http://madikwegamereserve.net/.
107 http://www.guardian.co.uk/environment/2009/oct/15/kew-millennium-seed-bank-hits-target.
108 http://independentsciencenews.org/news/goodbye-dolly-hello-synthia/.

Further reading and useful websites

Keller, D. R. (ed.) (2010) *Environmental Ethics: The Big Questions.* Oxford: Wiley Blackwell.

Specter, M. (2009) *Denialism: How Irrational Thinking Hinders Scientific Progress, Harms the Planet and Threatens Our Lives.* London: Penguin.

Wilson, E. O. (2002) *The Future of Life.* New York: Knopf.

http://plato.stanford.edu/entries/ethics-environmental/. The *Stanford Encyclopedia of Philosophy* on environmental ethics.

http://www.beep.ac.uk/content/174.0.html. The Bioethics Education Project on biodiversity.

http://www.beep.ac.uk/content/215.0.html. The Bioethics Education Project on climate change.

http://www.metoffice.gov.uk/climatechange/. The UK Meteorological Office on climate change.

22 Reflection, speculation and points to ponder

Objectives

In reading this final chapter you will be:

- reflecting on what you have read in this book;
- speculating on how social decisions may affect the future;
- thinking creatively about participative democracy.

You might be reading this before you read anything else. Well, why not? It is often a good way to discover whether you are going to enjoy a book. Or you might be reading it having worked your way through the rest of the book. If so, in reading this final chapter you will be pulling together everything you have read, and reflecting on how it might be of benefit, not just to you but to society as a whole.

We are going to engage in some speculation. In this book we have considered many controversial issues. As we saw in Chapter 3, where we discussed ethics in the context of society, when an issue is controversial – when equally rational people can come to different conclusions – governments must make hard decisions. The decisions they make will push society in one direction or another. If we are lucky enough to live in a democratic society we can, by participating in the decision-making process, affect these decisions.

So let's reflect on what we have read in this book, and on the decisions we might make regarding the issues we have discussed, to see how society might look in the future. We'll consider three different scenarios. The first concentrates on decisions made regarding reproduction and death, the second on the aftermath of war and the third on bio-information and health. After each scenario questions are provided to stimulate reflection. Having read and thought about all the scenarios, you might like to use these questions as prompts to stimulate your thinking at an even more general level:

- Do you think life in any of these imaginary societies sounds appealing? What do you like about them? What don't you like about them?
- By which decisions might society have become as it is depicted in each scenario? Which other decisions might have been made? If you think the decisions made were wrong, which decisions would have been the right ones?

- Do you think the scenarios are realistic? If not what do you think would prevent them coming about?
- Which images from each scenario impact on you particularly? Why? To what sort of governmental decision might they be traced? Do you think the decision made was the right one?
- Is there anything you can do *now* to help bring about or prevent the aspects of the scenarios about which you are uncomfortable? Are you inclined to do something? What should be your first step?

You might think that the scenarios omit reference to some of the ethical and/or social issues discussed in the book. If so, please write your own scenario. All you have to do is reflect on some of the hard decisions you have come across in this book, and on the possible consequences of such decisions. Let your imagination go!

Here is our first scenario:

Scenario one: AD 2320

James awoke with a start: today was his 122nd birthday and he was going to choose his children! He was due at the child library at 10. He was excited at the thought of the two hours or so he would spend with the quaintly named 'midwife' whose job it was to talk him through the genomes of each of the embryos he had had made.

With two of these embryos this would be an easy task. They were James' clones. The child library always suggests prospective parents add clones to the mix from which they make their choice. Although no one these days is unsophisticated enough to think that their clones will turn out exactly as they have turned out, many people like the idea of bringing into the world children who are as like them as they can possibly be.

The other embryos are the product of IVF, each the result of James' sperm, and eggs matured in an artificial ovary.[1] James had bought the eggs from a catalogue. Nowadays every female had her reproductive organs removed at birth, and all her eggs frozen. This not only relieved women of the 'periods' that used to be such a nuisance during their 'child-rearing years', it also relieved them of the need actually to give birth (thank goodness for artificial wombs!). Every woman – and every man come to that – could now have the two children they were allowed whenever they wanted to have them (though neither men nor women were allowed to have children after 250 years of age). Most women kept several spare eggs in case of accidents, but then sold the rest on the open market. Artificial sperm had been available for years.

Childlessness, therefore, was a thing of the past, as was accidental pregnancy and indeed pregnancy, abortion, the menarche, the menopause and discrimination against women on the basis of the fact they bear children.

Disability and disease (other than annoying ones such as the common cold) had also faded into history. James couldn't imagine a world in which parents might be told, after the birth of a child, that something was wrong with it. Embryos were placed in a womb only if they were disease- and disability-free, and if a problem occurred in the womb it was easy just to terminate that foetus and get started on another. Occasionally, of course, as the result of an accident a person would sustain a disability.

But since the euthanasia act of 2100 nearly all chose to end their lives quickly and painlessly (or had this chosen for them by their parent). Those who didn't rarely lived for more than a few months; disability being so frowned upon and uncatered for, suicide quickly became preferable.

James knew there were people who argued that differences were a good thing. He couldn't see it himself. Certainly not differences of ability or attractiveness.

Nowadays that old saying 'everybody is good at something' was simply a fact. Actually everyone was good at most things. The only problem with this was the fact that everyone had to spend some of their time doing society's 'grunt work'. Someone, after all, has to assist the suicides, do the boring admin, look after the crops in the crop dome, the animals in the animal zone and monitor the environmental parameters of the domes. At least the powers that be had got the annual stint down to two weeks. The rest of the time everyone did whatever suited them.

Not only was everyone good at most things, everyone was also attractive. Until the very day they chose to die (usually around 350 years of age) people could be confident in their ability to attract anyone. Brown, black, blonde and red hair, brown, black, grey and blue eyes had gone the way of disability With blue hair and yellow eyes being universally preferred, what was the loss? As for brown, white and black skin. . . well James wasn't one of those who mourned their loss: nowadays everyone was green-skinned.

Race, therefore, was no longer an issue. That this was a good thing is surely obvious after the devastating wars of 2060–85 had nearly destroyed the planet and everyone on it.

The wars had been racially motivated. At least this was what children learned during their 70 years of compulsory education. Many believed they were as motivated by poverty as by race, but as race and poverty were linked, the difference didn't seem important. Anyway poverty was eliminated along with race. GM technology now ensures, together with in vitro meat and proper global distribution, that everyone has enough to eat and drink and that the food they eat is nutritious and pharmacologically suitable for their genome and whichever dome they live in.

But thank goodness that the global government had had enough foresight to invest in geotechnology and nuclear fusion. Once the umbrellas were up, shielding us from the fierce heat of the sun, and the domes in place to protect us from the radiation consequent on the meltdown of the world's fission reactors, and once the much safer, cheaper and greener nuclear fusion was up and running, we were not only safe but also comfortable. The elimination of racial and economic differences, and indeed as far as possible all other differences, can only make the world even more comfortable.

Crime is also a thing of the past. As everyone's DNA is held on a central database from birth, no one can rely on misbehaviour going undetected. But few are inclined, anyway, to misbehave. The genes associated with criminal tendencies have long been eliminated. Families having been abolished in 2150, every child's upbringing is supervised by the state in such a way that child abuse is impossible. With no excuse for criminal behaviour, anyone engaging in anti-social behaviour is deemed to be disabled, and treated accordingly. They soon decide life isn't worth living.

No, James reflected, 2320 is a good time to live. It is also a good time to bring children into the world. He had decided to have his two 100 years apart so he could devote himself to one at a time. He was particularly looking forward to visiting them. He had never been in the children's dome. Even in this crime-free society it was decreed that children were safer isolated from all adults other than those who had brought them into the world, and those men and women who, for the moment at least, were choosing to devote their time to bringing up children and had undergone the appropriate surgery. He also looked forward to introducing them to the animal dome (or at least those parts of it where the tamer animals were to be found), and taking them to see the crop dome.

Once his children were out of the children's dome (at a startling 75; in James' view children grow up far too early nowadays), he looked forward to guiding them towards making the choices that would give them the life they wanted, so that when he got to around 350 he too could choose the day of his death, knowing he had lived a fulfilled and happy life.

Here are some questions to prompt your reflection on scenario one:

- What do you think about choosing your children from a 'child library'? What do you think a child library is?

- People in this imaginary society often choose clones for children. Do you think this is realistic? Why (not)? What would be the advantages and disadvantages of bringing up your clone as your child?

- Do you think it would be a good idea for females to have all their eggs frozen, and reproductive organs removed at birth, eliminating the need for periods and pregnancy? Are you happy about the idea of spare eggs being sold? Do you like the idea of artificial sperm?

- According to this scenario each adult is allowed two children who will be brought up by others in the 'child dome'. Does this sound like a good idea? Why (not)?

- There is no disease or disability in the society depicted. Why not? Is it a good thing that such disorders have been eliminated? What happens to those who sustain disabilities accidentally?

- There appears to be no natural death in this society. Instead people choose to die at 350 years of age. Do you think this is realistic? Why might people choose to die? Do you think the choice is a real one? Would you like to choose the day of your death?

- Everyone in this society is good at nearly everything. This means that everyone must take turns at society's 'grunt work'. How might this have come about? Is it a good thing?

- Everyone in this society is attractive (though their idea of attractiveness might not suit us!). They all sound very similar, if not identical, with their green skin, blue hair and yellow eyes: they are certainly all of the same race. How might this have come about? Do you think it is a good thing?

- There is no hunger in the world depicted in this scenario. Why not? Do you think that if it really became possible to eliminate hunger in this way we should do it? Do you think it will ever become possible (or even that it is possible now)?

- There is very little crime in this society. How was it eliminated? What happens to those few who do commit crimes? Do you think we should eliminate crime in this way were it to become possible?

- Families were abolished in this society. What is the implied reason for eliminating families? Do you think it is a good reason for eliminating families?
- Children in this society live in the 'child dome' and are brought up by people who have had 'appropriate surgery'. What sort of surgery do you think might be meant? Why do you think it is required? Adults other than those who have had this surgery, or are parents, are not permitted in the child dome. Why do you imagine this is? Is it a good idea?
- Some environmental disaster seems to have befallen the world by the time of this scenario. What do you think it was? Why do you think it happened? What are the remedies mentioned?

Having read and reflected on this scenario, you will probably have identified some things that fail to convince you. If so why not try to write your own scenario about the world as you imagine it will be in AD 2320?

Here is our second scenario:

Scenario two: AD 2070

There were two of them. Both men. Sara crouched further into the shadows. She'd lost contact with Damon, but felt secure in the rendezvous they'd agreed on earlier. They preferred to scavenge together – it wasn't much safer but at least they'd know if anything had happened to the other. Separately, though, they were more likely to find food enough to keep going. Today she'd been lucky: six tins of baked beans in the rucksack of a corpse that had somehow gone un-ransacked. She held them closer as she watched the two men rummage through the rubble of a ruined house. She could tell that they were sighted. She longed to hail them in the hope they were 'co-operators' but didn't dare; the cost, if they were not, could be too high.

Half an hour later, having watched the men leave empty-handed, Sara made her tentative way to their latest hiding place. Damon was pleased with her haul. He had found only a battered tin of sardines. In the half-light she could see the pockmarks on his face and knew that hers was as bad. But they were lucky. They had survived. Many others – most others – hadn't. And of those who had most were blind. They didn't survive for long.

Sara sometimes wished that she and Damon had stayed with the others. But the rules chafed. Imposed by a group whose strength (and willingness to use it) enabled them to appoint themselves leaders, there was no possibility of questioning them. Sara had tried, only to be told that if she didn't like it she could leave. They didn't think she would, of course, but when she met Damon, who felt as she did, they gave each other courage, agreeing that they would rather take the risk than 'co-operate' on the terms laid down. They hoped to find another group whose rules suited them better: some sort of democracy would be ideal. But how to find such a group? How to do so, furthermore, without falling foul of the solitaries, whose need for food mandated a form of co-operation, but not one that Sara or Damon could countenance?

Sara was 45, Damon 49. They had been in their mid-teens when a little known group of 'freedom fighters' calling themselves the 'Liberators' had made it their business to recruit a group of disaffected scientists with the aim of recreating the smallpox virus. They didn't find it difficult. The economic crises of the 2010s and 2020s had led to great unemployment. There were, in particular, a lot of unemployed scientists: so many had stayed in education, despite the cost, in the forlorn hope of riding out the economic downturn. Unemployed PhDs were ten a penny. At such times it is always easy to find people who feel that others should have been laid off first or who felt that their particular talents had been overlooked.

When you pay such people well (with funds provided by rich supporters), support them in their envious cynicism, isolate them from each other and lie to them about your goal, it isn't hard to keep them sweet. Especially when all almost of them want to do is solve whatever problem it is that they have been set (believing, of course, that they have set it themselves).

It would have been impossible of course without the trend for 'open source' wetware and resources. The papers of those who had recreated the polio, mouse pox and cowpox viruses proved invaluable. Despite the fact that in 2003[2] the editors of the main science journals had agreed to withhold from open publication the methodological section of papers describing the results of experiments with security implications, the fact that such papers had been published openly before made it a case of shutting the stable door...

Not content with recreating *Variola major*, the fatality rate of which was 30%, they recreated the haemorrhagic form of smallpox. In this form the characteristic rash is accompanied by bleeding into the mucous membranes and the skin. In this form smallpox is invariably fatal. It is every bit as infectious as the other forms of smallpox.

The aim of the Liberators was to decapitate the governments of the western world and the major corporations, especially big pharma. In the opinion of the Liberators both were guilty of crimes against humanity, of putting profit before people.

But they made a major error. They assumed that the vaccine stockpiled in the aftermath of 9/11 would soon stop the virus in its tracks. They hoped to cause the sort of chaos that would enable 'right-thinking' people, the sort of people who cared for others, to take power. They did not intend to unleash an epidemic that would kill 95% of the world's population. But this is what they did.

In laying their plans they hadn't allowed for the fact that the genome of the virus they created was not quite that against which the vaccine was efficacious.

The first to die were the very people whose job it was to co-ordinate a response to such an event: heads of government and of the major industries. Those who might have taken over from them died next. The food ran out even before the shops closed. People first boarded themselves up in their houses. For fear of starving, however, they soon took to their cars. But then the fuel ran out. Communications held up for a while, but the mobile phones started to go dead. Then the internet went down. Without leadership no company can manage for long.

Within 2 years humanity – or what was left of it – had largely reverted to a 'state of nature'. There were no functioning schools, hospitals or public transport. The only trading that went on was between individuals who were, for a while, able to swap possessions for others they wanted more. Money had ceased to have value because there was nothing to buy. Local government had gone the way of national government: no one was in charge unless by force of personality or strength. Now all there was were lots of independent groups, usually run by those able to shout down or outfight the others.

Sara and Damon dearly wanted society to rise again from the ashes. But they were both realists: if it didn't happen before the death of those who had been educated, it might not happen at all. Yes, groups like the one to which they had been attached made it their business to save as many books as they could. But it was increasingly difficult to hold out against those who argued that warmth was more important than knowledge.

Shivering, Sara snuggled closer to Damon, whose turn it was to keep watch. It was good to have had something more substantial than grass to eat. Her dream was to live in a group strong enough to have successfully guarded enough land to cultivate crops and vegetables, possibly even to have found and nurtured some chickens, sheep or goats, maybe a cow or two: some fresh milk would be so good.

Oh well, she thought as sleep overtook her, at least we can still dream.

Here are some questions to prompt your reflection on scenario two:

- Sara seems to be worried that the men she is watching are not 'co-operators'. What do you think this means? Why is it important to Sara?

- If you were in a similar situation, but on your own, can you think of a way to determine whether the men you were watching were co-operators or not?

- Sara doesn't seem fazed by the fact she took the baked beans from the rucksack of a corpse. Why not? Do you think this is realistic?

- The society imagined seems to be constituted of lots of small groups of people. Why is this the case? Do you think this is realistic? What characterises these groups? Why would they differ from each other in this way?

- Do you think the smallpox virus, if it were released into society, could have the effects described, or do you think this is far-fetched?

- Could society as we know it disintegrate so comprehensively? If not for the reason described for some other reason?

- What *would* happen if 'no one was in charge'? Can you imagine consequences other than those described?

- Would it help to prevent such a situation if the publication of certain (parts of) scientific papers was censored? Should papers with safety and/or security implications be censored?

- What would be the downside of censoring scientific papers?

- Sara and Damon are concerned about the death of those who had been educated. Why? Would you share their concern?

- If it was for you a choice between books and warmth what would you decide?

- Do you think society as *we* know it could rise again from the ashes? How?

Having read and reflected on this second scenario, you will probably again have identified some things that fail to convince you. If so why not try to write your own scenario about the world as you imagine it will be in AD 2070?

Here is our third scenario:

Scenario three: AD 2190

The bell rang loudly. Everyone sighed. Time for their medication. A queue started to form. The pills were dispensed. Then everyone, including Stig, returned to their rooms to complete their video blogs. It was important they record everything regularly; how else would anyone be sure whether or not the drugs were working?

Stig couldn't wait until his turn as a guinea pig was over. Only 3 more months. Then he wouldn't be required to do it again for 15 years or so. Then, like everyone else, he'd have to do another 6 month stint.

There was no chance of getting away with it. Stig had learned his lessons well: in the days when 'juries' were needed to decide whether people had committed criminal acts, people often got away without serving. Not only were the government's files poorly maintained, so people were often never even called up, if they were called up, they only had to plead a prior engagement and they'd be excused.

No chance of that for drug service. These days the government could find you in the time it took to key in your citizen number. In seconds they'd know where you were, who you were talking to, what you had eaten that day, the current state of your health, and whether you were happy, sad or anxious. If you didn't turn up at the appointed time in the appointed place, you would be found and brought in immediately. Then your stint time would be doubled. No other commitment was deemed as important as your time on drug duty.

It may seem a bit draconian, Stig reflected, but he wouldn't want to go back to the old days. It was only fair that everyone should take turns to try out new drugs. How else were the pharmaceutical companies to discover whether or not the drugs they were developing worked? There simply weren't enough volunteers.

It was undeniably good, of course, that there was no more 'third world' to exploit. There was a time, Stig understood, when drugs were invariably tested on poor people in India or Africa. Such people were unpaid, uninformed and often suffered as a result of having 'volunteered' to test drugs, often in exchange for nothing more than 'free' medical treatment. But the economic boom in the third world put paid to that, thankfully. The whole world was wealthy now. No one needed to test drugs for money or healthcare. But drugs still needed to be tested.

Some hankered after the days when animals were used. But that simply wasn't on any more. Animals had had rights – including the right to life – since 2150. Many people were vociferous in their defence of these rights and no one dared touch the hair of the head of an animal.

It hadn't done animals much good, reflected Stig. Since the pets had been freed they largely lived a life of scavenging. Natural selection had soon weeded out the weakest and now one wouldn't dare approach a cat, never mind stroke it. Eyes were lost that way.

No, nowadays the animal stage of drug testing had been eliminated in favour of cell cultures, computer simulations and human tests. But these days the pre-human tests were far better than they had been in the days of animals. They had to be. Unlike animals, humans knew what was going on when they were used to test drugs: the government would have a revolt on its hands if too many drug tests went wrong. The elimination of the animal part of testing hadn't half focused the drug companies' minds on safety.

Results had, on the whole, been excellent. It was whispered that governments, with the help of the drug companies, hushed up many disasters but, reflected Stig, it was undeniably the case that everyone was far healthier these days.

No one, for example, died unnecessarily. 'Crash' teams left the hospitals in 2111. A heart attack, for example, or stroke, would now sound the alarm in some control room, the appropriate drugs and, if necessary, an electric shock, would be administered internally via the implants everyone was given at birth, nano-machines in your blood stream would rush to the site of any blockage and get to work on it immediately. The flying doctor would be with you as soon as the turbo chargers on his backpack could get him there, sometimes whilst you were still thinking it was indigestion!

The idea of 'compliance' was gone too. Drug taking was too important to leave to the memories or whims of individuals. As soon as it was determined, by the monitors, that you needed some drug, the right dose would be administered at the right time and in the right place. No one needed to remember their medication anymore. No one was allowed to refuse to take it: health, like education, was made compulsory in 2125.

But it was amazing, Stig supposed, that health could be made compulsory. The drug companies had been hugely instrumental in this. But the development of substitutes for human organs and tissue had also been instrumental. As soon as the monitors detected that an organ had started to fail, the blood of your umbilical cord would be taken out of storage, a clone would be produced, and its stem cells used to grow whatever it was you needed. Any problem with your skeleton was made good with one of the many new materials produced by nanotechnologists and physicists.

No one's health suffered through a poor lifestyle, either. As soon as your genome was sequenced, at birth it was known to which diseases and disorders you would be susceptible, and your parents knew immediately what you should or shouldn't eat. All the food manufacturers produced food to which substances had been added or subtracted to suit every possible diet. So long as you scanned your irises at the supermarket check-in, you would not be allowed to buy anything unsuitable. There was a black market of course but Stig couldn't understand why anyone would want to risk their health for, for example, a pizza with real pepperoni, when the substitute pepperoni was almost as good.

But to be healthy was a tremendous boon. Everyone knew it. Those who used to agitate about governmental interference were long gone. They lived on their islands allowing themselves to succumb to every disease under the sun. Their lifespans were pitifully short, and they often suffered from some disability. No, on the whole, Stig decided, he'd just have to put up with his drug stints: life may not be perfect, but it was surely the best possible?

Here are some questions to prompt your reflection on scenario three:

- Why do citizens in this society have to take turns at being guinea pigs? Do you think this could happen? If not why not?

- Do you think the analogies between jury service and the drug service, and between compulsory education and compulsory health are good ones? If not why not?
- In this scenario the government apparently knows everything about you. How might this have come about? What do you think about it?
- The government will fetch you if you fail to turn up for your drug service, and double your time there. Do you think this could happen? How do you feel about it?
- Animals in this society have been given rights, including the right to life. Do you think that this might have the consequences described? If not why not?
- The economic woes of the third world have been eliminated in this society. Do you think this is possible? How might it have come about? Would this have the impact on drug development imagined?
- If drugs had to be tested on human beings why might the government try to 'hush up' situations in which drugs had adverse effects? Is it likely to succeed in this? Why (not)?
- In this society drug compliance is no longer an issue. What is 'compliance'? Why is it no longer an issue? If this were possible would it be a good thing?
- What do you think of the idea that a heart attack could be treated even before you knew you were having one? Would this be a good thing? Why (not)?
- In this society citizens' health is monitored constantly, so the powers that be know and act immediately if anything is wrong. Would this be a good reason to be sanguine about being monitored constantly?
- Do you think that you would put up with being monitored constantly in exchange for guaranteed health?
- What do you think of the idea of being unable to buy or eat anything that wasn't good for you? Would you be happy to be relieved of the responsibility for your own lifestyle, or would you be outraged to be coerced?
- There appear to be some outlaws in this society, people who live on islands and put up with the downside of not being monitored. Would you want to join these people? If not why not? If so, why?

Having read and reflected on this third scenario, you will probably again have identified some things that fail to convince you. If so why not try to write your own scenario about the world as you imagine it will be in 2190 AD?

Attempts to predict what will happen in the future have often been notoriously wide of the mark. Here are a few, taken from the website 'Top 87 Bad Predictions about the Future':[3]

- 1878: Sir William Preece, Chief Engineer, British Post Office:
  'The Americans have need of the telephone, but we do not. We have plenty of messenger boys.'
- 1880: Sir William Siemens said of Edison's light bulb: 'Such startling announcements as these should be deprecated as being unworthy of science and mischievous to its true progress.'

- 1883: Lord Kelvin, President of the Royal Society: 'X-rays will prove to be a hoax.'
- 1901: Wilbur Wright whose first successful flight was in 1903, said: 'Man will not fly for 50 years.'
- 1936: The *New York Times* said: 'A rocket will never be able to leave the Earth's atmosphere.'
- 1955: Alex Lewyt, president of vacuum cleaner company Lewyt Corp said: 'Nuclear-powered vacuum cleaners will probably be a reality in 10 years.'
- 1977: Ken Olson, president, chairman and founder of Digital Equipment Corp. (DEC), maker of big business mainframe computers said: 'There is no reason anyone would want a computer in their home.'
- 1988: Dr Peter Duesberg, a professor of molecular biology at UC Berkeley said, of HIV: 'That virus is a pussycat.'

But of course individuals can be wrong about virtually anything. Governments have to be more careful. This is why they convene committees of the great and the good to advise them on the making of decisions about issues that are controversial, and that could have serious ramifications for the future. It is hoped by the use of such committees to avoid the sort of disasters that could befall society as a result of erroneous decision-making.

Such committees nearly always start the process of decision-making by launching a public consultation so that concerned individuals and organisations can submit their arguments. Responding to such a public consultation is one of the ways in which you, as an individual, can have an impact on democratic decision-making.

There are other ways of having an impact on issues that concern you. Here are just a few:

- write to a newspaper;
- organise a petition;
- attract followers to a Twitter feed and tweet about what concerns you;
- start a Facebook page;
- join an organisation (or start one);
- offer yourself as a speaker.

Before you do any such thing, however, it is important that you have thought through your arguments. It is not, of course, simply the arguments *for* your case that you should have thought through. Throughout this book it has been suggested that it is just as important to think through the arguments *against* your case. By playing devil's advocate to yourself you will:

- give yourself the chance to discover you are making a mistake – and we *all* make mistakes;
- identify the weak points in your own arguments – giving yourself the opportunity to strengthen your argument;
- enhance your chances of constructing the strongest argument possible – one that takes into account the strengths of your opponents' case.

It is also important that you listen to the arguments of others. They might have thought of an argument that has escaped you. The use of charity in argument (see pages 62–69) is vital: in treating the appearance of falsehood and stupidity in your opponent as evidence of *your* bad interpretation, you can guarantee that the likelihood of making a mistake is small. Your aim is always to understand *why* your opponent is saying whatever it is he is saying. If you can't see why, then assume you haven't yet understood.

Biotechnology is a fast moving discipline. By the time this book is in print it is likely already to be out of date on the latest advances in biotechnology (which is why there is an associated website). But the nature of argument does not change: everything you have learned about arguments in this book, from how to identify them to how to evaluate them, will stand you in as good stead in 30 years' time as it will now.

We have now completed our survey of the ethical and social issues of biotechnology. As the author I hope this book has succeeded in achieving the aim stated in the preface, that it would help you, the reader:

- understand the key issues in bioethics and the different positions people take on them;
- appreciate the arguments for and against the differing positions;
- discuss the issues with confidence;
- think productively about the issues that might arise in the future;
- come to your own considered positions on various issues, understanding the arguments for and against those positions.

The website will enable you to keep up to date on these issues, and on issues that arise in the future. I hope you have enjoyed the journey and I wish you the very best of luck in your cogitations!

Marianne Talbot, 2012.

Notes

1 http://www.sciencedaily.com/releases/2010/09/100914102108.htm.
2 'Statement on Scientific Publication and Security', February 2003, the editors of *Science, Nature,* and *The Proceedings of the National Academy of Sciences* together with the America Society for Microbiology. *Science,* 21 February 2003, 1149.
3 http://www.2spare.com/item_50221.aspx.

INDEX

Printed in the United States
by Thotmasters

Printed in the United States
By Bookmasters